ADVANCES IN

Pharmacology and Chemotherapy

VOLUME 18

ADVANCES IN

Pharmacology and Chemotherapy

EDITED BY

Silvio Garattini

Istituto di Ricerche Farmacologiche "Mario Negri" Milano, Italy

A. Goldin

National Cancer Institute Bethesda, Maryland

F. Hawking

Commonwealth Institute of Helminthology St. Albans, Herts., England

I. J. Kopin

National Institute of Mental Health Bethesda, Maryland

Consulting Editor

R. J. Schnitzer

Mount Sinai School of Medicine New York, New York

VOLUME 18—1981

ACADEMIC PRESS

A Subsidiary of Harcourt Brace Jovanovich, Publishers

New York London Toronto Sydney San Francisco

ACADEMIC PRESS, INC.
111 Fifth Avenue, New York, New York 10003

United Kingdom Edition published by
ACADEMIC PRESS, INC. (LONDON) LTD.
24/28 Oval Road, London NW1 7DX

LIBRARY OF CONGRESS CATALOG CARD NUMBER: 61–18298

ISBN 0–12–032918–2

PRINTED IN THE UNITED STATES OF AMERICA

81 82 83 84 9 8 7 6 5 4 3 2 1

CONTENTS

The Action of Metronidazole on Anaerobic Bacilli and Similar Organisms

E. J. BAINES AND J. A. MCFADZEAN

Chemotherapeutic Inhibitors of the Enzymes of the *de Novo* Pyrimidine Pathway

THOMAS W. KENSLER AND DAVID A. COONEY

CONTRIBUTORS TO THIS VOLUME

Numbers in parentheses indicate the pages on which the authors' contributions begin.

E. J. BAINES (223), *Pharmaceutical Division, May & Baker Ltd., Dagenham, Essex RM10 7XS, England*

DAVID A. COONEY (273), *Laboratory of Medicinal Chemistry and Biology, National Cancer Institute, National Institutes of Health, Bethesda, Maryland 20205*

MICHAEL B. GRAVESTOCK (49), *Imperial Chemical Industries Ltd., Pharmaceuticals Division, Mereside, Alderley Park, Macclesfield, Cheshire SK10 4TG, England*

ROBERT L. JONES (177), *Department of Chemistry and Laboratory for Microbial and Biochemical Sciences, Georgia State University, Atlanta, Georgia 30303*

THOMAS W. KENSLER (273), *Laboratory of Medicinal Chemistry and Biology, National Cancer Institute, National Institutes of Health, Bethesda, Maryland 20205, and Division of Toxicology, Department of Environmental Health Sciences, Johns Hopkins University School of Hygiene and Public Health, Baltimore, Maryland 21205*

J. A. MCFADZEAN (223), *Pharmaceutical Division, May & Baker Ltd., Dagenham, Essex RM10 7XS, England*

J. PHILIP POYSER (49), *Imperial Chemical Industries Ltd., Pharmaceuticals Division, Mereside, Alderley Park, Macclesfield, Cheshire SK10 4TG, England*

JOHN F. RYLEY (49), *Imperial Chemical Industries Ltd., Pharmaceuticals Division, Mereside, Alderley Park, Macclesfield, Cheshire SK10 4TG, England*

MELVIN J. SILVER (1), *Cardeza Foundation and Department of Pharmacology, Thomas Jefferson University, Philadelphia, Pennsylvania 19107*

ROBERT G. WILSON (49), *Imperial Chemical Industries Ltd., Pharmaceuticals Division, Mereside, Alderley Park, Macclesfield, Cheshire SK10 4TG, England*

W. DAVID WILSON (177), *Department of Chemistry and Laboratory for Microbial and Biochemical Sciences, Georgia State University, Atlanta, Georgia 30303*

ADVANCES IN

Pharmacology and Chemotherapy

VOLUME 18

ADVANCES IN PHARMACOLOGY AND CHEMOTHERAPY, VOL. 18

Mechanisms of Hemostasis and Therapy of Thrombosis: New Concepts Based on the Metabolism of Arachidonic Acid by Platelets and Endothelial Cells

MELVIN J. SILVER

Cardeza Foundation and Department of Pharmacology
Thomas Jefferson University
Philadelphia, Pennsylvania

ISBN 0-12-032918-2

I. Introduction

During the 10 years between 1970 and 1980 a number of new and outstanding findings were made which increased our understanding of hemostasis and thrombosis by showing how metabolites of arachidonic acid, formed by platelets or cells of the walls of blood vessels, may influence these processes. This period will surely be viewed by future investigators of hemostasis and thrombosis as the decade of the blossoming of knowledge concerning the metabolism of arachidonic acid by cells in the cardiovascular system. It is the purpose of this article to review these developments and to point out some of the ways in which they are being used and will be used to treat or prevent thrombosis. (For more detailed information in some of the areas mentioned in this article see Smith and Silver, 1976; Silver *et al.,* 1977, 1978, 1980c; Samuelsson *et al.,* 1978; Nicolaou and Smith, 1979; Dusting *et al.,* 1979; Moncada and Vane, 1978, 1979; Burch and Majerus, 1979; Marcus, 1978; Smith, 1980; Lands, 1979; Harris *et al.,* 1979.) This article consists of two major sections, one entitled hemostasis (Section II) and the other thrombosis (Section III). The section on hemostasis begins by defining hemostasis and proceeds to discuss the hemostatic process in terms of the general physiological events that occur and the mechanisms involved, with special emphasis on the role of prostaglandin synthesis by platelets and blood vessels. The section on thrombosis, in similar fashion, begins with a discussion of the thrombotic process and then considers the ways in which various aspects of normal prostaglandin synthesis by platelets or blood vessels may become abnormal and lead to a hemorrhagic or thrombotic diathesis. This progresses to a discussion of how our newer knowledge of the metabolism of arachidonic acid by platelets or blood vessels has given us rationales for the prevention and treatment of thrombosis.

II. Hemostasis

Hemostasis is the physiological response to injury of blood vessels. The net result of the hemostatic process is the arrest of bleeding and the initiation of the repair of the injured vessel wall. It is a dynamic process which involves the blood vessel wall, blood platelets, the blood clotting system, and the fibrinolytic system. The initial event in hemostasis as well as inflammation, thrombosis, and atherosclerosis is injury to the wall of a blood vessel. The consequence of the injury may depend on its severity, the conditions in the local environment, the general health of the subject, and his nutritional status.

When a blood vessel wall is damaged in normal individuals the immediate and late responses will depend on the extent (minor injury, complete cut) of the damage, the contents of the circulating blood, the pressure and flow rate, as well as local hydrodynamics.

A. Transection of Large Vessels

Obviously, if a large vessel (with high pressure and rapid flow) is transected it will be extremely difficult to arrest the bleeding. Vasoconstriction and blood coagulation may be assisted by external pressure on the cut ends, the application of a tourniquet to arrest flow in the vessel, and surgical intervention to repair the vessel.

B. Puncture of Small Vessels

Most physical damage to blood vessels involves injury to smaller vessels (venules, arterioles, and capillaries). If the vessel wall is punctured, bleeding occurs. As blood flows through the opening and contacts the damaged tissues, platelets, but not white cells or red cells, immediately cling to the exposed subendothelial tissue. This adherence of platelets to subendothelial tissue is rapidly followed by adherence of more platelets to those already sticking to subendothelium and an amplified reaction then ensues resulting in rapid aggregation of many platelets in the region. The growth of this aggregating mass of platelets culminates in the formation of a clump of aggregated platelets called the hemostatic platelet plug, which plugs the opening and stops bleeding from the vessel. The morphology of the hemostatic platelet plug has been the subject of extensive study (Wester *et al.*, 1978). During the aggregation process the blood clotting and the inflammatory process are also initiated. Their major effects occur later in time—progressing over a period of minutes, hours, and days—and involve consolidation of the platelet plug by the fibrin network of the coagulum, so that rebleeding does not occur. Slow healing of the wound ensues. During the coagulation process thrombin is formed. This enzyme, besides converting the soluble fibrinogen in blood plasma to fibrin, can also cause platelet aggregation. There is little doubt that the larger amounts of thrombin formed, as coagulation proceeds, may cause further aggregation of platelets on the outer surface of the already well advanced platelet plug. The possibility that trace amounts of thrombin, insufficient to induce coagulation, may contribute to the induction of platelet aggregation in the initial stages of the formation of the platelet plug has been suggested (Ardlie and Han, 1974). At present it is not possible to test the validity of this hypothesis because it is not possible to measure the trace amounts of thrombin present in the region of the forming platelet plug (for example, at 1–10 seconds after injury). In any event, it is not necessary to invoke trace amounts of thrombin since the initial platelet aggregation can be, to a great extent, accounted for by contact of the platelets with collagen in the subendothelium, which triggers platelet phospholipase activity and the release of arachidonic acid. This is followed by the formation of cyclic endoperoxides and thromboxane A_2 whose role in platelet aggregation is discussed below.

C. Lesser Damage to Blood Vessels

While transection and puncturing of blood vessels may result in bleeding which can be arrested by normal hemostatic processes, failure to arrest such bleeding may result in losses of large amounts of blood culminating in shock or death. However, when lesser injuries occur without bleeding, thromboembolic problems may develop if physiologic responses or proper treatment are not effective. Minor damage to blood vessels may provoke injury to smooth muscle cells and other subendothelial components. Varying degrees of endothelial damage may occur when vessels are crushed by accidental injury or even by clamps used in surgery (Richling *et al.,* 1979).

D. Injuries within Blood Vessels

In straight segments of normal blood vessels, where smooth, laminar flow of blood occurs, endothelium is apparently undisturbed. However, endothelial damage may be occurring constantly at sites of branching of blood vessels. Such repeated insults are probably among the initial causes of atherosclerosis in man. Aggravating factors may include the presence of various agents in the blood such as high levels of fatty acids, cholesterol, other lipids, or lipoproteins.

E. The Role of Platelets and Blood Vessel Walls

The walls of blood vessels are covered with a layer of endothelial cells only one cell thick. In normal, healthy individuals, *except at points of branching,* blood tends to flow in arteries with a laminar flow. The formed elements tend to flow in a central column with platelets and white cells on the outside and erythrocytes in the center. A clear layer of blood plasma is on the outside in contact with the endothelium of the vessel wall. When injury occurs endothelial cells may be damaged and stripped from the vessel wall, the smooth flow is disturbed, and the local hydrodynamics are changed. This may result in further damage to endothelial cells and also allow for contact of platelets with subendothelial tissue.

F. Adhesion of Platelets

The earliest visible response to injury of a blood vessel is the adhesion of blood platelets to exposed subendothelial tissue. Recent evidence suggests that a plasma factor called Factor VIII–Von Willebrand factor is necessary for adhesion of platelets to subendothelium (Sakariassen *et al.*, 1979). It is believed that collagen is the major component in the subendothelial tissue to which platelets adhere. Only platelets adhere to exposed subendothelial tissue, white cells and red cells do not. The factors involved in adhesion and various approaches to measuring adhesion have been reviewed by Baumgartner and Muggli (1976) and more specific discussion of the adhesion of platelets to various types of collagen may be found in the reviews of Jaffe (1976) and Legrand *et al.* (1979).

G. Shape Change, Aggregation, the Release Reaction, and Formation of the Hemostatic Platelet Plug

Within seconds after adhesion of some platelets to subendothelial tissue other platelets stick to those already stuck. Then many platelets in the region of the damaged vessel begin to aggregate with each other and a progressively larger and larger mass of clumped platelets forms the hemostatic platelet plug. Prior to, and occurring progressively during aggregation, the normally disc-shaped platelets change their shape. They tend to become spherical and extend pseudopods which intertwine with those of other platelets during aggregation. At a very early stage (probably shortly after the first contact of platelets with subendothelial collagen) a subprocess known as the "platelet-release reaction" occurs. During this reaction the contents of platelet granules are released to the surrounding blood: the dense bodies of the platelets release serotonin, calcium, ATP, and ADP which are normally stored there and lysosomal enzymes are released from subcellular particles of platelets called α-granules. The release of ADP, a potent aggregating agent in its own right, may amplify platelet aggregation in vicinal platelets. The release reaction has been reviewed by Macintyre (1976).

Platelet prostaglandin synthesis probably begins immediately in response to contact with collagen when arachidonic acid is released from platelet phospholipids by stimulated phospholipase activity. Products formed from arachidonic acid include cyclic endoperoxides and thromboxane A_2 which can induce the platelet release reaction and aggregation.

The discovery that human platelet aggregation may be induced by the prostaglandin precursor, arachidonic acid, came about 8 years ago and is discussed further below. Prior to this it was known that several naturally occurring agents may induce platelet aggregation. The principal ones are ADP, collagen, epinephrine, and thrombin. It now appears that while prostaglandin synthesis may partially explain platelet aggregation in response to these agents other pathways are also involved since some platelet aggregation may be induced by them even when inhibitors of prostaglandin synthesis are present. These other mechanisms are the subject of intensive investigation and have been reviewed by Packham *et al.* (1977).

Platelets as well as vessel walls (see further) can form prostaglandins and other metabolites of arachidonic acid, while newly formed thrombin may further stimulate the formation of these products by platelets.

The biological activities of the potent substances known to be formed by platelets or vessel walls fall roughly into three main categories: (1) induction or inhibition of platelet aggregation and the release reaction; (2) vasoconstriction or vasodilation; (3) chemotaxis or increased vascular permeability, thus influencing the inflammatory process (see Table I). In the ensuing sections we shall consider the roles of platelets and blood vessels in the hemostatic process with special reference to the formation of prostaglandins and other metabolites of arachidonic acid.

TABLE I

BIOLOGICAL ACTIVITIES[a] OF METABOLITES OF ARACHIDONIC ACID PRODUCED BY PLATELETS OR ENDOTHELIAL CELLS

	Metabolite	
	Platelets	Endothelial cells
Induction of platelet aggregation	PGG_2, PGH_2 Thromboxane A_2	PGG_2, PGH_2 Thromboxane A_2
Inhibition of platelet aggregation	PGD_2	PGI_2
Vasoconstriction	PGG_2, PGH_2, $PGF_{2\alpha}$ Thromboxane A_2	PGG_2, PGH_2 Thromboxane A_2
Vasodilation	PGE_2	PGI_2

[a] The activities listed in this table are related to hemostasis and thrombosis. Other activities of some of these metabolites indicate their possible role in inflammatory processes. For example, HETE and thromboxane B_2 are chemotactic while PGE_2 and PGD_2 are known to increase vascular permeability which is a hallmark of inflammation.

A review of the role of other factors in hemostasis and thrombosis such as rheology and the influence of red cells and white cells has appeared recently (Mason and Saba, 1978).

H. Prostaglandin Synthesis by Platelets and Endothelial Cells

1. *Platelets*

Important recent advances in our understanding of hemostasis and thrombosis are derived from studies on prostaglandin synthesis by blood platelets and endothelial cells. Our current knowledge in these areas is summarized in Figs. 1, 2, and 3. These figures may also be referred to for the structures of some of the compounds mentioned below. The very exciting series of findings in this field of research began in 1970 with the original discoveries of Smith and Willis (1971) who showed that washed, human platelets, when treated with thrombin, formed PGE_2 and $PGF_{2\alpha}$ which were measured by bioassay. They further showed that aspirin and indomethacin could inhibit such platelet prostaglandin production *in vitro* and that platelets obtained from individuals who had previously ingested either of these drugs did not produce prostaglandins in response to thrombin *ex vivo*. It is now recognized that aspirin and other nonsteroidal antiinflammatory agents will interfere with stimulated prostaglandin formation of most cells by inhibiting cyclooxygenase activity. Since it had previously been known that aspirin inhibited platelet aggregation (Weiss *et al.*, 1968) and caused a prolongation of the skin bleeding time (Mielke *et al.*, 1969) it became evident that a close relationship existed between hemostatic or thrombotic events and platelet prostaglandin synthesis. The next advance connecting platelet prostaglandin synthesis to a hemostatic event (namely blood coagulation) came in 1972 when it was shown that prostaglandins were formed by platelets during blood clotting and that they could be detected in the serum after whole blood had been allowed to clot (Silver *et al.*, 1972a). In the hemostatic process, platelet aggregation is an earlier event than blood clotting and in 1973 it was shown that PGE_2 and $PGF_{2\alpha}$ were formed during platelet aggregation *in vitro* in response to the well-known aggregating agents collagen, ADP, and adrenaline (Smith *et al.*, 1973). It was now quite clear that platelet prostaglandin synthesis must play a role in platelet aggregation and since arachidonic acid, the precursor of the platelet prostaglandins, was not present as the free acid in platelets, but esterified in platelet phospholipids, the first step in platelet prostaglandin synthesis was probably the release of free arachidonic acid from the phospholipids. The possibility of bypassing the phospholipase

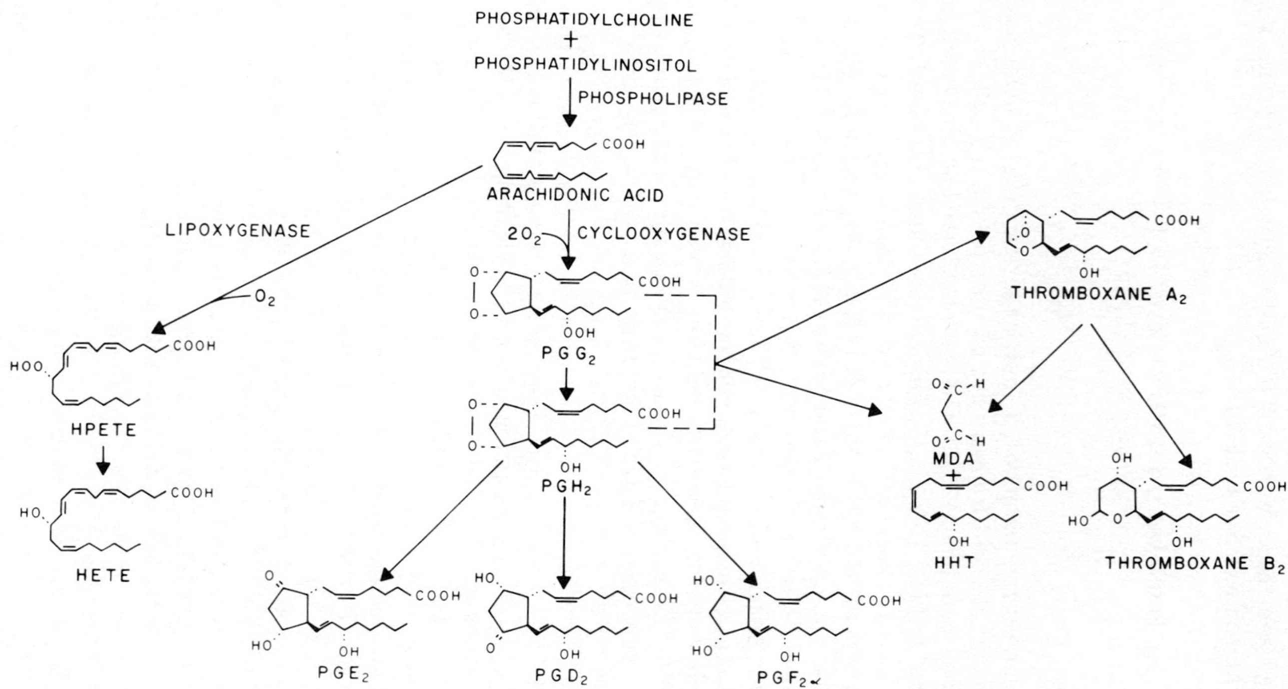

FIG. 1. Metabolism of arachidonic acid by human blood platelets.

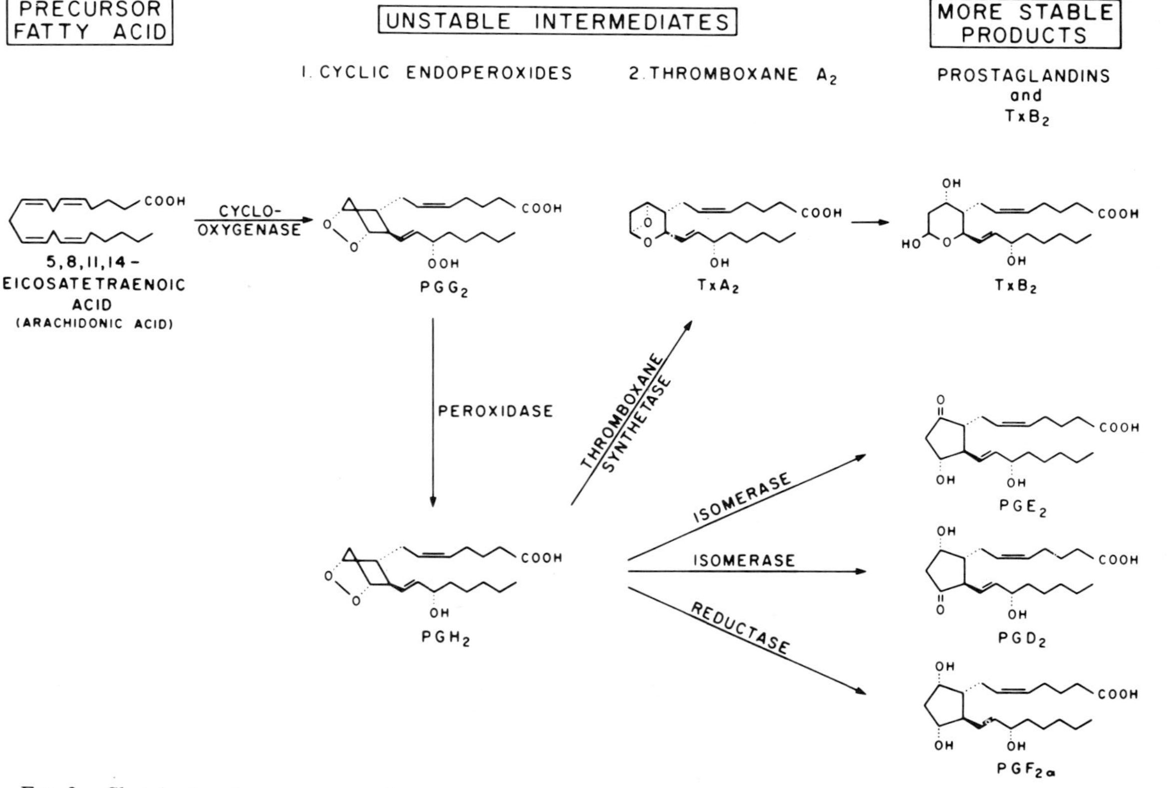

FIG. 2. Sketch of cyclooxygenase and thromboxane synthetase pathways in human blood platelets. (From Silver *et al.*, 1980, with permission.)

step by adding exogenous arachidonic acid to platelet-rich plasma was then considered. Indeed it was demonstrated that the addition of arachidonic acid induced both platelet aggregation and prostaglandin synthesis and both were inhibited by aspirin (Silver *et al.,* 1972b, 1973; Vargaftig and Zirinis, 1973). If exogenous arachidonic acid could indeed bypass the endogenous platelet phospholipase step, become substrate for the platelet cyclooxygenase, be converted to prostaglandins and cause platelet aggregation *in vitro,* could it do so *in vivo?* This question was answered by experiments in which arachidonic acid was injected into the marginal ear veins of rabbits (Silver *et al.,* 1974). It was anticipated that such injections would result in arachidonic acid contacting platelets in the blood flowing by and, if aggregation did occur, the platelet aggregates would be carried downstream to the heart via the jugular vein and then into the microcirculation of the lungs via the pulmonary artery. One minute after the injection of arachidonic acid (1.4 mg/kg) platelet aggregates were found in blood samples obtained from the heart and the animal appeared to have great difficulty in breathing. Within 2 to 3 minutes after the injection the animal was dead and samples of all the organs were rapidly removed for histological examination. Many vessels of the microvasculature of the lungs were seen to be occluded with platelet aggregates. It was concluded then that the animals could have died from physical obstruction of the lung microvasculature coupled with the local release of a vasoconstrictor such as $PGF_{2\alpha}$ coming from platelets or lung tissue. Other fatty acids did not cause such effects. Since then, in similar experiments, with arachidonic acid, it has been shown that the potent vasoconstrictor thromboxane A_2 may become available and most likely plays a role (Cerskus *et al.,* 1978).

By late 1973, it was evident that there was indeed a very close association, if not a cause and effect relationship, between platelet prostaglandin synthesis and platelet aggregation. The then known end-products of platelet prostaglandin synthesis, PGE_2 and $PGF_{2\alpha}$, could not induce platelet aggregation whereas the precursor, arachidonic acid, could. In addition, platelet prostaglandin synthesis induced by arachidonic acid in platelet-rich plasma was inhibited by aspirin and indomethacin. Since neither the end-products nor the precursor could directly induce platelet aggregation it became clear that the inducer of aggregation was either an intermediate in platelet prostaglandin synthesis or an unknown product. At this point attention was focused on the cyclic endoperoxide intermediates in PG synthesis whose formation by seminal vesicles had previously been discovered by Nugteren and Hazelhof (1973) and Hamberg and Samuelsson (1973). These cyclic endoperoxides were named PGG_2 (which has an hydroperoxy group at the 15 position) and PGH_2 (which has an hydroxy group at the 15 position). Using methods similar to those that had been employed for seminal vesicles, Smith *et al.* (1974b) educed evidence that cyclic endoperoxides were formed during platelet aggregation and suggested that they could induce platelet aggregation. Willis and Kuhn (1973) first showed that an intermediate in PG biosynthesis by sheep vesicular glands could induce platelet aggregation and Hamberg and Samuelsson (1974) as well as Willis *et al.* (1974) showed that cyclic endoperoxides are indeed formed by platelets during aggregation. Finally, definitive evidence that both PGG_2 and PGH_2 can induce platelet aggregation came from the work of Hamberg *et al.* (1974).

In 1975 there were several noteworthy advances. An outstanding achievement was that of Hamberg *et al.* (1975) who showed that a previously recognized hemiacetal compound produced by platelets, and now named thromboxane B_2, was derived from the cyclic endoperoxides via another unstable intermediate named thromboxane A_2. They also gave evidence that thromboxane A_2 was a potent vasoconstrictor as well as an inducer of platelet aggregation. Another important development at that time was the report of Bills *et al.* (1976) who showed that human platelets may incorporate radioactive arachidonic acid into their phospholipids from plasma and that thrombin stimulates platelet phospholipase A_2 activity which liberates free arachidonic acid from certain platelet phospholipids. This free radioactive arachidonic acid was then shown to be converted via the cyclooxygenase pathway to the complex endoperoxides or thromboxane A_2, which are potent inducers of platelet aggregation. The importance of phospholipase A_2 and other phospholipases has been reviewed elsewhere (Silver *et al.*, 1978, 1980c; Smith, 1980). The mechanism by which aspirin inhibits platelet prostaglandin synthesis and so inhibits platelet aggregation was elucidated by Roth and Majerus (1975) who showed, by using radioactive aspirin, that this compound actually acetylates the platelet cyclooxygenase enzyme.

In 1976 Smith *et al.* showed that human platelets may form PGD_2 from added PGH_2 during platelet aggregation. Since PGD_2 had previously been shown to be a potent inhibitor of human platelet aggregation (Smith *et al.*, 1974a) they concluded that the formation of this prostaglandin during platelet aggregation could serve to limit thrombus formation via a negative feedback mechanism.

2. *Blood Vessels—Endothelial Cells*

Turning from the platelets to blood vessel walls, it was reported in 1976 by Moncada *et al.* that blood vessels could produce an unknown, unstable prostaglandin which was an extremely potent inhibitor of platelet aggregation as well as a vasodilator. This was a major breakthrough and inspired a tremendous amount of new research on the role of blood vessels in hemostasis and thrombosis.

Prior to this, Saba and Mason (1974) reported that endothelial cells produced an inhibitor of platelet aggregation, suggesting a role for blood vessels in hemostasis and thrombosis. Moncada *et al.* (1976) showed that microsomes, prepared from aortas of animals, when incubated with cyclic endoperoxides or arachidonic acid, produced a very potent inhibitor of platelet aggregation and a vasodilator. The active substance was highly unstable, rapidly losing these activities at room temperature and at physiological pH. They also showed that segments of blood vessels could produce, *in vitro,* a substance with these activities and characteristics. The purification and determination of the structure of this new prostaglandin was first reported by Johnson *et al.* (1976). The structure and a proposed metabolic pathway from arachidonic acid is shown in Fig. 3. The compound was given the trivial name prostacyclin and the designation PGI_2. This highly unstable substance is rapidly converted in aqueous media at pH 7.4 to the more stable 6-keto-$PGF_{1\alpha}$ (see Fig. 3). Thus the measurement of the formation of 6-keto-$PGF_{1\alpha}$ is an indirect measure of the prior formation of PGI_2.

The discovery that PGI_2 may be formed by the walls of blood vessels was an important advance in the quest for knowledge about the role of blood vessels in hemostasis, thrombosis, atherosclerosis, and inflammation. An exciting finding was the very great potency of this naturally occurring prostaglandin. However, the unqualified early statements and conclusions as to its remarkable inhibitory activity in platelet aggregation need to be tempered. This is especially important when comparing the inhibitory activity of PGI_2 to that of PGE_1 or PGD_2 because slowly metabolized stable analogs of all three of these substances may turn out to be valuable antithrombotic agents. In contrast to general statements such as PGI_2 "is 30–40 times more potent than PGE_1" (Moncada and Vane, 1978) as an inhibitor of platelet aggregation, systematic studies comparing the inhibitory activity of PGI_2, PGD_2, and PGE_1 have shown that the differences in potency between these prostaglandins is not so great and that one must consider their effects against each specific aggregating agent separately (Di Minno *et al.,* 1979).

Besides its inhibitory effect on platelet aggregation, PGI_2 has been shown to inhibit adhesion of platelets to subendothelial tissue on strips of deendothelialized rabbit aorta (Higgs *et al.,* 1978). Considering the similarities of the effects of PGI_2, PGD_2, and PGE_1 on platelet aggregation it would be interesting to see how the latter two prostaglandins compare to PGI_2 in inhibiting platelet adhesion.

Other tissues, besides blood vessels, have been shown to be capable of

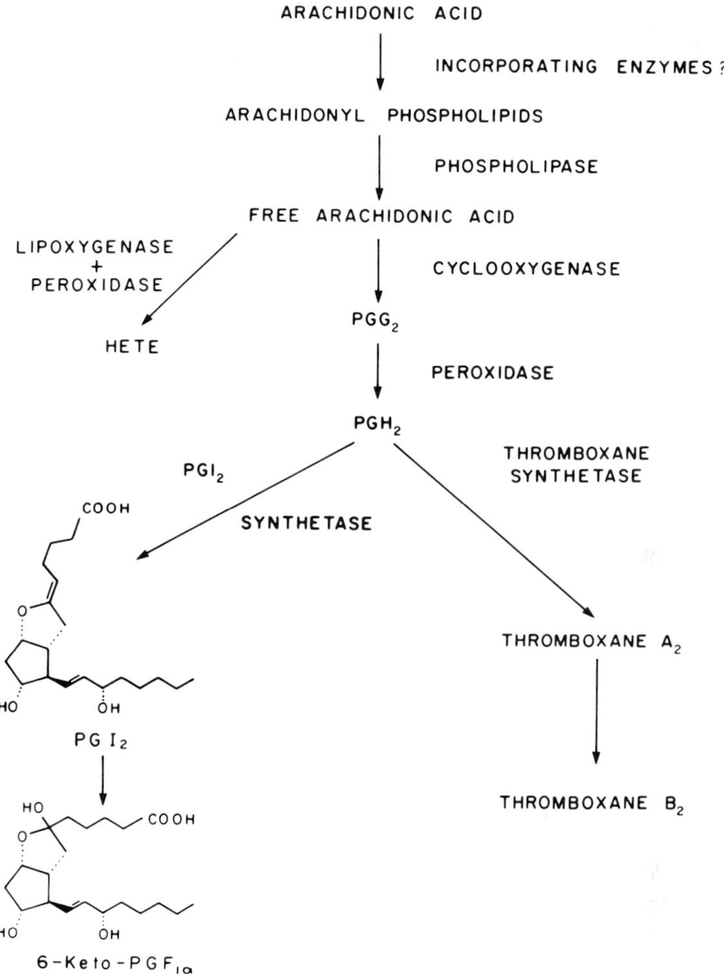

FIG. 3. Proposed pathways for the metabolism of arachidonic acid by endothelial cells.

producing PGI_2, whose formation has been inferred by detection of the stable end product 6-keto-$PGF_{1\alpha}$. This, as well as the pharmacological actions of PGI_2, has recently been reviewed (Weeks, 1978) and will only be touched on here. 6-keto-$PGF_{1\alpha}$ has been shown to be formed by microsomes from the rat stomach, bull and sheep seminal vesicles, guinea pig and rabbit lung, human and rabbit kidney, rat, rabbit, monkey, and human uterus, as well as cow and horse corpus luteum. Its pharmacological actions include a bronchodilatory effect, a vasodepressor effect on the systemic and pulmonary circulation, and inhibition of gastric secretion.

It was soon shown that *endothelial cells* (Baenziger *et al.*, 1977; Weksler *et al.*, 1977) and perhaps other cells in the deeper layers of blood vessels can form PGI_2. The early work suggested several hypotheses concerning the possible role of PGI_2 in hemostasis or thrombosis (Moncada *et al.*, 1976) which led many to believe that hemostasis simply required a balance between the aggregating effects of metabolites of arachidonic acid formed by platelets and the inhibitory effects on platelet aggregation of prostacyclin coming from endothelial cells.

I. Endothelial Cells Produce Thromboxane A_2 as well as Prostacyclin

Recently it has been shown that human, arterial, or venous rings *in vitro* and rabbit arteries *in situ* as well as cultured endothelial cells from bovine aorta can form thromboxane A_2 in response to arachidonic acid (Ingerman *et al.*, 1980, 1981; Silver *et al.*, 1980a,b). The production of thromboxane A_2 and PGI_2 was monitored by specific radioimmunoassays for their stable products thromboxane B_2 and 6-keto-$PGF_{1\alpha}$, respectively. Aspirin and indomethacin inhibited formation of both 6-keto-$PGF_{1\alpha}$ and thromboxane B_2, indicating that these products were formed via a cyclooxygenase in endothelial cells. Strong supporting evidence that the compound detected in the thromboxane B_2 assay was indeed thromboxane B_2 was provided by the fact that imidazole, a known inhibitor of thromboxane synthetase, inhibited the suspected thromboxane B_2 production, without inhibiting the 6-keto-$PGF_{1\alpha}$ production. That the endothelial cells of the blood vessels, rather than the smooth muscle cells, were indeed making thromboxane was indicated by the fact that while endothelial cells in culture produced relatively large amounts of both 6-keto-$PGF_{1\alpha}$ and thromboxane B_2, smooth muscle cells produced only small amounts of PGI_2 and no detectable thromboxane B_2. It would therefore be highly unlikely that thromboxane B_2 could come from smooth muscle cells in the intact blood vessels and most likely that it comes from endothelial cells. Since endothelial cells can make thromboxane A_2, a powerful aggregating agent and vasoconstrictor, we must revise our thinking about the possible role of blood vessels in hemostasis and thrombosis.

J. Hemostasis, Thrombosis, and the Balance between Inhibitors and Accelerators of Platelet Aggregation and between Vasodilators and Vasoconstrictors

Prior to the discovery that PGI_2 could be produced by blood vessels it was difficult to say much about the role of blood vessel walls in hemostasis. It was considered and rejected that the vasoconstrictor serotonin, coming from platelets, might cause the early transient vasoconstriction seen when a blood vessel is injured (see Barkhan and Silver, 1962). Later, with the discovery of the production of $PGF_{2\alpha}$ by platelets, it was considered that this vasoconstrictor might be the agent (Silver *et al.*, 1974). Finally, with the discovery of the formation of thromboxane A_2 by platelets this vasoconstrictor must be given serious consideration. A simplistic line of reasoning led many to believe that only events favoring hemostasis or thrombosis, including vasoconstriction and platelet aggregation, were related to the synthesis of prostaglandins by platelets while only antihemostatic or antithrombotic events were related to prostaglandin synthesis by blood vessels. In spite of the fact that PGD_2 was shown to be a potent inhibitor of human platelet aggregation (Smith *et al.*, 1974b) and was formed by human platelets in significant amounts (Oelz *et al.*, 1977) it was not seriously considered as making a significant contribution in hemostasis or thrombosis. This was probably due to the fact that the discovery of PGD_2 formed by platelets was overshadowed by the discovery that the somewhat more potent PGI_2 was formed by blood vessels.

Hemostasis and thrombosis are obviously very complex processes and the simple concept of viewing platelets as the sole source of inducers of aggregation and vasoconstrictors, while considering blood vessels as the sole source of inhibitors of aggregation and vasodilators, is not tenable. The inhibitory role in platelet aggregation of PGD_2 formed by platelets must be seriously considered. The fact that the well-known inducer of platelet aggregation, ADP, may be secreted by endothelial cells and converted in plasma to the vasodilator adenosine (Pearson and Gordon, 1979) cannot be ignored. It is difficult to understand why the possible potent proaggregating and vasoconstrictor activity of PGG_2 and PGH_2, made by endothelial cells, has been dismissed up to now. Obviously, these compounds are obligatory intermediates for the formation of PGI_2 and must be formed and be present, at least momentarily, in larger amounts than PGI_2 itself because they also serve as intermediates for the formation of thromboxane A_2. It is now clear that endothelial cells, as well as platelets, can produce an aggregating agent and vasoconstrictor. The possible interaction of all of these hemostatic and antihemostatic agents must be very complex. Not only the relative amounts of each of them present at any particular time but also the sequence of their appearance and the duration of their production and local availability after a stimulus or damage to endothelium, could determine the resultant biological effect—normal hemostasis, bleeding, thrombosis, or emboli of platelet aggregates. Possible roles of various components of blood vessel walls in hemostasis and thrombosis are listed in Table II. An intriguing variety of possibilities are suggested there. Most of the items presented are purely speculative at this

TABLE II

SOME POSSIBLE ROLES OF ENDOTHELIAL CELLS AND SUBENDOTHELIAL TISSUE IN HEMOSTASIS AND THROMBOSIS

	Possible effect
A. Endothelial cells (EC)	
1. Basic output of PGI_2?	Normally prevents adhesion and aggregation?
2. Stimulated output of PGI_2	Prevents adhesion and aggregation when EC receive mild stimulus?
3. Damage to EC inhibits production of PGI_2?	Allows for adhesion and aggregation?
4. PGI_2 from EC, on the periphery of growing platelet plug, terminates aggregation?	Local antithrombotic effect?
(Endoperoxides from aggregating platelets or white cells may feed the PGI_2 synthetase of EC?)	Related to inflammatory process?
5. PGI_2 causes vasodilation	Antithrombotic effect, reduces ischemia?
6. Basic output of PGG_2, PGH_2, TxA_2?	Balances basic output of PGI_2?
7. Stimulated output of PGG_2 PGH_2, TxA_2	Causes initial vasoconstriction and platelet aggregation? Elevated production could favor thrombosis?
8. Damage to EC inhibits production of PGG_2, PGH_2, TxA_2?	Antihemostatic or antithrombotic effect?
9. PGG_2, PGH_2, TxA_2 cause prolonged vasoconstriction?	Thrombotic effect, increases ischemia?
B. Exposed Subendothelial tissue	
1. Collagen in basement membrane	Promotes hemostasis by initiating adhesion of platelets and consequent release and aggregation
2. Smooth muscle cells	
Initial constriction	Promotes hemostasis
Spasm	Causes ischemia, promotes thrombosis
PGI_2 production?	Causes vasodilation, relaxes vessel, and relieves ischemia?

time. Those which are followed by question marks lack strong supporting evidence, are controversial, and are being actively investigated or merit investigation. The statements not followed by question marks are somewhat less controversial and would be accepted as being likely occurrences by most workers in the field. The possibility that under physiological or pathological circumstances, endoperoxides coming from platelets could be used as substrate by the prostacyclin synthetase or thromboxane synthetase of nearby endothelial cells or vice versa is highly speculative, controversial, and surely will be extremely difficult to prove.

K. Interaction between Platelet and Endothelial Cell Prostaglandin Synthesis and Its Relationship to Hemostasis and Thrombosis

The exact mechanisms of the important early events occurring during hemostatic or thromboembolic processes remain to be clarified. However, the physical proximity that develops between damaged endothelial cells and platelets on the one hand and exposed subendothelial tissue and platelets on the other strongly indicates the possibility of interaction between these various components of hemostasis and thrombosis. I would offer the following working hypothesis for the sequence of events in hemostasis related to the metabolism of arachidonic acid by platelets and endothelial cells:

1. Trauma to a blood vessel by a physical or chemical agent causes damage to or removal of some endothelial cells and exposure of subendothelial tissue.
2. Contact of platelets with subendothelial collagen, in the presence of Factor VIII–von Willebrand factor initiates adhesion of platelets and triggers stimulated platelet phospholipase activities.
3. Platelet phospholipase A_2 and phospholipase C cause rapid breakdown of membrane arachidonylphosphatidylinositol resulting in platelet shape change.
4. Platelet phospholipase A_2 causes release of arachidonic acid from platelet phospholipids (mainly from phosphatidylcholine and phosphatidylinositol, but also from phosphatidylethanolamine) and formation of lysophosphatides. Some arachidonic acid may also come from the action of platelet diglyceride lipase on arachidonyl diglyceride released after phospholipase C activity on phosphatidylinositol.
5. Similar early metabolism of arachidonic acid probably occurs in endothelial cells as well as platelets. This remains to be studied in detail.
6. Arachidonic acid released from platelet and endothelial cell phospholipids is converted into cyclic endoperoxides and thromboxane A_2. These agents may induce platelet aggregation and the platelet release reaction which amplifies platelet aggregation by causing the aggregation of other platelets. These same agents are also vasoactive and no doubt contribute to the vasoconstriction seen soon after injury to the blood vessel. The relative contribution of these agents, coming either from platelets or from endothelial cells, in platelet aggregation or vasoconstriction is not known.
7. The logical sequence of events in hemostasis should now involve the production and availability of sufficient amounts of agents which would (a) inhibit platelet aggregation so that the newly formed hemostatic platelet

plug is limited and does not continue to add platelet aggregates to form a pathological thrombus and (b) have vasodilatory activity to overcome the prior vasoconstrictor activity and so prevent ischemia and allow continued flow in the vessel. These agents are of course PGD_2 coming from the platelets and PGI_2 coming from the endothelial cells. Their relative contributions in limiting the size of the platelet plug or keeping the blood vessel open are unknown.

8. One of the intermediate metabolites of the lipoxygenase pathway (Fig. 1) is 12-L-hydroperoxy-5,8,10,14-eicosatetraenoic acid (HPETE). This compound has been shown to inhibit thromboxane synthetase (Hammarström and Falardeau, 1977). Therefore, its production may be of importance in modulating the hemostatic process.

L. Importance of Enzymes Involved in the Metabolism of Arachidonic Acid by Platelets or Endothelial Cells

1. *Platelets*

The role of the major enzymes involved in the metabolism of arachidonic acid becomes evident by noting their substrates and products in Fig. 1 and Table III. The key role of *phospholipase* activity in liberating arachidonic acid from phospholipids is apparent because without it free

TABLE III

Enzymes Involved in Metabolism of Arachidonic Acid by Platelets or Endothelial Cells

Enzymes	Action and products
1. Incorporating enzymes	Arachidonic acid → arachidonyl-phosphatides
2. Phospholipase A_2	Arachidonyl-phosphatides → arachidonic acid + lysophosphatides
3. Phospholipase C	Arachidonyl-phosphatidylinositol → arachidonyl-diglyceride + phosphorylinositol
4. Diglyceride lipase	Arachidonyl-diglyceride → arachidonic acid + monoglyceride?
5. Lipoxygenase	AA → HPETE
6. Cyclooxygenase	AA → PGG_2
7. Peroxidases	HPETE → HETE PGG_2 → PGH_2
8. Thromboxane synthetase	Cyclic endoperoxides → thromboxane A_2
9. Prostacyclin synthetase (endothelial cells, not platelets)	Cyclic endoperosides → PGI_2

arachidonic acid would not become available to serve as substrate for the two consequent enzyme activities, namely *cyclooxygenase* and *lipoxygenase*. *Cyclooxygenase* activity is important because it results in the conversion of arachidonic acid to the cyclic endoperoxides PGG_2 and PGH_2 which are highly unstable, biologically active (induce platelet aggregation and the release reaction) substances which are then converted to a variety of compounds some of which have potent biological activities. Some of the newly formed endoperoxides may be rapidly converted to small amounts of prostaglandins in platelets via chemical reduction or platelet *isomerases*. These prostaglandins are the potent inhibitor of aggregation, PGD_2; a possible modulator of aggregation and a vasodilator, PGE_2; a vasoconstrictor, $PGF_{2\alpha}$. A major part of the cyclic endoperoxides is converted via the enzyme *thromboxane synthetase* to the highly unstable thromboxane A_2, which apparently is a potent inducer of platelet aggregation and a potent vasoconstrictor. However, thromboxane A_2 still remains to be isolated in stable form and tested. Until then we shall not be certain of its true biological activity. It is rapidly transformed into the more stable thromboxane B_2 which is chemotactic for polymorphonuclear leukocytes. Other substances formed from the cyclic endoperoxides are the 3-carbon moiety malondialdehyde and the 17-carbon, hydroxy fatty acid, HHT whose possible biological activities are yet to be determined.

The remainder of the free arachidonic acid is metabolized via the platelet lipoxygenase pathway, which leads to the formation of considerable amounts of 12-L-hydroperoxy-5,8,10,14-eicosatetraenoic acid (HPETE) which is reduced to 12-L-hydroxy-eicosatetraenoic acid (HETE) (Hamberg and Samuelsson, 1974; Nugteren and Hazelhof, 1975) as well as to di- and tri-hydroxy fatty acids (Jones *et al.*, 1978; Bryant and Bailey, 1979). Neither aspirin nor indomethacin inhibits lipoxygenase activity. In fact, HETE formation by platelets appears to be stimulated in the presence of aspirin but this is probably because the cyclooxygenase is inhibited, allowing more free arachidonic acid to become available as substrate for the lipoxygenase (Hamberg *et al.*, 1974; Bills *et al.*, 1976). The enzyme is present in the soluble fraction of platelets. The bovine enzyme prefers arachidonic acid as substrate but can also use other C-20 fatty acids which have cis double bonds at C-9 and C-12 (Nugteren and Hazelhof, 1975). Recent studies from our laboratory show that a soluble, cytoplasmic, lipoxygenase fraction of sonicated human platelets was potently inhibited by the ferric iron chelating agent, toluene-3,4-dithiol and not by a ferrous iron chelating agent, suggesting that its activity depends on ferric iron (Aharony *et al.*, 1980, 1981). HETE has been reported to be chemotactic for polymorphonuclear leukocytes *in vitro* (Turner *et al.*, 1975). Since HPETE may inhibit thromboxane synthetase (Hammarström and Falardeau, 1977), the lipoxygenase pathway, through production of HPETE, could modulate hemostasis.

2. *Endothelial Cells*

Endothelial cells obviously have the enzymatic machinery to form the cyclic endoperoxides. An important pathway for the metabolism of the endoperoxides appears to be via an enzyme which converts them into the unstable PGI_2, an inhibitor of platelet aggregation and a vasodilator. PGI_2 is inactivated by conversion into 6-keto-$PGF_{1\alpha}$ (see Fig. 3) and 6,15-diketo-$PGF_{1\alpha}$. The possibility that endothelial cells may metabolize arachidonic acid in other ways is being intensively investigated. It has recently been shown that the lipoxygenase pathway is operative in blood vessels (Greenwald *et al.,* 1979; Herman *et al.,* 1979). Our findings that bovine aorta endothelial cells in culture, excised strips of human arteries or veins, as well as rabbit arteries *in situ* can make thromboxane B_2 clearly indicates the presence of thromboxane synthetase in endothelial cells. Thus, inhibition of one or more of these enzymatic pathways may result in augmenting or inhibiting platelet aggregation or vasoconstriction and so influence hemostasis or thrombosis. The biological activities of the various metabolites of arachidonic acid formed by platelets or endothelial cells are summarized in Table I.

M. The Modulating Role of Plasma Albumin in Platelet Aggregation and Prostaglandin Synthesis

In normal individuals the plasma albumin concentrations are between 4 and 5 gm/100 (4–5%) and the arachidonic acid content of normal plasma has been reported to be as high as 30 μM. However, ordinarily, this circulating arachidonic acid does not cause platelet aggregation because it is bound by albumin. In 1973 we found that prostglandin production, in response to added arachidonic acid, by washed platelets, in the absence of albumin, was much greater than by platelets in plasma (Silver *et al.,* 1973). Later, we found that if radioactive arachidonic acid were added to washed platelets in the absence of albumin it was immediately oxidized to all of the metabolites that we have previously discussed. On the other hand, if 1% albumin were present, then the only event noted was that the radioactive arachidonic acid was incorporated into the platelet phospholipids (Bills *et al.,* 1976). This suggests that similar incorporation of free arachidonic acid into the platelet phospholipids may occur in the circulating blood. Finally, platelet aggregation may be induced *in vitro* by *micromolar* amounts of AA in the *absence of albumin,* but almost *millimolar amounts* are needed to induce aggregation in *platelet-rich plasma.* Furthermore, albumin in higher concentrations can inhibit platelet aggregation induced by arachidonic acid, collagen, or ADP (Silver *et al.*, 1973). These are some examples of how albumin can regulate platelet prostaglandin and thromboxane synthesis as well as platelet aggregation. They suggest that competition for free arachidonic acid in the vicinity of the platelet membrane exists between plasma albumin and the platelet enzymes that metabolize it.

III. Thrombosis

Thrombosis may be viewed as a pathological extension of hemostasis. Indeed the pathological thrombus in arteries has been reported to be similar in structure and content to the physiological hemostatic platelet plug and the underlying mechanisms and modulating influences in hemostasis and thrombosis are similar. The formation of the hemostatic platelet plug is often life-saving. Bleeding will be arrested, and the flow of blood often will continue in the injured vessel. However, under pathological conditions, when a thrombus develops, what starts out like a hemostatic platelet plug may grow until it becomes so big as to occlude vessels and cut off the blood supply to tissues. If the occluded vessels are serving vital organs like the heart or the brain, death may occur.

A. Interrelationship between Atherosclerosis and Thrombosis: The Role of Repeated Minor Damage to the Endothelium

Repeated injury to a blood vessel, which in itself is not enough to cause a thrombotic episode, may eventually result in the formation of an atherosclerotic plaque which can be a nidus for thrombotic events on the vessel wall. Therefore, individuals with atherosclerosis are prone to thrombotic episodes.

Speculation concerning the initial consequences of varying kinds of minor damage to the endothelium can be based on studies in which morphological changes in the blood vessel walls of experimental animals have been observed by electron microscopy following an insult to the endothelium or in response to an atherogenic diet. For example, in studies in which fatty acids were injected into veins in rabbits (Sedar *et al.*, 1978) the first signs of injury noted included swelling of the nuclei and loss of the rhomboidal shape of the endothelial cells (Figs. 4 and 5). Platelets were not seen to be adhering to the damaged endothelium. It is possible that such minimal morphological damage is reversible, without functional changes and that these cells recover. Further damage to the endothelial cells in-

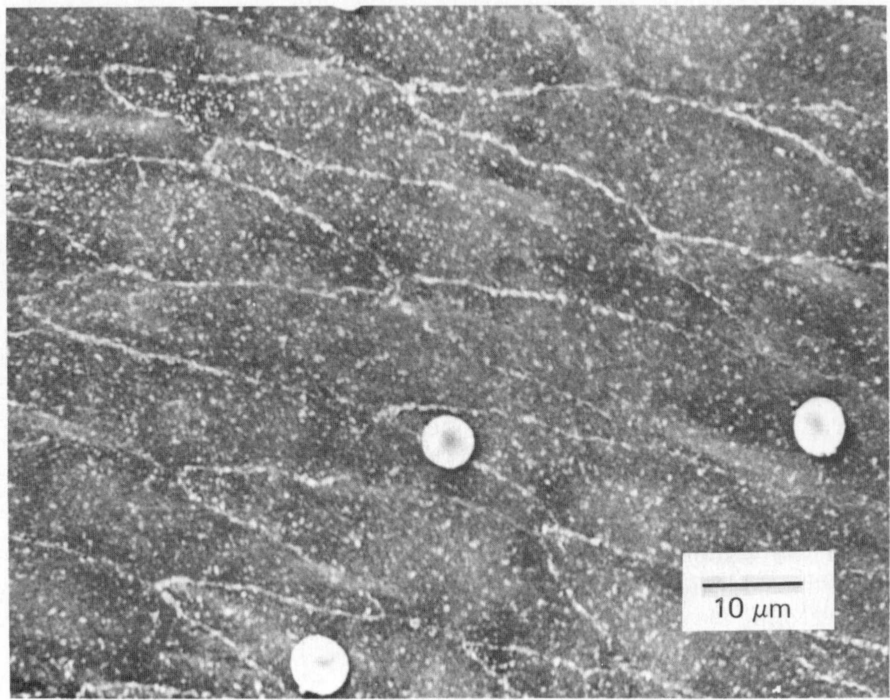

FIG. 4. Endothelium of rabbit ear vein. Control. (From Sedar *et al.*, 1978, with permission.)

cluded the tearing away of the nucleus from the endothelial cell and sometimes complete enucleation of the cell, leaving behind a "nuclear crater" (Fig. 6). In those cases where the endothelium was damaged, but the injured cells remained *in situ*, platelets were not seen adhering to the endothelium in experiments in which blood was allowed to flow by, following the injury. Such partially damaged cells may recover and be replaced by new endothelial cells, or the damaged area could become a focus for future thrombi. In the studies reported by Sedar *et al.* (1978) specimens for scanning electron microscopy were taken only at 3 minutes after the damaging event and not at later times. Similar damage to *arterial* endothelial cells in rabbits was reported more recently (Sedar *et al.*, 1980).

Progressive damage to the endothelium involves the separation of the cells from each other and opening up of intercellular clefts. Platelets, presumably in contact with subendothelial tissue, may be seen adhering in these gaps (Fig. 7). Such platelets have changed shape from disc-like to spherical with pseudopods. This damaged blood vessel wall, with exposed

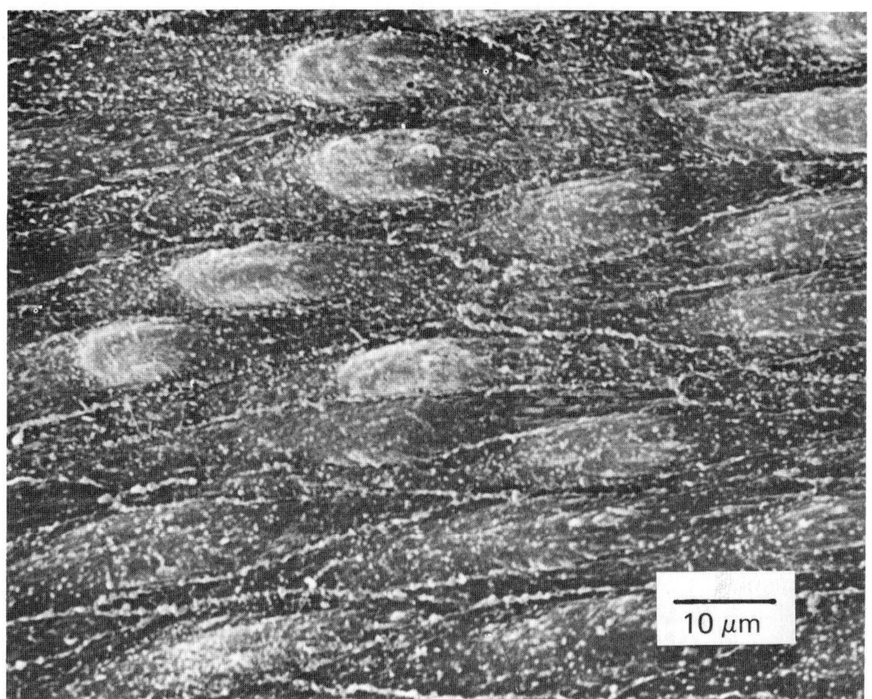

FIG. 5. Endothelium of rabbit ear vein. First signs of injury after injection of arachidonate (low concentration). Nuclei of endothelial cells are clearly outlined and are of greater intensity than in controls. (From Sedar *et al.*, 1978, with permission.)

subendothelium, may now be a focal point for possible thromboembolic events. For example, in a fast flowing blood stream, pieces of platelet aggregates forming on the exposed subendothelium may be broken off to flow down stream and occlude a vessel of smaller diameter. If the vessel is injured in a region of laminar flow and receives only one injury, healing, involving regeneration of endothelium, most likely occurs without the formation of a large thrombus or excessive thickening of the intima and serious ischemia does not occur (Poole *et al.*, 1958; Fishman *et al.*, 1975; Sholley *et al.*, 1977). However, if the injury is repeated or is in a region of turbulent hydrodynamics the damaged vessel wall may become a nidus for the formation of a large growing thrombus and intimal thickening, resulting in ischemia, reduced flow of blood, stasis, and finally, complete occlusion of the vessel. An example of this would be an atherosclerotic lesion in a coronary artery which would culminate in cutting off the blood supply to a portion of the myocardium and an infarct.

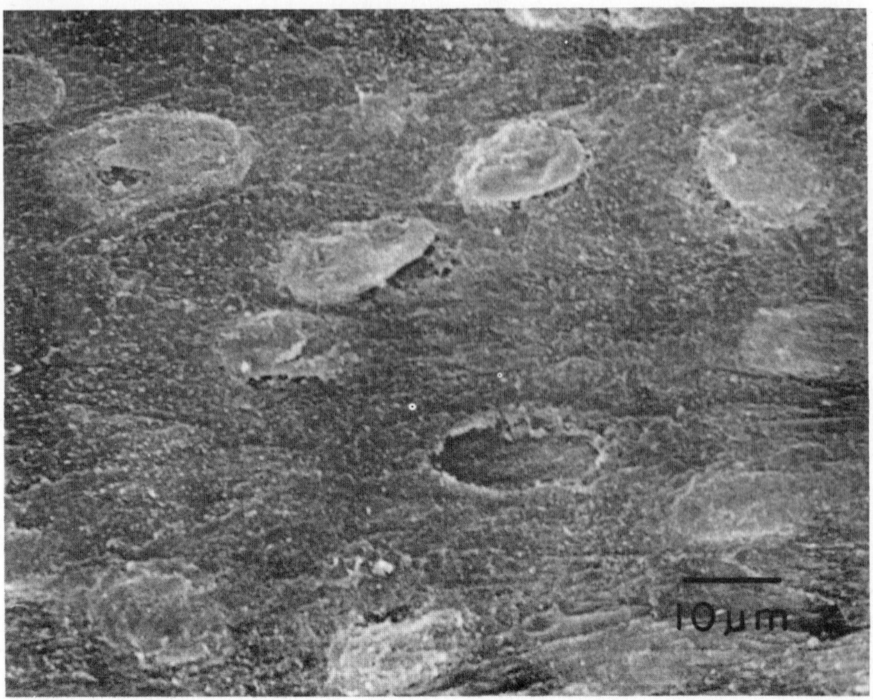

FIG. 6. Further damage to endothelium after injection of arachidonate (higher concentration). Damaged nuclei and a nuclear crater can be seen. (From Sedar *et al.*, 1978, with permission.)

B. Abnormal Metabolism of Arachidonic Acid by Platelets or Endothelial Cells

From the studies reviewed in Section II on hemostasis we are inexorably driven to the conclusion that the essential fatty acid, arachidonic acid, is unique among fatty acids in human physiology. Since this fatty acid is of such great importance it is possible that certain, heretofore, unexplained thrombotic problems may now be explained by abnormalities in the metabolism of arachidonic acid by platelets or by blood vessels and that certain thrombotic processes may be prevented or alleviated by controlling one or more steps in the metabolism of arachidonic acid.

The metabolites of arachidonic acid presently believed to influence hemostasis via platelet aggregation or vasoactivity are PGG_2, PGH_2, thromboxane A_2, PGD_2, PGE_2, PGI_2, and HPETE. The amounts of any one or several of these substances formed locally in response to injury to a blood vessel could be abnormally high or low in a variety of situations, including abnormal genetic problems or responses to foods or drugs.

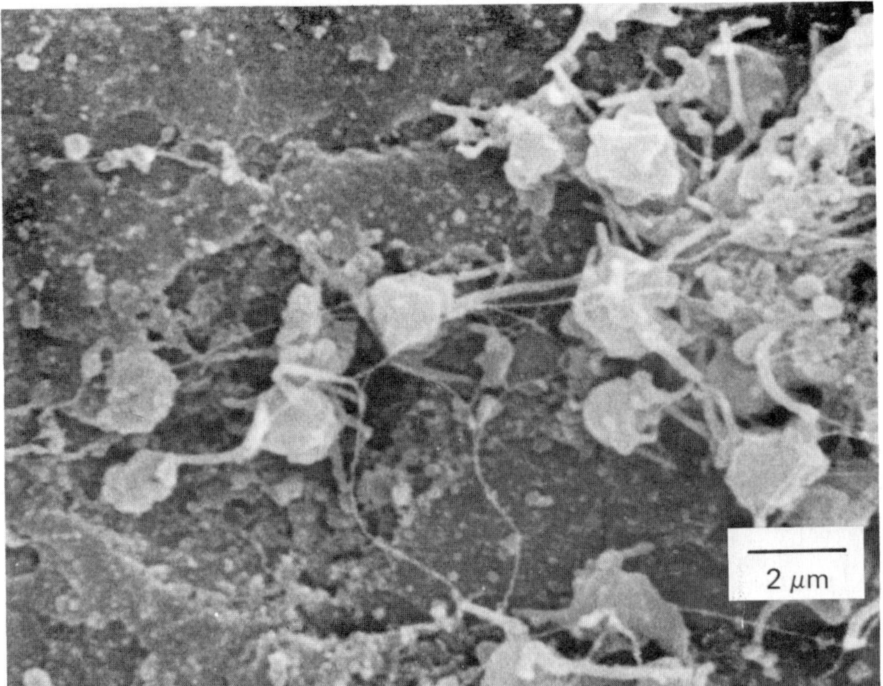

FIG. 7. Platelets adhering to exposed subendothelium after injection of arachidonate (high concentration). Platelets have undergone shape change and exhibit pseudopodia. (From Sedar *et al.*, 1978, with permission.)

1. *Abnormal Levels of Arachidonic Acid in Plasma or in Platelet or Endothelial Cell Phospholipids*

The levels of arachidonic acid present in plasma may be a controlling factor for the levels of arachidonic acid present in platelet phospholipids and this may be determined nutritionally. If abnormally large amounts of arachidonic acid are present in platelet and plasma lipids it is possible that abnormally high amounts may become available locally at a point of injury to a blood vessel and lead to a hyperthrombotic state. This concept is supported by the experiments of Seyberth *et al.* (1975) who showed that after the ingestion of 6 gm per day of ethyl arachidonate by four normal humans there was an elevation of the content of arachidonic acid in the plasma and platelet lipids and that the platelets in platelet-rich plasma of these individuals were hypersensitive to ADP in tests of platelet aggregation. The hyperactivity to platelet aggregation and the elevated levels of arachidonic acid returned to normal after the feeding of arachidonate was stopped. It also seems reasonable that abnormally low levels of arachidonic acid might bring about a hypothrombotic state. That this is so is suggested by the report of Friedman *et al.* (1976) who studied three infants who developed a deficiency in essential fatty acids while on a fat-free diet. They found that these infants were deficient in arachidonic and linoleic acids and that their platelet-rich plasma could not produce a second wave of aggregation in response to ADP. When the patients recovered, their platelet aggregation patterns were similar to those of normals. The authors suggested that platelet aggregation responses should be studied in infants with a hemorrhagic diathesis. Little is known about possible genetic defects involving abnormally high or low levels of arachidonic acid in platelet phospholipids which might be specifically attributed to a deficiency or high or low activity of the platelet enzymes involved in incorporating arachidonic acid into platelet phospholipids. There has been one report of a patient, apparently a variant case of the Hermansky–Pudlak syndrome, whose platelets incorporated significantly less [^{14}C]arachidonic acid into their phospholipids as compared to normal controls (Rendu *et al.*, 1978).

2. *Abnormal Phospholipase Activity*

Arachidonic acid might be released from platelet phospholipids via several possible pathways. Figure 8 indicates a variety of these possibilities. Obviously a deficit in phospholipase activity would result in a reduction of the release of arachidonic acid from platelet phospholipids and a subsequent diminution of the levels of metabolites of arachidonic acid that can induce platelet aggregation. This might result in a hypothrombotic tendency with diminished aggregability of platelets. On the other hand hyperactive phospholipase activity might result in the local release of abnormally large amounts of arachidonic acid, resulting in the formation of abnormally large amounts of metabolites which could lead to a thrombotic incident. A case has been reported of an individual whose platelets appeared to have less than normal phospholipase activity (Rendu *et al.*, 1978). However, the major defect in that individual's platelets was subnormal capacity to incorporate arachidonic acid into the platelet phospholipids, as mentioned above.

3. *Abnormal Cyclooxygenase Activity*

Arachidonic acid, when released from platelet phospholipids, becomes available to the enzyme cyclooxygenase which converts it into the cyclic endoperoxides PGG_2 and PGH_2. These cyclic endoperoxides may induce aggregation in their own right and are also largely and rapidly converted to thromboxane A_2, which is considered to be a potent inducer of platelet

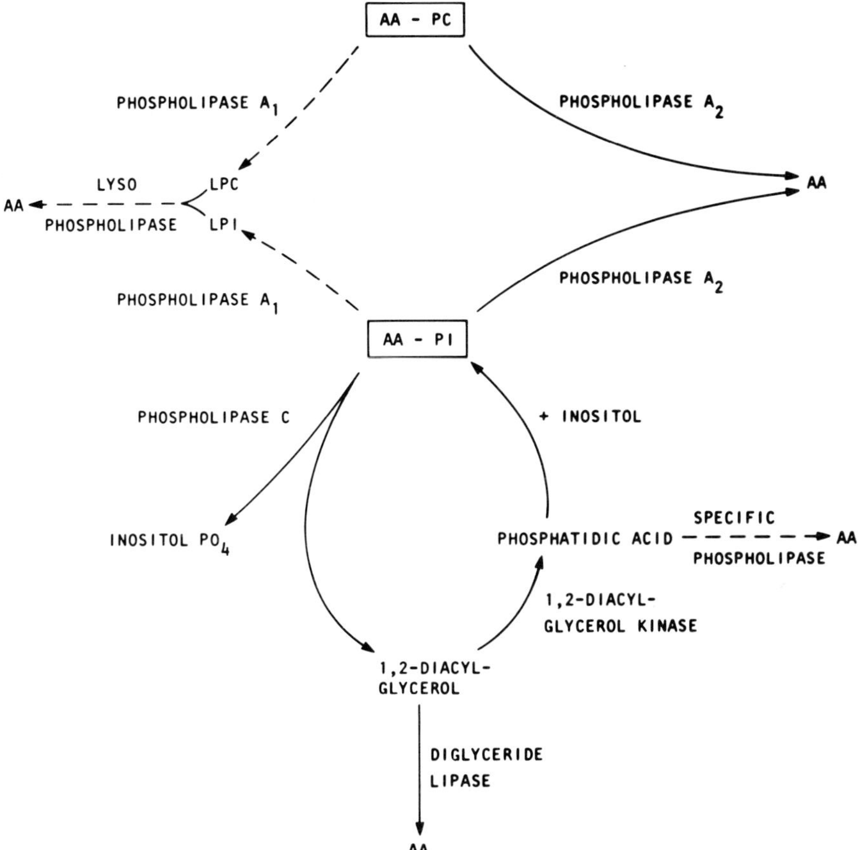

FIG. 8. Possible ways in which arachidonic acid could be released from phosphatidylcholine and phosphatidylinositol for further metabolism in human platelets (From Silver *et al.*, 1980, with permission.)

aggregation and a vasoconstrictor and which therefore may play an important role in thrombosis. Thus, abnormally elevated cyclooxygenase activity in platelets carries with it an elevated potential for thrombotic activity while abnormally low activity may result in an hypothrombotic state or cause a bleeding tendency. Since the findings in cyclooxygenase deficiency closely resemble those seen in normal individuals who have ingested aspirin, it is incumbent upon the investigator to completely eliminate the possibility of recent aspirin ingestion. Repeat studies should be done at several intervals. The first case of cyclooxygenase deficiency was reported by Malmsten and his associates at the Karolinska Institute (1975). In general, the data reported indicated a cyclooxygenase deficiency. The statement was made that aggregation could not be induced by arachidonic acid. Unfortunately, the response of the patients' platelets was tested only at 0.2 m*M* arachidonic acid. We have found that the threshold concentrations of arachidonic acid required for the induction of platelet aggregation in normal platelet-rich plasma vary between 0.2 and 1.0 m*M*, with most responses occurring at about 0.5 m*M*, and suggest that it cannot be stated that aggregation *cannot* be induced by arachidonic acid unless one has tried 1 m*M* arachidonic acid. The second case is that of Weiss and Lages (1977) and other cases are included in the reports of Lagarde *et al.* (1978) and Nyman *et al.* (1979). Their findings are consistent with a diagnosis of cyclooxygenase deficiency.

4. *Abnormal Thromboxane Synthetase Activity*

The paper by Weiss and Lages (1977) was primarily concerned with a case of a possible defect in thromboxane synthetase in the patient's platelets. Their findings appeared to be consistent with a deficit of thromboxane synthetase, but they were limited to aggregation tests. More definitive evidence is awaited.

5. *Abnormal Lipoxygenase Activity*

Okuma and Uchino (1979) have reported on a series of patients, with myeloproliferative disorders and a thrombotic tendency, whose platelets appear to have subnormal lipoxygenase activity and are hypersensitive to platelet aggregating agents. Perhaps low production of HPETE by the platelets of these individuals leads to unregulated thromboxane A_2 activity and thrombotic episodes.

6. *Abnormal Activity of Other Enzymes Involved in Arachidonate Metabolism*

At the time of this writing there were no reports in the literature with definitive evidence for abnormalities in platelet PGD_2 isomerase activity, or in PGI_2 synthetase in blood vessels. However, Remuzzi *et al.* (1978) reported abnormally high levels of PGI_2-like activity produced by pieces of vein from uremic patients with a bleeding tendency.

C. Abnormal Plasma Albumin Levels and Thrombosis in the Nephrotic Syndrome

The importance of plasma albumin as a modulator of the metabolism of arachidonic acid has been discussed in Section II on hemostasis. Recently it has been shown that in the nephrotic syndrome patients' platelets are hyperaggregable and they have a thrombotic tendency which correlates with abnormally low plasma albumin levels (Remuzzi *et al.*, 1979).

D. Decreased Sensitivity to PGD_2 by Platelets from Patients with Myeloproliferative Disorders and Thrombotic Tendency

Cooper *et al.* (1978) have shown less activation of platelet adenylate cyclase in 20 patients than in normal controls. In 5 patients they showed that the amount of PGD_2 required to inhibit collagen-induced [^{14}C]serotonin release from platelets was 10 times as great as in normals. This was specific for PGD_2. Stimulation of adenylate cyclase by PGE_1 and PGI_2 was normal for these patients, indicating that a binding site specific for PGD_2 was involved.

E. Vasoconstriction Caused by TxA_2 in Prinzmetal's Angina

Besides its ability to induce platelet aggregation and the release reaction thromboxane (TxA_2) is a potent vasoconstrictor. As little as 30 pmole was shown to cause marked constriction of the rabbit aorta (Needleman *et al.*, 1977). Coronary artery spasm has been well documented in Prinzmetal's variant angina and now appears to be a hallmark of this syndrome (Chahine, 1979). It has also been shown that TxA_2 coming from platelets can constrict the smooth muscle of coronary arteries. Recently, we have found elevated levels of TxB_2 in blood plasma from six patients with Prinzmetal's angina but not in the plasma of normal volunteers (Lewy et al., 1979). TxB_2 was not detected in the plasma of a patient while on aspirin and was detected when the aspirin was discontinued. These findings suggest that thromboxane A_2 coming from platelets or endothelial cells may be the cause of coronary vasospasm in these patients and possibly in other cases of vasospasm.

F. Prevention of Thrombosis

Why is it that in normal physiology, platelet aggregation proceeds to a certain point and then stops when the injured part of the vessel is plugged and bleeding stops? Is it because the stimulus causes production of enough of the aggregating agents and no more? Or, is it also because inhibitors of platelet aggregation are being formed near the site of the injury and they arrest further platelet aggregation when the hemostatic plug is formed? Rationales for the prophylaxis or therapy of thrombosis should consider that thrombosis may be due to an increase in production of aggregating agents such as PGG_2, PGH_2, or TxA_2, or a decrease in production of the naturally occurring inhibitors PGD_2, produced by platelets, or PGI_2, produced by blood vessels and that thrombotic episodes may be intensified or alleviated by local vasoconstrictor or vasodilatory actions of some of these agents. Possible differences in the metabolism of arachidonic acid between arteries and veins, between different portions of the same vessel and between straight pieces of a vessel and portions at branches or valves may prove to be of considerable interest and are being investigated. Accumulated knowledge in the study of thrombosis indicates the predominance of platelet aggregation in arterial thrombosis (which generally involves pulsatile, fast flow, and high pressure) whereas blood clotting tends to predominate in venous thrombosis (which generally involves slower flow, sometimes stasis, and lower pressures). As would be expected the anticoagulant drugs tend to be more effective in venous thrombosis whereas the drugs which inhibit platelet aggregation tend to be helpful in arterial thrombosis, which is our main concern here.

There are at least three important contributing factors to thrombosis that we should be considering here: (1) adhesion of platelets to exposed subendothelial tissue; (2) aggregation of platelets; (3) vasoconstriction. Each of these plays a role in the normal arrest of bleeding and abnormally high activity of one, two, or all three of these processes could contribute to a thrombotic event. The corollary is, of course, that agents or other means that can inhibit one or more of these processes should have an antithrombotic effect. It is also possible that the fluidity of the blood, the normal tone of blood vessels, and normal hemostasis may be promoted by basal formation of metabolites of arachidonic acid which are inhibitors of aggregation or of adhesion or are vasodilators. At present there is no solid evidence to support such contentions.

Approaches to the thrombosis problem related to the metabolism of arachidonic acid may be considered at several levels. (1) We can try to eliminate all metabolism of arachidonic acid starting with inhibition of its release from platelet or endothelial cell phospholipids. (2) We can try to specifically inhibit the formation of only one metabolite of arachidonic acid, e.g., thromboxane A_2. (3) We can try to inhibit an intermediary stage, e.g., cyclooxygenase or lipoxygenase.

In each case we must consider what the net effect may be on thrombosis and we must also consider what the effects may be on other processes such as inflammation. Other factors to be weighed are: (1) Antithrombotic agents may inhibit, to varying degrees, one or more stages of the metabolism of arachidonic acid by both platelets and endothelial cells. Therefore, it is important to consider the relative contributions of metabolites coming from each of these two types of cells and how an antithrombotic agent may influence the metabolism of arachidonic acid by these two important cells, *in vivo*. Presently this is extremely difficult to evaluate, but hopefully progress will be made as new methods are developed. (2) Antithrombotic agents may inhibit the formation of both inducers or inhibitors of platelet aggregation, on the one hand, as well as vasoconstrictors or vasodilators on the other. Therefore, the evaluation of the relative contributions of platelet aggregation or vasoconstriction is very important. (3) The possible contribution of increased numbers of smooth muscle cells, in a growing atherosclerotic plaque, to local thrombotic episodes needs to be evaluated, especially since smooth muscle cells (Harker *et al.*, 1978) as well as endothelial cells (Sage *et al.*, 1979), can make collagen and prostacyclin.

G. Approaches to Prevention or Therapy of Thrombosis Based on the Metabolism of Arachidonic Acid by Platelets or Endothelial Cells

The general approaches that are considered here include (1) inhibition of the formation of metabolites of arachidonic acid which may induce platelet aggregation or cause vasoconstriction; (2) promotion of the formation of inhibitors of platelet aggregation; (3) use of antagonists of the activity of metabolites which induce platelet aggregation or vasoconstriction.

An important advantage of these approaches to the thrombosis problem is that they probably involve little risk of hemorrhage, i.e., the effects should be antithrombotic without completely inhibiting hemostasis. The reason for this is that the metabolism of arachidonic acid is not the only pathway for the induction of platelet aggregation and when the arachidonate pathway is blocked some platelet aggregation may still occur via other mechanisms.

Since platelets and endothelial cells appear to have generally similar enzymatic pathways for the metabolism of arachidonic acid, the relative effects on these two cells of any agent employed in the circulation must be considered. For example, the net effect of an antithrombotic agent designed to inhibit the formation of metabolites of arachidonic acid which induce platelet aggregation or vasoconstriction will depend partly on its relative effects on the formation of these agents by platelets as well as endothelial cells. It will also depend on its effects on the formation of *inhibitors* of aggregation and *vasodilators* by these two cells. With the caveat that none of the approaches suggested below will be simple and that rigorous proof of efficacy will be required, we can consider some of them.

1. *Antithrombotic Agents*

a. Inhibitors of the Activity of Phospholipase A_2, Other Phospholipases, or Diglyceride Lipase. Inhibition of phospholipase activity may be partial or complete. If it is complete, no free arachidonic acid would become available to be converted into biologically active metabolites. The major effects related to hemostasis or thrombosis would be lack of formation of the metabolites which induce platelet aggregation or cause vasoconstriction. This might result in a net antithrombotic tendency. Would it also promote an antihemostatic tendency which might result in hemorrhage rather than hemostasis in response to injury to blood vessels? Hopefully any antihemostatic tendency would be minimal because some aggregation could still occur by mechanisms which do not involve the metabolism of arachidonic acid. Of course, another factor to be considered is that agents such as PGD_2 from platelets and PGI_2 from endothelial cells which, probably, normally limit platelet aggregation would also not be formed. A further complicating eventuality would be that no substrate arachidonic acid would be available for the lipoxygenase pathway. It is therefore difficult to predict the net consequences in hemostasis or thrombosis of the absolute inhibition of the release of free arachidonic acid from platelets or endothelial cells. The possible consequences of partial inhibition of platelet or endothelial cell phospholipase activity are even more unpredictable. The reason for this is that we do not presently know what proportions of subnormal amounts of available arachidonic acid, after injury to a blood vessel, would be utilized by the lipoxygenase pathway or the cyclooxygenase pathway. At present there is no known inhibitor of platelet or endothelial cell phospholipase activity which causes an antithrombotic tendency *in vivo*.

Elevated platelet cyclic AMP levels, inhibition of platelet aggregation, and inhibition of platelet phospholipase A_2. Three naturally occurring prostaglandins PGI_2, PGD_2, and PGE_1 are potent inhibitors of human platelet aggregation (Moncada *et al.*, 1976; Smith *et al.*, 1974; Kloeze, 1967) and cause elevation of platelet cAMP (Best *et al.*, 1977; Mills and Macfarlane, 1974; Robison *et al.*, 1969). In addition, dibutyryl cAMP inhibits platelet phospholipase activity (Minkes *et al.*, 1977; Gerrard *et al.*, 1977; Lapetina *et al.*, 1977; Bills *et al.*, 1978).

It thus seems likely that an important factor in the mechanisms of inhibition of platelet aggregation by these prostaglandins involves elevation of intracellular cAMP levels, resulting in inhibition of phospholipase activity normally occurring in response to aggregating agents.

b. Inhibitors of Cyclooxygenase Activity. i. Aspirin. Early recognition that the initial steps in the endogenous formation of PGI_2 were probably similar to those involved in prostaglandin and thromboxane synthesis in a variety of tissues, i.e., via endoperoxide formation by a cyclooxygenase, raised doubts about the use of aspirin as an antithrombotic agent. While it is always possible that aspirin could be thrombogenic in some circumstances by inhibiting PGI_2 formation by blood vessels, several studies on this question (Jaffe and Weksler, 1979; Czervionke *et al.*, 1979; Burch *et al.*, 1978) suggested that at low therapeutic doses there is probably little to fear. It appears that inhibition of the endothelial cell cyclooxygenase requires a much higher concentration of aspirin than that of the platelet enzyme and that the effect of aspirin on endothelial cells is of short duration (hours) while that on platelets lasts for days. On the other hand, there has been a recent preliminary study (Pareti *et al.*, 1979) reporting that PGI_2 production in biopsy specimens of human veins taken 2 hours after the individual had ingested 300 mg of aspirin was inhibited. This question should be resolved in the near future. Certainly, after many years of clinical experience with aspirin, there is little evidence that it is thrombogenic in humans.

Inhibition of cyclooxygenase activity in platelets or endothelial cells should decrease the production of the potent aggregating agents PGG_2, PGH_2, and TxA_2. Aspirin does this effectively *in vivo,* with negligible side effects at the therapeutic dose. Aspirin inhibits platelet cyclooxygenase and the second wave of platelet aggregation with little effect on the first wave. Since primary aggregation occurs, a platelet plug, albeit less stable than in the absence of aspirin (Wester *et al.*, 1978), may be formed and this should reduce the risk of bleeding during aspirin therapy. For this reason, aspirin should have a mild antithrombotic effect without being antihemostatic. This is borne out by the clinical experience of hundreds of millions of users of aspirin for more than 50 years. The clinical pharmacology of aspirin has been reviewed by Cohen (1976).

ii. Dosage of aspirin. One gram of aspirin per day was used in some of the clinical trials mentioned below and is a fairly high dose, certainly much more than is needed to significantly inhibit human platelet aggregation and cyclooxygenase activity. This probably can be achieved in most individuals with one quarter or less of that dose. Since prostacyclin formation by endothelial cells may also be inhibited by aspirin it would defeat the purpose of aspirin treatment to use a high dose of the drug which would also inhibit prostacyclin synthesis by endothelial cells. It would obviously be better to find a dose of aspirin which would cause maximum inhibition of platelet aggregation and thromboxane formation and minimal or no inhibition of PGI_2 production by endothelial cells. It is not going to be a simple matter to find the ideal, antithrombotic, dose of aspirin or any other drug which may inhibit the cyclooxygenase activity of platelets but not endothelial cells.

iii. Antithrombotic and antiatherosclerotic effects of aspirin in experimental animals. Aspirin has been shown to protect against thromboembolic episodes and death induced by the intravascular injection of arachidonic acid in rabbits (Silver *et al.,* 1974) and to inhibit the formation of atherosclerotic lesions in the coronary arteries of monkeys on an atherogenic diet (Pick *et al.,* 1979).

iv. Clinical trials of aspirin. The easy availability of pharmaceutical preparations containing aspirin complicates matters. Over 200 of such "over-the-counter" preparations have been listed by Cohen (1976) and it is quite possible that there are many more. The consumption of aspirin by Americans is enormous and may have beneficial or sometimes detrimental effects related to thrombosis. An example of a possible beneficial effect may be that, unbeknownst to them, those Americans consuming aspirin for analgesic purposes may also be reducing the number of transient ischemic attacks (TIAs) (see below under Stroke) or other thromboembolic episodes that they would otherwise be subjected to. An example of a possible detrimental effect relates to the possible use of aspirin containing compounds by patients assigned to the placebo group in a clinical trial of aspirin. If compliance is not rigidly controlled, and some placebo patients do take "over-the-counter" medicaments containing aspirin during the trial, the results might suggest that there was no difference between the aspirin and placebo groups when in actual fact both groups may have benefited from aspirin. Absolute compliance is difficult but essential in such clinical trials.

In recent years there have been a number of clinical trials of aspirin as an antithrombotic agent. An extensive review of this subject will not be made here. However, some of the highlights will be mentioned. Clinical trials of aspirin which were done prior to 1975 have been reviewed by Harker *et al.* (1975). The studies reviewed there involved the possible reduction in the thromboembolic events in patients with artificial heart valves or arteriovenous Silastic cannulas (used as shunts), the possible reduction of such events during dialysis, and the long term antithrombotic effects in cerebrovascular disorders or coronary artery disease. They noted a correlation between platelet consumption and frequency of thromboembolic events, suggesting that the measurement of platelet survival may help to predict the efficacy of antithrombotic agents *in vivo.* Harker and Schlichter (1970) showed that in patients with prosthetic heart valves or recurrent thromboembolism aspirin potentiated the reduction of platelet consumption by dipyridamole but had no effect alone. Lindsay *et al.* (1972) showed that aspirin reduced thrombus formation as well as the fall in numbers of circulating platelets seen in chronic uremia patients during dialysis.

Harris *et al.* (1977) assessed the prophylactic effects of aspirin against venous thromboembolism in patients over 40 years old undergoing total hip replacement. This was a carefully controlled, double-blind study in which radiographic phlebography was used to detect thromboembolism. Their data indicated that 600 mg of aspirin twice daily protected the male patients. Female patients were not protected. This remains to be explained. Recently, Harter *et al.* (1979) ran a randomized double-blind trial of aspirin on patients undergoing chronic hemodialysis. They used a low dose of aspirin (160 mg per day) and found that aspirin prevented shunt thrombosis. They observed thrombosis in 72% of the patients on placebo and 32% of patients treated with aspirin.

v. Stroke. The efficacy of aspirin now appears to be established for the prophylaxis of TIAs. The findings of the Canadian Cooperative Stroke Study Group (1978) have been reviewed by Barnett (1979). Patients in the study included individuals who had one or more minor ischemic events within 3 months of entry into the study. Only those who had TIA lasting 24 hours or less or those with minor nonprogressing, nondisabling, neurological effects were accepted. Patients on aspirin took 1300 mg per day. Other patients in the study received placebo or sulfinpyrazone (800 mg per day) or both drugs. The administration of aspirin caused a 19% reduction in the risk of continuing TIA, stroke, or death. Sulfinpyrazone was ineffective and did not have a synergistic effect in combination with aspirin. Aspirin caused a 31% reduction of the risk for stroke or death when they were considered apart from TIA and this was increased to 48% when only the male patients were considered. Aspirin did not reduce the risk of stroke or death among female patients. The reason for the apparently different effects of aspirin on male patients as compared to women remains to be explored.

vi. Myocardial infarction. Several clinical trials have been run to see whether aspirin could reduce the incidence of mortality due to coronary heart disease or of a second myocardial infarct in patients that have already had one infarct. None of these has shown a statistically significant difference between the effects of aspirin and the effects of placebo. In the latest big study, sponsored by the Aspirin Myocardial Infarction Study Research Group (1979), it was found that the incidence of mortality or second infarcts over a 3-year period was 14.1% in the aspirin group and 14.8% in the placebo group. The patients receiving aspirin took 1 gm per day.

It may be that these results were obtained because certain aspects of the study were not well conceived or carried out and that a better study would give different results. On the other hand it is quite possible that the wrong population was chosen for the study. Individuals who have already had a myocardial infarct would presumably also have fairly advanced atherosclerosis and since aspirin is only a mild antithrombotic agent there was little chance that aspirin would be effective. It is not readily apparent why a population with advanced atherosclerosis was chosen for this study. On the other hand, aspirin may prove to be an effective, prophylactic, antithrombotic agent, when the degree of atherosclerosis is not too far advanced. The value of aspirin as an antithrombotic agent most likely lies in its ability to suppress thrombotic and thromboembolic episodes and its potential to suppress the further development of atherosclerotic plaques beginning to form in individuals who have not yet had a myocardial infarct.

vii. Sulfinpyrazone. Results of the Anturane Reinfarction Trial (1978) suggest that sulfinpyrazone is "effective in reducing cardiac deaths during the first year after myocardial infarction." In this limited study the patients selected were between 45 and 70 years old and had had at least one myocardial infarction which occurred 25 to 35 days before enrollment in the study. The patients taking sulfinpyrazone received 200 mg four times a day. The annual death rate for cardiac deaths was 9.5% in the placebo group and 4.9% in the sulfinpyrazone group or a reduction of 48.5%. When the annual sudden-cardiac death rate was considered the reduction was 57.2%. The exact mechanism for the effectiveness of sulfinpyrazone in these studies is not known. This drug is known to inhibit platelet aggregation and prostaglandin synthesis (cyclooxygenase activity) but it may also be effective in preventing abnormal heart rhythms. The combined antiplatelet and antiarrhythmic activity may explain its effectiveness. Following the publication of the results of the Anturane Reinfarction Trial a controversy developed in which the design of the study and the analysis of the results were seriously questioned. This resulted in disapproval of the drug by the United States Food and Drug Administration for use in the prevention of sudden death in patients that had already had a myocardial infarct. Details on various aspects of this controversy have been reviewed by Kolata (1980).

c. Inhibitors of Thromboxane Synthetase and Antagonists of the Biological Activities of Thromboxane A_2. The apparent potency of thromboxane A_2 as an inducer of platelet aggregation and a vasoconstrictor suggests that substances which specifically inhibit its formation or activity might be good antithrombotic agents. Some approaches which may be used for screening such agents *in vitro* are suggested by Gryglewski (1978). Several agents have been shown to be selective inhibitors of thromboxane synthesis *in vitro*. These include imidazole and several of its analogs (see Moncada *et al.*, 1977; Needleman *et al.*, 1977; Nijkamp *et al.*, 1977); L 8027, 1'-(isopropyl-2-indolyl)-3-pyridyl-3 ketone (Gryglewski *et al.*, 1977); 9,11-azoprosta-5,13-dienoic acid (Gorman *et al.*, 1977). Hydralazine, dipyridamole, and diazoxide were also shown to be selective inhibitors of thromboxane synthesis (Greenwald *et al.*, 1978). Hammarström and Falardeau (1977) purified thromboxane synthetase from human platelet microsomes and showed that it was inhibited by HPETE, a product of the platelet lipoxygenase pathway. Recently, 9,11-azo-13-oxa-15-hydroxyprostanoic acid has been shown to be a potent inhibitor of thromboxane synthetase as well as an antagonist of thromboxane A_2 and PGH_2 (Kam *et al.*, 1979). Other antagonists of thromboxane A_2 include 9,11-epoxyiminoprosta-5,13-dienoic acid (Fitzpatrick *et al.*, 1978) and pinane thromboxane A_2 (Nicolaou *et al.*, 1978). For further discussion of agents of this type see Nicolaou and Smith (1979) and Smith (1980). It remains to be seen whether any of these agents or others with similar activities will be effective antithrombotic agents *in vivo*.

d. Agents which Increase the Production of PGD_2 by Platelets or PGI_2 by Endothelial Cells. Although this is a potentially interesting approach to the thrombosis problem there has only been one report of this kind. Vermylen *et al.* (1979) proposed that the antithrombotic effect of Bay g 6575 might be caused by its ability to stimulate PGI_2 formation by blood vessels.

e. Slowly Metabolized Analogs of PGD_2, PGE_1, or PGI_2. Prostaglandin D_2, E_1, and I_2 are all potent inhibitors of platelet aggregation *in vitro* (see Di Minno *et al.*, 1979). As indicated in Section III,G,1,a, they apparently inhibit platelet aggregation by stimulating the formation of cyclic AMP by platelets. cAMP, in turn, may inhibit platelet phospholipase activity. The effect would be no release of arachidonic acid from phospholipids and no production of the metabolites which induce platelet aggregation. Whether these prostaglandins may also inhibit aggregation by other mechanisms remains to be determined. Unfortunately their effects *in vivo* are of short duration because they are very rapidly metabolized in the body. Sustained inhibition of platelet aggregation, *in vivo,* by these prostaglandins can be attained only by constant infusion, which raises other problems mostly related to their vasoactive effects. Perhaps slowly metabolized, more active, analogs of these prostaglandins might prove to be of value. Nishizawa (1977) and Smith *et al.* (1979) have discussed the use in experimental animals of analogs of prostaglandins which inhibit platelet aggregation. There are still no reports of the efficacy of such analogs in humans. Recently, Whitaker *et al.* (1979) have shown that PGD_3 is a potent inhibitor of platelet aggregation suggesting that it, or an appropriate analog, also merit consideration.

f. Albumin. Sections II,M and III,C discussed the role of plasma albumin as a modulator of arachidonate metabolism and the fact that low levels of circulating plasma albumin correlated with hyperaggregable platelets and a thrombotic tendency in patients with the nephrotic syndrome. Remuzzi *et al.* (1979) further showed that the response of these patients' platelets to aggregating agents could be normalized by addition of albumin to their platelet-rich plasma *in vitro;* but, more important than this, infusion of albumin corrected the hyperaggregable state of the patients' platelets *ex vivo.* This strongly suggests that infusions of albumin might diminish the thrombotic tendency in patients with the nephrotic syndrome.

2. *Replacement of Arachidonic Acid in Platelet Phospholipids by 8,11,14-Eicosatrienoic Acid or 5,8,11,14,17-Eicosapentaenollic Acid*

In 1973 it was reported that both 8,11,14-eicosatrienoic acid and 5,8,11,14,17-eicosapentaenoic acid could inhibit the aggregation of human platelets (Silver *et al.,* 1973). These fatty acids are known precursors of prostaglandins of the 1 or 3 series, respectively (e.g., PGE_1; PGD_3) which would tend to inhibit aggregation. Compared to arachidonic acid these fatty acids make up a small and often insignificant portion of the prostaglandin precursor fatty acids consumed in the diet of most Americans and Europeans and their platelet phospholipids would contain little of these fatty acids. A reasonable approach to the thrombosis problem therefore suggests itself: Change the ratio of arachidonic acid to one or the other of these fatty acids in the phospholipids of circulating platelets. This might be accomplished by reducing the dietary intake of arachidonic and increasing that of 8,11,14-eicosatrienoic acid or 5,8,11,14,17-eicosapentaenoic acid or administering one of these in pure form as a prophylactic agent. Such a regime would have to be continued for relatively long periods of time or over a lifetime since the life span of human platelets is only about 10 days. The hoped-for prophylactic result would be to have platelets that, in response to stimulated phospholipase activity resulting from injury to a blood vessel, would release fatty acids which would be converted to a variety of metabolites whose resultant biological activity would tend to be antithrombotic rather than prothrombotic. Thus, the potent induction of aggregation and vasoconstriction caused by certain metabolites of arachidonic acid would be tempered by the inhibitory effects of the metabolites coming from the other precursor fatty acids. The diminution in the absolute amounts of arachidonic acid present in the platelet phospholipids might also result in release of less arachidonic acid in response to phospholipase activity and therefore formation of lesser amounts of potentially prothrombotic metabolites.

This approach to the thrombosis problem is attractive and merits careful investigation to determine whether it may be successful. Assuming that there are no toxic effects of such regimens, unrelated to hemostasis, there are still a variety of possible complications that might arise and are being considered by workers in this field. These include, at least, the following: (1) Arachidonic acid in platelet phospholipids might be diminished to such a degree that the overwhelming effect of the metabolites of the other fatty acid might lead to a bleeding tendency. (2) The amounts and biological activities of metabolites of the other two prostaglandin precursor fatty acids formed via the lipoxygenase, prostaglandin, or thromboxane pathways have been little studied and might cause unsuspected complications.

The studies that have been done with 8,11,14-eicosatrienoic acid and 5,8,11,14,17-eicosapentaenoic acid will be considered separately.

a. 8,11,14-Eicosatrienoic Acid (Also Called Dihomo-γ-linolenic Acid). *i. In vitro studies.* It is possible that 8,11,14-eicosatrienoic acid may have inherent ability to inhibit platelet aggregation, but its possible conversion to inhibitory metabolites has been given more consideration. In 1973 it was shown that human platelets could convert 8,11,14-eicosatrienoic acid into PGE_1, a known inhibitor of platelet aggregation (Silver *et al.*, 1973). Later, Gorman and Miller (1977) reported that PGH_1, the endoperoxide formed from 8,11,14-eicosatrienoic acid, can inhibit the aggregation of platelets in plasma and elevate platelet cAMP. This apparently occurs because it can be converted to PGE_1. Needleman *et al.* (1980) have shown that, when the inhibitory effect of formed PGE_1 is blocked in a washed platelet system, PGH_1 can induce aggregation. The other metabolites of 8,11,14-eicosatrienoic acid which might inhibit platelet aggregation are PGE_1 and PGD_1. Since washed platelets do not produce much PGD_1 it is likely that PGE_1 is the metabolite that could play an antithrombotic role. However, it is often difficult to predict what may happen *in vivo* by extrapolating from *in vitro* or *ex vivo* experiments, especially with washed platelets. We have already stressed the modulatory role of albumin in the metabolism of arachidonic acid. To properly evaluate the effectiveness of these fatty acids as antithrombotic agents one must test them in animals and humans.

ii. In vivo studies. If oral administration of prostaglandin precursors is to be used effectively to prevent thrombosis these fatty acids must be esterified into the platelet pool of phosphatidylcholine and phosphatidylinositol. It was first shown by Bills *et al.* (1976, 1977) that arachidonic acid as well as 8,11,14-eicosatrienoic acid could be rapidly incorporated from blood plasma into human platelet phospholipids *in vitro*. This indicates that such incorporation might occur in circulating blood. In fact, Seyberth *et al.* had previously (1975) shown that the oral administration of ethyl arachidonate to humans resulted in an increase in the relative and absolute amount of arachidonate in the triglycerides, phospholipids, and cholesteryl esters of the blood platelets as well as the plasma. This was accompanied by an increase in the sensitivity of the platelets to induction of aggregation by ADP. Thus it was shown that one risked the development of a thrombotic tendency by increasing the ingestion of arachidonic acid. Could a thrombotic tendency be reversed by oral administration of 8,11,14-eicosatrienoic acid? In a detailed study of the changes in fatty acid composition of many tissues, including platelets, Danon *et al.* (1975) reported a 6-fold increase in the 8,11,14-eicosatrienoic acid content of the platelet phospholipids of rats receiving a diet supplemented with ethyl dihomo-γ-linolenate. Willis *et al.* (1977) reported a significant reduction in platelet aggregation in response to ADP and collagen in rats fed free 8,11,14-eicosatrienoic acid for 8 days at a dose of 400 mg/kg. However, Oelz *et al.* (1976) found that rabbits responded differently. They fed rabbits with the ethyl ester of 8,11,14-eicosatrienoic acid (1 gm/kg/day) for 25 days and found that the platelet phospholipids, as well as all plasma lipid classes, were highly enriched in this fatty acid whereas the arachidonic acid content in platelet phospholipids was significantly lower than in the controls. They also found that platelet aggregation in these rabbits in response to ADP, collagen, or arachidonic acid, did not differ from that seen in the controls. This shows that there may be important species differences and the important question is "What happens in man"? In a limited study (Sim and McCraw, 1977) the methyl ester of 8,11,14-eicosatrienoic acid was administered orally to three human volunteers. A single dose of 1.5 mg/kg was given to one female. Aggregation of her platelets in platelet-rich plasma was markedly reduced in response to ADP at 2 and 4 hours after the dose with a return to normal at 6 hours. Two male volunteers were given single sequential daily doses of 1.5 mg/kg for 3 or 5 days. Except for a tendency to return to a normal aggregation response 24 hours after a dose, the responses to aggregation by ADP were markedly reduced at the other times studied. In another study, Kernoff *et al.* (1977) fed either the ethyl ester or free 8,11,14-eicosatrienoic acid to eight human volunteers. They used a variety of dosage schedules, sometimes going as high as 1 gm, twice a day, for 10 days. In general there was a decreased sensitivity of the platelets to aggregate in response to ADP. However, there appeared to be variability of response from individual to individual. For example, in one individual receiving 1 gm/day there was a sustained response showing diminished sensitivity to aggregation by ADP, adrenaline, and ristocetin; in another individual this could not be shown. In all cases it was shown that platelets from the experimental subjects had an increased capacity to produce PGE_1 which may be made only in trace amounts by individuals not consuming 8,11,14-eicosatrienoic acid. Possible adverse effects appeared to be minimal in these studies. Obviously considerably more work has to be done in humans to determine the value of this fatty acid as an antithrombotic agent.

b. 5,8,11,14,17-Eicosapentaenoic Acid. i. In vitro studies. That 5,8,11,-14,17-eicosapentaenoic acid (as well as 4,7,10,13,16,19-docosahexaenoic acid) could inhibit the aggregation of human platelets was first reported by Silver *et al.* (1973). Detailed studies of the inhibition of platelet aggregation have been done only recently. Jakubowski and Ardlie (1979) showed inhibition of platelet aggregation and the release reaction induced by collagen, ADP, adrenaline, thrombin, the ionophore A23187, and arachidonic acid. In addition Gryglewski *et al.* (1979) showed that this fatty acid could also inhibit aggregation induced by the compound U46619 the stable 9-11 methano-oxy analog of PGH_2. Whitaker *et al.* (1979) showed that PGH_3 was rapidly converted to PGD_3 in plasma and that both metabolites of 5,8,11,14,17-eicosapentaenoic acid inhibited human platelet aggregation induced by arachidonic acid and caused an elevation of platelet cAMP levels. They further showed that a PGD antiserum blocked the inhibitory activity of both PGH_3 and PGD_3, suggesting that the inhibition of platelet aggregation by PGH_3 was due to its rapid conversion to PGD_3.

ii. In vivo studies. Radioactive eicosapentaenoic acid may be incorporated into platelet phospholipids (Needleman *et al.*, 1979; McKean *et al.*, 1981), suggesting that such incorporation may occur *in vivo.* The normal dietary intake of the Greenland Eskimos consists of seafoods rich in eicosapentaenoic acid while their Danish compatriots consume a Western European diet, relatively rich in arachidonic acid and deficient in eicosapentaenoic acid. This sets the scene for what might appear to be an almost preconceived nutritional experiment with a control group. Realizing this, Dyerberg *et al.* (1978) observed that there was a low incidence of acute myocardial infarction among these Eskimos and that their blood lipids contained high levels of eicosapentaenoic and low levels of arachidonic acid while in Danish volunteers the reverse was true. Later, Dyerberg and Bang (1979) showed that the Eskimos had significantly longer bleeding times than the Danes, lower platelet counts, a tendency toward reduced sensitivity to platelet aggregation induced by ADP, and high levels of eicosapentaenoic acid with low levels of arachidonic acid in their platelet lipids.

Siess *et al.* (1980) put seven healthy men on a diet containing 500–800 gm of mackerel per day. This contained 7 to 11 gm of eicosapentaenoic acid. Studies on blood samples were done before and on the third and sixth day after starting the diet. There was a decrease in their platelet aggregation, *in vitro,* in response to a low concentration of collagen, which correlated with decreased formation of thromboxane B_2 by the platelets and an increase in the ratio of eicosapentaenoic acid to arachidonic acid in the platelet phospholipids. Decreases in platelet aggregation in response to a high concentration of collagen or ADP were not significant. The concentration of arachidonic acid used for inducing aggregation (1.8 m*M*) was unfortunately much too high. However, Dyerberg and Bang (1979) showed that aggregation responses to arachidonic acid at 0.6 m*M* were normal in the platelet-rich plasma of 10 different Greenland Eskimos.

IV. Conclusions

Millions of deaths due to myocardial infarction and other thrombotic disorders occur every year in the Western world. Thrombus formation, which involves platelet aggregation, plays an important role in these deaths. In recent years important discoveries have been made pertaining to the metabolism of arachidonic acid and other prostaglandin precursors by platelets and endothelial cells. They have advanced our understanding of platelet aggregation as well as hemostasis and thrombosis. Some of the metabolites formed can induce, inhibit, or modulate platelet aggregation; some are also vasoconstrictors or vasodilators. This new knowledge has provided the information to develop rationales to prevent or treat thrombosis. Aspirin, which inhibits platelet aggregation and platelet cyclooxygenase, may be a good antithrombotic agent when used properly. Several of the other approaches suggested here may turn out to be valuable approaches to the thrombosis problem. This area of investigation is being pursued intensively and we may look forward to new discoveries and new approaches to the prevention and treatment of thrombosis in the near future.

Acknowledgments

Much of this material was conceived and written during the author's tenure of the Johananoff fellowship at the Mario Negri Institute, Milan, Italy in 1978. The work was supported in part by grant HLB-14890 of the National Institutes of Health.

References

Aharony, D., Smith, J. B., and Silver, M. J. (1980). *Fed. Proc. Fed. Am. Soc. Exp. Biol.* **39,** 424.

Aharony, D., Smith, J. B., and Silver, M. J. (1981). *Prostaglandins Med.,* in press.

Anturane Reinfarction Trial (1978). *New Engl. J. Med.* **298,** 289.

Ardlie, N. G., and Han, P. (1974). *Br. J. Haematol.* **26**, 331.

Aspirin Myocardial Infarction Study Research Group (1979). *J. Am. Med. Assoc.* **243**, 661.

Baenziger, N. L., Dillender, M. J., and Majerus, P. W. (1977). *Biochem. Biophys. Res. Commun.* **78**, 294.

Barkhan, P., and Silver, M. J. (1962). *In* "Progress in Hematology" (L. M. Tocantins, ed.), Vol. III, pp. 170–202. Grune & Stratton, New York.

Barnett, H. J. M. (1979). *In* "Cerebrovascular Diseases" (T. R. Price and E. Nelson, eds.), pp. 221–236. Raven, New York.

Baumgartner, N. R., and Muggli, R. (1976). *In* "Platelets in Biology and Pathology" (J. L. Gordon, ed.), pp. 23–60. North-Holland Publ., Amsterdam.

Best, L. C., Martin, T. J., Russel, R. G. G., and Preston, F. E. (1977). *Nature (London)* **267**, 850.

Bills, T. K., Smith, J. B., and Silver, M. J. (1976). *Biochim. Biophys. Acta* **424**, 303.

Bills, T. K., Smith, J. B., and Silver, M. J. (1977). *J. Clin. Invest.* **60**, 1.

Bills, T. K., Smith, J. B., and Silver, M. J. (1978). *Thromb. Res.* **40**, 219.

Bryant, R. W., and Bailey, J. M. (1979). *Prostaglandins* **17**, 9.

Burch, J. W., and Majerus (1979). *Semin. Hematol.* **16**, 196.

Burch, J. W., Baenziger, N. L., Stanford, N., and Majerus, P. W. (1978). *Proc. Natl. Acad. Sci. U.S.A.* **75**, 5181.

Canadian Cooperative Stroke Study Group (1978). *New Engl. J. Med.* **299**, 53–59.

Cerskus, A. L., Ali, M., Zamecnik, J., and McDonald, J. W. D. (1978). *Thromb. Res.* **12**, 549.

Chahine, R. A. (1979). *Arch. Intern. Med.* **139**, 26.

Cohen, L. S. (1976). *Semin. Thromb. Hemostasis* **2**, 146.

Cooper, B., Schafer, A., Pucholsky, D., and Handin, R. I. (1978). *Blood* **52**, 618.

Czervionke, R. L., Smith, J. B., Fry, G. L., Hoak, J. C., and Haycraft, D. L. (1979). *J. Clin. Invest.* **63**, 1089.

Danon, A., Heimberg, M., and Oates, J. A. (1975). *Biochim. Biophys. Acta* **388**, 318.

Di Minno, G., Silver, M. J., and de Gaetano, G. (1979). *Br. J. Haematol.* **43**, 637.

Dusting, G. J., Moncada, S., and Vane, J. R. (1979). *Prog. Cardiovasc. Dis.* **21**, 405.

Dyerberg, J., and Bang, H. O. (1979). *Lancet* **1**, 433.

Dyerberg, J., Bang, H. O., Stoffersen, E., Moncada, S., and Vane, J. R. (1978). *Lancet* **15**, 117.

Fishman, J. A., Ryan, G. B., and Karnovsky, M. J. (1975). *Lab. Invest.* **32**, 339.

Fitzpatrick, F. A., Bundy, G. L., Gorman, R. R., and Honohan, T. (1978). *Nature (London)* **275**, 764.

Friedman, Z., Lamberth, E. L., Stahlman, M. T., and Oates, J. A. (1976). *Adv. Prostaglandin Thromboxane Res.* **2**, 852.

Gerrard, J. M., Peller, J. D., Krick, T. P., and White, J. G. (1977). *Prostaglandins* **14**, 39.

Gorman, R. R., and Miller, O. V. (1977). *In* "Prostaglandins in Hematology" (M. J. Silver, J. B. Smith, and J. J. Kocsis, eds.), pp. 235–246. Spectrum, New York.

Gorman, R., Bundy, G. L., Peterson, D. C., Sun, F. F., Miller, O. V., and Fitzpatrick, F. A. (1977). *Proc. Natl. Acad. Sci. U.S.A.* **74**, 4007.

Greenwald, J. E., Wong, L. K., Rao, M., Bianchine, J. R., and Panganamala, R. V. (1978). *Biochem. Biophys. Res. Commun.* **84**, 1112.

Greenwald, J. E., Bianchine, J. R., and Wong, L. K. (1979). *Nature (London)* **281**, 588.

Gryglewski, R. J. (1978). *In* "Advances in Lipid Research" (R. Paoletti and D. Kritchevsky, eds.), Vol. 16, pp. 327–344. Academic Press, New York.

Gryglewski, R. J., Zmuda, A., Dembinska-Kiec, A., and Krecioch, E. (1977). *Pharmacol. Res. Commun.* **9**, 109.

Gryglewski, R. J., Salmon, J. A., Ubatuba, F. B., Weatherly, B. C., Moncada, S., and Vane, J. R. (1979). *Prostaglandins* **18**, 453.

Hamberg, M., and Samuelsson, B. (1973). *Proc. Natl. Acad. Sci. U.S.A.* **70,** 899.

Hamberg, M., and Samuelsson, B. (1974). *Proc. Natl. Acad. Sci. U.S.A.* **71,** 3400.

Hamberg, M., Svensson, J., and Samuelsson, B. (1974). *Proc. Natl. Acad. Sci. U.S.A.* **71,** 3824.

Hamberg, M., Svensson, J., and Samuelsson, B. (1975). *Proc. Natl. Acad. Sci. U.S.A.* **72,** 2994.

Hammarström, S., and Falardeau, P. (1977). *Proc. Natl. Acad. Sci. U.S.A.* **74,** 3691.

Harker, L. A., and Schlichter, S. J. (1970). *New Engl. J. Med.* **283,** 1302.

Harker, L. A., Hirsh, J., Gent, M., and Genton, E. (1975). *Prog. Hematol.* **9,** 229.

Harker, L. A., Ross, R., and Glomset, J. A. (1978). *In* "Platelets: A Multidisciplinary Approach" (G. de Gaetano and J. Garattini, eds.), pp. 89–102. Raven, New York.

Harris, W. H., Salzman, E. W., Athanasoulis, C. A., Waltman, C. A., and De Sanctis, R. W. (1977). *New Engl. J. Med.* **297,** 1246.

Harris, R. H., Ramwell, P. W., and Gilmer, P. J. (1979). *Annu. Rev. Physiol.* **41,** 653.

Harter, H. R., Burch, J. W., Majerus, P. W., Stanford, N., Delmez, J. A., Anderson, C. B., and Weerts, C. A. (1979). *New Engl. J. Med.* **301,** 577.

Herman, A. G., Claeys, M., Moncada, S., and Vane, J. R. (1979). *Prostaglandins* **18,** 439.

Higgs, E. A., Moncada, S., and Vane, J. R. (1978). *Prostaglandins* **16,** 17.

Ingerman, C. M., Aharony, D., Silver, M. J., Smith, J. B., Nissenbaum, M., Sedar, A. W., and Macarak, E. (1980). *Fed. Proc. Fed. Am. Soc. Exp. Biol.* **39,** 391.

Ingerman, C. M., Silver, M., J., and Smith, J. B. (1981). *J. Clin. Invest.* **67,** 1293.

Jaffe, R. M. (1976). *In* "Platelets in Biology and Pathology" (J. L. Gordon, ed.), pp. 261–292. North-Holland Publ., Amsterdam.

Jaffe, E., and Weksler, B. B. (1979). *J. Clin. Invest.* **63,** 532.

Jakubowski, J. A., and Ardlie, N. G. (1979). *Thromb. Res.* **16,** 205.

Johnson, R. A., Morton, D. R., Kinner, J. H., Gorman, R. R., McGuire, J. C., Sun, F. F., Whitaker, N., Bunting, S., Salmon, J., Moncada, S., and Vane, J. R. (1976). *Prostaglandins* **12,** 915.

Jones, R. L., Kerry, P. J., Poyser, N. L., Walker, T. C., and Wilson, N. J. (1978). *Prostaglandins* **16,** 583.

Kam, S. T., Portoghese, P. S., Dunham, E. W., and Gerrard, J. M. (1979). *Prostaglandins Med.* **3,** 279.

Kernoff, P. B. A., Willis, A. L., Stone, K. J., Davies, J. A., and McNicol, G. P. (1977). *Br. Med. J.* **3,** 1441.

Kloeze, J. (1967). *In* "Second Nobel Symposium: Prostaglandins" (S. Berström and B. Samuelsson, eds.), pp. 243–252. Almquist & Wiksell, Stockholm.

Kolata, G. B. (1980). *Science* **208,** 1130.

Lagarde, M., Byron, P. A., Vargaftig, B., and Dechavanne, M. (1978). *Br. J. Haematol.* **38,** 251.

Lands, W. E. M. (1979). *Annu. Rev. Physiol.* **41,** 633.

Lapetina, E. G., Schmitges, C. G., Chandrabose, K., and Cuatrecasas, P. (1977). *Biochem. Biophys. Res. Commun.* **76,** 828.

Legrand, Y. G., Faurel, F., and Caen, J. B. (1979). *In* "Frontiers of Matrix Biology" (L. Robert, ed.), pp. 235–245. Karger, Basel.

Lewy, R. I., Smith, J. B., Silver, M. J., Saia, J., Walinsky, P., and Wiener, L. (1979). *Prostaglandins Med.* **2,** 243.

Lindsay, R. M., Prentice, C. R. M., Ferguson, D., Burton, J. A., and McNicol, G. P. (1972). *Lancet* **2,** 1287.

Macintyre, D. E. (1976). *In* "Platelets in Biology and Pathology" (J. L. Gordon, ed.), pp. 61–85. Elsevier, Amsterdam.

McKean, M. L., Smith, J. B., and Silver, M. J. (1981). *Prog. Lipid Res.*, in press.
Malmsten, C., Hamberg, M., Svensson, J., and Samuelsson, B. (1975). *Proc. Natl. Acad. Sci. U.S.A.* **72**, 1446.
Marcus, A. J. (1978). *J. Lipid Res.* **19**, 793.
Mason, R. G., and Saba, H. I. (1978). *Am. J. Pathol.* **92**, 775.
Mielke, C. H., Kaneshiro, M. M., Maher, I. A., Wiener, J. M., and Rapaport, S. I. (1969). *Blood* **34**, 204.
Mills, D. C. B., and Macfarlane, D. E. (1974). *Thromb. Res.* **5**, 401.
Minkes, M., Stanford, N., Chi, M. M., Roth, G., Raz, A., Needleman, P., and Majerus, P. (1977). *J. Clin. Invest.* **59**, 449.
Moncada, S., and Vane, J. R. (1978). *In* "Platelets: A Multidisciplinary Approach" (G. de Gaetano and S. Garattini, eds.), pp. 239–258. Raven, New York.
Moncada, S., and Vane, J. R. (1979). *New Engl. J. Med.* **300**, 1142.
Moncada, S., Gryglewski, R., Bunting, S., and Vane, J. R. (1976). *Nature (London)* **263**, 663.
Moncada, S., Bunting, S., Mullane, K., Thorogood, P., and Vane, J. R. (1977). *Prostaglandins* **13**, 611.
Needleman, P., Raz, A., Ferrendelli, J. A., and Minkes, M. (1977). *Proc. Natl. Acad. Sci. U.S.A.* **74**, 1716.
Needleman, P., Raz, A., Minkes, M. S., Ferrendelli, J. A., and Sprecher, H. (1979). *Proc. Natl. Acad. Sci. U.S.A.* **76**, 944.
Needleman, P., Whitaker, M. O., Wyche, A., Watters, K., Sprecher, H., and Raz, A. (1980). *Prostaglandins* **19**, 165.
Nicolaou, K. C., and Smith, J. B. (1979). *Annu. Rep. Med. Chem.* **14**, 178.
Nicolaou, K. C., Barnette, W. W., Magolda, R. L., Grieco, P. A., Owens, W., Wong, C. L. J., Smith, J. B., Ogletree, M., and Lefer, A. M. (1978). *Prostaglandins* **16**, 789.
Nijkamp, F. P., Moncada, S., White, H. L., and Vane, J. R. (1977). *Eur. J. Pharmacol.* **44**, 179.
Nishizawa, E. E. (1977). *In* "Prostaglandins in Hematology" (M. J. Silver, J. B. Smith, and J. J. Kocsis, eds.), pp. 321–329. Spectrum, New York.
Nugteren, D. H., and Hazelhof, E. (1973). *Biochim. Biophys. Acta* **326:L25**, 448.
Nugteren, D. H., and Hazelhof, E. (1975). *Biochim. Biophys. Acta* **380**, 299.
Nyman, D., Eriksson, A. W., Lehmann, W., and Blombäck, M. (1979). *Thromb. Res.* **14**, 739.
Oelz, O., Seyberth, H. W., Knopp, H. R., Sweetman, B. J., and Oates, J. A. (1976). *Biochim. Biophys. Acta* **431**, 268.
Oelz, O., Oelz, R., and Knopp, H. R. (1977). *Prostaglandins* **13**, 225.
Okuma, M., and Uchino, H. (1979). *Blood* **54**, 1258.
Packham, M. A., Kinlough-Rathbone, R. L., Reimers, H. J., Scott, S., and Mustard, J. F. (1977). *In* "Prostaglandins in Hematology" (M. J. Silver, J. B. Smith, and J. J. Kocsis, eds.), pp. 247–276. Spectrum, New York.
Pareti, F. I., Smith, J. B., D'Angelo, A., and Manucci, P. M. (1979). *Thromb. Haemostasis* **42**, 156.
Pearson, J. D., and Gordon, J. L. (1979). *Nature (London)* **281**, 384.
Pick, R., Chediak, J., and Glick, G. (1979). *J. Clin. Invest.* **63**, 158.
Poole, J. C. F., Sanders, A. G., and Florey, H. W. (1958). *J. Pathol. Bacteriol.* **75**, 133.
Remuzzi, G., Marchesi, D., Tino, M., Cavenaghi, D., Mecca, G., Donati, M. B., and de Gaetano, G. (1978). *Thromb. Res.* **13**, 1007.
Remuzzi, G., Mecca, G., Marchesi, D., Livio, M., de Gaetano, G., Donati, M. B., and Silver, M. J. (1979). *Thromb. Res.* **16**, 345.

Rendu, F., Breton-Gorius, J., Trugnan, G., Castro-Malaspina, H., Andrieu, J., Bereziat, G., Lebret, M., and Caen, J. G. (1978). *Am. J. Hematol.* **4**, 387.
Richling, M. D., Griesmayr, G., Lametschwander, A., and Scheiblbrandner, W. (1979). *J. Neurosurg.* **51**, 654.
Robison, G. A., Arnold, A., and Hartman, R. C. (1969). *Pharmacol. Res. Commun.* **1**, 325.
Roth, G. J., and Majerus, P. W. (1975). *J. Clin. Invest.* **56**, 624.
Saba, S. R., and Mason, R. G. (1974). *Thromb. Res.* **5**, 747.
Sage, H., Crouch, E., and Bornstein, P. (1979). *Biochemistry* **24**, 5433.
Sakariassen, K. S., Bolhuis, P. A., and Sixma, J. J. (1979). *Nature (London)* **279**, 636.
Samuelsson, B., Goldyne, M., Granström, E., Hamberg, M., Hammarström, S., and Malmsten, C. (1978). *Annu. Rev. Biochem.* **47**, 997.
Sedar, A. W., Silver, M. J., Kocsis, J. J., and Smith, J. B. (1978). *Atherosclerosis* **30**, 273.
Sedar, A. W., Silver, M. J., Ingerman, C. M., Nissenbaum, M., and Smith, J. B. (1980). *Scan. Electron Microsc.* **3**, 235.
Seyberth, H. W., Oelz, O., Kennedy, T., Sweetman, B. J., Danon, A., Frölich, J. C., Heimberg, M., and Oates, J. A. (1975). *J. Clin. Pharmacol. Ther.* **18**, 521.
Sholley, M. M., Gimbrone, M. A., and Cotran, R. S. (1977). *Lab. Invest.* **36**, 18.
Siess, W., Scherer, B., Böhlig, Roth, P., Kurzmann, I., and Weber, P. C. (1980). *Lancet* **1**, 441.
Silver, M. J., Smith, J. B., Ingerman, C., and Kocsis, J. J. (1972a). *Prostaglandins* **1**, 429.
Silver, M. J., Hernandovich, J., Ingerman, C. M., Kocsis, J. J., and Smith, J. B. (1972b). *In* "Platelets and Thrombosis" (S. Sherry and A. Scriabine, eds.), pp. 91–98. Univ. Park Press, Philadelphia, Pennsylvania.
Silver, M. J., Smith, J. B., Ingerman, C. M., and Kocsis, J. J. (1973). *Prostaglandins* **4**, 863.
Silver, M. J., Hoch, W., Kocsis, J. J., Ingerman, C. M., and Smith, J. B. (1974). *Science* **183**, 1085.
Silver, M. J., Smith, J. B., and Kocsis, J. J. (1977). "Prostaglandins in Hematology," pp. 27–56. Spectrum, New York.
Silver, M. J., Bills, T. K., and Smith, J. B. (1978). *In* "Platelets: A Multidisciplinary Approach" (G. de Gaetano and S. Garattini, eds.), pp. 213–255. Raven, New York.
Silver, M. J., Ingerman, C. M., Smith, J. B., Nissenbaum, M., and Sedar, A. W. (1980a). *Fed. Proc. Fed. Am. Soc. Exp. Biol.* **39**, 428.
Silver, M. J., Sedar, A. W., Nissenbaum, M., and Smith, J. B. (1980b). *Artery* **8**, 80.
Silver, M. J., Smith, J. B., McKean, M. L., and Bills, T. K. (1980c). *In* "Hemostasis, Prostaglandins and Renal Diseases" (G. Remuzzi, G. Meca, and G. de Gaetano, eds.). Raven, New York.
Sim, A. K., and McCraw, A. P. (1977). *Thromb. Res.* **10**, 385.
Smith, J. B. (1980). *Am. J. Clin. Pathol.* **99**, 741.
Smith, J. B., and Silver, M. J. (1976). *In* "Platelets in Biology and Pathology" (J. L. Gordon, ed.), pp. 331–352. Elsevier, Amsterdam.
Smith, J. B., and Willis, A. L. (1970). *Br. J. Pharmacol.* **40**, 545P.
Smith, J. B., and Willis, A. L. (1971). *Nature (London)* **231**, 235.
Smith, J. B., Ingerman, C. M., Kocsis, J. J., and Silver, M. J. (1973). *J. Clin. Invest.* **52**, 965.
Smith, J. B., Silver, M. J., Ingerman, C. M., and Kocsis, J. J. (1974a). *Thromb. Res.* **5**, 291.
Smith, J. B., Ingerman, C., Kocsis, J. J., and Silver, M. J. (1974b). *J. Clin. Invest.* **53**, 1468.
Smith, J. B., Ingerman, C. M., and Silver, M. J. (1976). *Thromb. Res.* **9**, 413.
Smith, J. B., Ingerman, C. M., and Silver, M. J. (1979). *In* "Haemostasis and Thrombosis" (G. G. Neri Serneri and C. R. M. Prentice, eds.), pp. 103–112. Academic Press, New York.
Turner, S. R., Tainer, J. A., and Lynn, W. S. (1975). *Nature (London)* **257**, 680.

Vargaftig, B. B., and Zirinis, P. (1973). *Nature (London)* **244,** 114.

Verymylen, J., Chamone, D. A. F., and Verstraete, M. (1979). *Lancet* **1,** 518.

Weeks, J. R. (1978). *Acta Biol. Med. Ger.* **37,** 707.

Weiss, H. J., and Lages, B. A. (1977). *Lancet* April 2, 760.

Weiss, H. J., Aledort, L. M., and Kochwa, S. (1968). *J. Clin. Invest.* **47,** 2169.

Weksler, B. B., Marcus, A. J., and Jaffe, E. A. (1977). *Proc. Natl. Acad. Sci. U.S.A.* **74,** 3922.

Wester, J., Sixma, J. J., Geuze, J. J., and van der Veen, J. (1978). *Lab. Invest.* **39,** 298.

Whitaker, M. O., Wyche, A., Fitzpatrick, F., Sprecher, H., and Needleman, P. (1979). *Proc. Natl. Acad. Sci. U.S.A.* **76,** 5919.

Willis, A. L., and Kuhn, D. C. (1973). *Prostaglandins* **4,** 127.

Willis, A. L., Vane, F. M., Kuhn, D. C., Scott, C. G., and Petrin, M. (1974). *Prostaglandins* **8,** 453.

Willis, A. L., Stone, K. J., Hart, M., Gibson, V., Marples, P., and Botfield, E. (1977). *In* "Prostaglandins in Hematology" (M. J. Silver, J. B. Smith, and J. J. Kocsis, eds.), pp. 371–410. Spectrum, New York.

ADVANCES IN PHARMACOLOGY AND CHEMOTHERAPY, VOL. 18

Experimental Approaches to Antifungal Chemotherapy

JOHN F. RYLEY, ROBERT G. WILSON, MICHAEL B. GRAVESTOCK, AND J. PHILIP POYSER

Imperial Chemical Industries Ltd.
Pharmaceuticals Division
Mereside, Alderley Park, Macclesfield
Cheshire, England

ISBN 0-12-032918-2

I. Introduction

A. Infections—Superficial and Systemic

Of the thousands of fungal species named, well over 100 are potentially pathogenic in man (Emmons *et al.,* 1977). As leafing through such a textbook of medical mycology will indicate, some are capable of producing grossly disfiguring lesions (e.g., the causative agents of blastomycosis, chromomycosis, lobomycosis, ètc.), others can lead to incapacitating deformities (such as Madura foot), many will cause irritating but not necessarily serious lesions of the skin (e.g., ringworm fungi), while some under certain conditions may prove fatal. Fungal diseases in general occur in all parts of the world and affect all ages, though a number of particular species are restricted geographically in their incidence. Although some forms of mycosis can be attributed to modern medicine—systemic mycotic disease may develop following the use of immunosuppressive or cytotoxic drugs—paracoccidioidomycosis has recently been described from a third century AD Chilean mummy (Allison *et al.,* 1979), and doubtless some of the blemishes described in the Bible and elsewhere as "leprosy" could well have had a fungal etiology. In spite of recent advances in chemotherapy, treatment of most fungal diseases is far from satisfactory.

B. Inadequacy of Present Drugs

Potassium iodide for the treatment of sporotrichosis or Whitfield's ointment (a mixture of benzoic and salicylic acids in an emulsifying base) for the treatment of ringworm infections of the skin are old established remedies; it says little for modern antifungals that as far as efficacy is concerned, there is not much to choose between them and Whitfield's ointment (Clayton and Connor, 1973)! A number of drugs developed in other fields have limited and specific applications in mycology: sulfonamides are the agents of choice for nocardiosis, penicillin is the best treatment for actinomycosis, while aromatic diamidines (e.g., hydroxystilbamidine; I) may be useful in the treatment of cutaneous blastomycosis. Griseofulvin (II) has for more than 20 years been used successfully in the treatment of dermatophyte infections. The drug is unusual in that it is active when given by mouth, but unless special tricks of formulation are employed, it is not active topically. Although rapidly effective in simple superficial infections (excluding *Candida*), treatment in other instances may have to be prolonged, and in the case of foot and toenail infections, treatment for a year or more may be necessary with no guarantee of success. 5-Fluorocytosine (5-FC; III) is another antifungal having systemic activity, but is effective only against certain yeasts, *Aspergillus,* and some of the dematiaceous fungi causing chromomycosis. Even with these

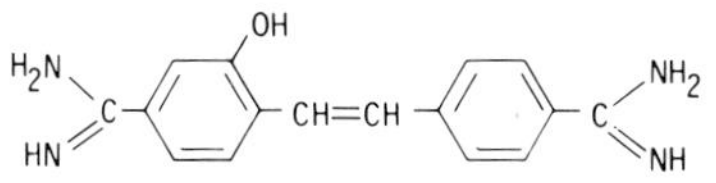

(I) hydroxystilbamidine 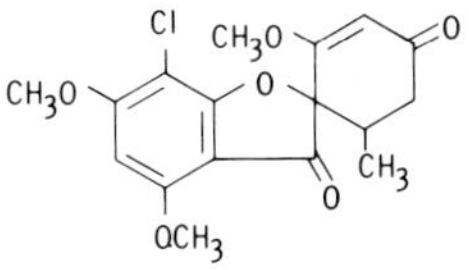 (II) griseofulvin 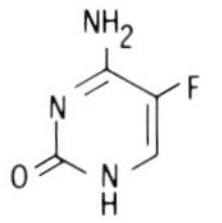 (III) 5 - fluorocytosine

limited species, there are marked strain differences in susceptibility; some strains may be naturally resistant, while others can readily develop drug resistance during the course of treatment. A recent useful development has been the combination of 5-FC with amphotericin B (IV) in the treatment of life-threatening mycoses (Utz *et al.,* 1975; Bennett *et al.,* 1976). Use of such a combination allows a reduction in the dose of amphotericin resulting in a reduction in the degree of kidney damage; nevertheless kidney function needs to be monitored and the dose of 5-FC adjusted in the light of any inhibition of excretion. Amphotericin B is a unique member of the polyene group of drugs which originated with nystatin (V). These are in general potentially active against a wide variety of fungi, but are not absorbed from the intestinal tract of man and are extremely toxic when administered parenterally. A number of polyenes are used in topical preparations for treatment of the skin or for candidosis of the vagina or gastrointestinal tract. Amphotericin B is absorbed from the gut of the

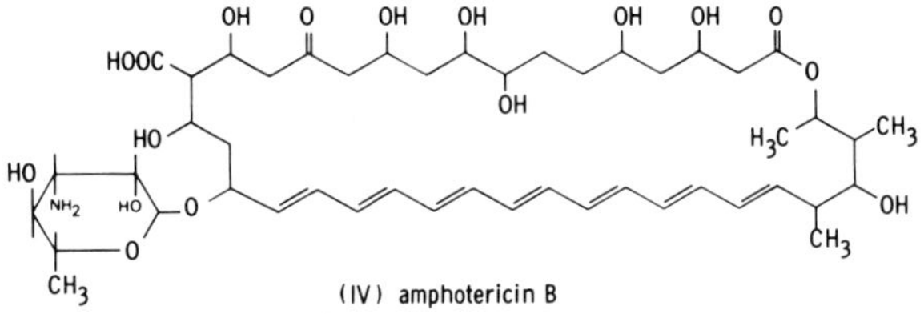

(IV) amphotericin B

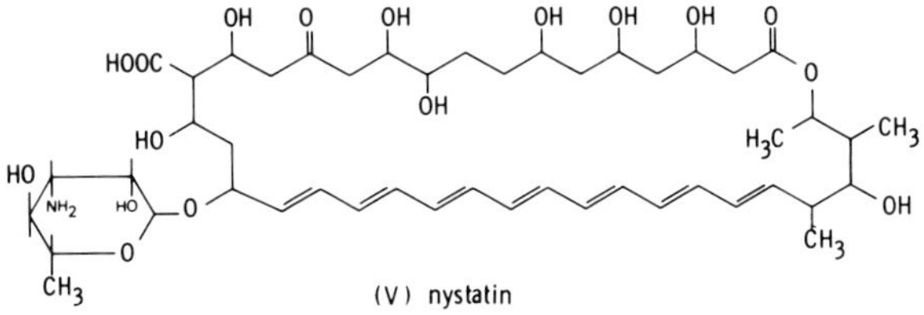

(V) nystatin

mouse, but not higher mammals. It can be administered to man by slow intravenous infusion to produce blood levels adequate to treat a number of systemic mycoses. The drug is undoubtedly toxic; although some would play down this toxicity (see Baum, 1979), others claim permanent kidney damage in the majority of patients treated, and we have heard of patients who preferred to die of coccidioidomycosis rather than continue amphotericin treatment! A realistic assessment of the situation is given by Medoff and Kobayashi (1980a,b). More recently introduced to antifungal chemotherapy are the imidazoles. Clotrimazole (VI), miconazole (VII), econazole (VIII), and a number of other derivatives at various stages of development have wide-spectrum antifungal activity, and find ready utility in topical preparations for the treatment of skin and vaginal infections. Absorption of these imidazoles from the intestinal tract is limited, and some of them at least are potentially too toxic to consider for parenteral use. Miconazole has been used intravenously in the treatment of serious deep-seated mycoses, but obviously this form of administration is far from

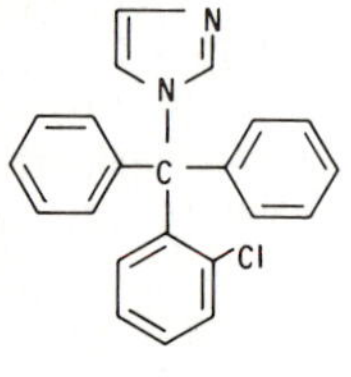

(VI) clotrimazole

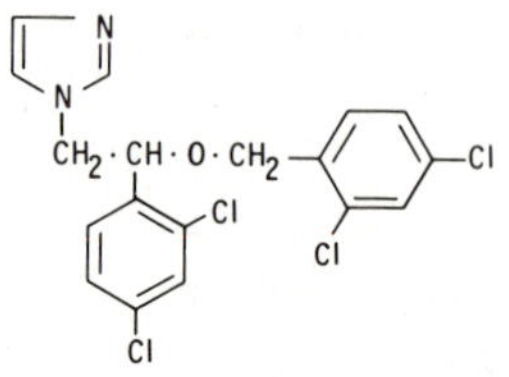

(VII) miconazole

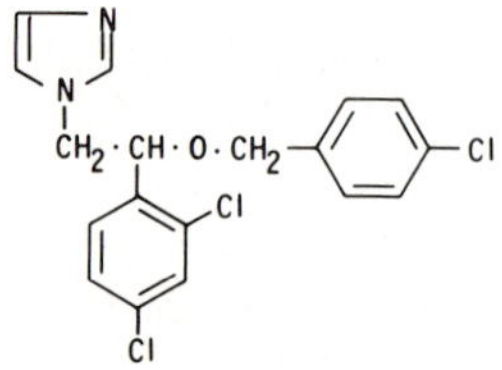

(VIII) econazole

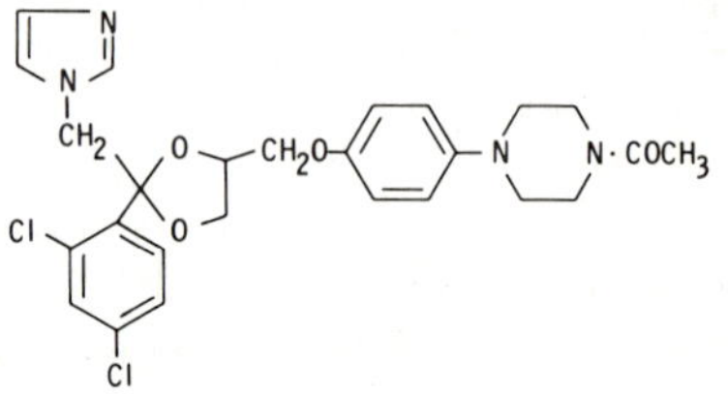

(IX) ketoconazole

convenient. An orally active imidazole, ketoconazole (IX), is currently under development, and would appear to be free from toxicity at therapeutically active doses; activity against vaginal candidosis, skin and nail mycoses (Botter *et al.*, 1979), and a variety of systemic infections has been shown. Whether activity and toxicity are adequate to make ketoconazole an acceptable antimycotic remains to be seen.

Ketoconazole apart, drugs currently available for the treatment of superficial or systemic mycoses leave much to be desired. Wide-spectrum activity, the possibility of oral administration with freedom from toxicity, and cheapness are all necessary in a new drug, and it would be good to get away from the polyenes and imidazoles! It is the purpose of this article to discuss experimental approaches to the discovery of antifungal drugs and to survey synthetic chemical and natural product types of compound reported in both the scientific and the patent literature with claims of antifungal activity, irrespective of whether this has led to clinical utility. An excellent book edited by Speller (1980) is now available covering all aspects of *established* antifungal agents and their use in clinical practice.

C. Systemic versus Topical Treatment

It goes without saying that a systemic fungal infection will require systemic treatment. When however the fungus is confined to the skin or mucosal membranes, then the possibility exists of applying a topical treatment to the affected area, or alternatively treating the infection systemically, getting the parasite from "behind." With a topical treatment the patient may feel he is doing something positive by applying the medication to the lesion whereas an oral treatment may give the feeling of irrelevance. On the other hand there would seem little point in applying a messy treatment to an already messy lesion if an alternative oral treatment were available. It is held by many that compounds too toxic for systemic administration are safe to use topically. In many cases this may be so, but sight should never be lost of the possibility of absorption through the skin or mucous membranes; after all, some penetration is going to be necessary to achieve an antifungal effect. Topical medication requires the identification and treatment of all lesions, including small and developing ones; systemic medication on the other hand will take care of both recognized *and* unrecognized foci of infection. It is this latter aspect that could be so important in the treatment of a disease such as vaginal candidosis. Although the use of pessaries and/or creams can result in the relief of clinical symptoms and even the elimination of *Candida* from the vagina, cessation of treatment may well be followed by the recurrence of symptoms due to reinvasion of the vagina by organisms from extravaginal sites such as the gut, or even the sexual partner. It was the discovery of the orally active metronidazole and related nitro-imidazoles which transformed the treatment of vaginal trichomoniasis by virtue of the drugs' ability to reach extravaginal protozoa, and achieve radical cure. We believe that, provided complete freedom from toxicity is possible, by far the best treatment for superficial fungal infections would be one which could be given by mouth.

D. Cost of Drug Research and Development

Drug design, discovery, and development is an extremely costly procedure; many hundreds of compounds may need to be synthesized and many thousands of compounds screened before worthwhile activity is found. This is only the start of the problem! In the unlikely event of useful activity being found, this activity has to be investigated to see what the compound will and will not do, and how it does it. It is little use killing the fungus if at the same time the compound kills or damages the host! Studies of great complexity on metabolism and toxicity have to be carried out to make sure the proposed treatment is safe for the patient, as well as to satisfy the ever escalating demands of a host of regulatory authorities. Clinical trials have then to be organized and run to make sure that the laboratory findings on antifungal activity have been adequately predictive of behavior in the clinic. Only then, when a clean bill of health as regards activity and safety of the compound has been established, can the new drug be made generally available. All this costs money! We estimate that were we to discover a new drug today, it would cost £25,000,000 in research and development before that drug could be made available for use in man. It is obvious that few enterprises can commit themselves to such a program of work. The most likely candidates are the larger pharmaceutical companies of the western world. These companies, for better or for worse, are financed entirely out of profits made from the sale of drugs. As a result they can only afford to work on problems of sufficient magnitude that they hold out a prospect of eventual return on the investment made. Where activity of a potential drug is restricted to the less common fungi, or problems with production make costs too high, the demise of the compound is assured; such has been the fate of saramycetin, hamycin (Baum, 1979), and more recently, ambruticin (CXLVII).

We find it interesting that much emphasis at meetings and in the literature is placed on the unusual and obscure, and that the ever recurring mundane problems get little attention. Surveys indicate however that by far the most frequent mycological problem is vaginal candidosis, with dermatophyte infections being a smaller, but still significant problem. Although many other fungal infections may be grossly disfiguring in consequence, or even fatal in outcome, it is a fact of life that the *numbers* of such cases are relatively small. Our ambition is to find a new antifungal agent which when given by mouth would control both vaginal candidosis and superficial dermatophyte infections—and so justify the research expenditure—and yet at the same time would have a sufficiently broad spectrum of antifungal activity to make possible effective treatment of the less frequent but more severe fungal infections.

II. Experimental

…CH TO DRUG DISCOVERY AND EVALUATION

… intellectually very satisfying to study the biochemistry or physiology of the target organism and then sit down and design a drug to combat it. This may be the pattern for the remote future, but with the present state of knowledge in the area of infectious diseases it is an approach with little chance of success. Not only do we need to find a compound which will interfere with some vital function in the fungus, and so kill it; it must also have the right pharmacological properties in the host—i.e., be absorbed from the gut and reach the site of fungal parasitization without being metabolically inactivated—and at the same time not interfere with any vital processes in that host. Nevertheless it would be wrong not to attempt any synthetic work if inspiration can be found from some unique aspect of fungal metabolism. Another source of inspiration for synthesis must be currently available antifungal drugs, with a view to increasing potency, safety, and spectrum of activity. One of the purposes of this article is to try to identify chemical structures having limited antifungal activity, which may be improved upon by the synthesis of analogs or more distantly related compounds which retain the key features associated with that activity. But in any realistic drug-hunting enterprise an empirical element is necessary, involving the screening of very large numbers of compounds prepared for a whole variety of reasons, in the search for a novel lead. Once activity in a new class of chemical is found, then more rational synthesis can be employed in an attempt to improve upon that activity. Many compounds useful in the treatment of infectious diseases are natural products, and of course the discovery of such compounds can only be by the empirical approach (although screening systems may be adapted to exclude certain unwanted types of activity).

If a large number of compounds is to be tested, the initial test must be very simple. Its purpose is simply to provide a yes/no answer to the question "is there sufficient interaction between this compound and the fungus to warrant more detailed investigation?" This is screening. The essentials of a screening procedure include such features as simplicity of operation, unambiguity of interpretation, and high throughput of compounds week after week. It matters little if a screen lets through moderate numbers of compounds which will be rejected at a later stage of evaluation; it is important however that the reverse does *not* occur, i.e., the screen rejects compounds of potential interest in the final disease situation (false negatives). Most compounds will initially be available only in small quantities, and synthesis of larger quantities will require evidence of activity to stimulate the chemist concerned! *In vitro* testing will allow examination of large numbers of compounds against a wide spectrum of organisms and will require very small samples of compounds. It must however be borne in mind that *in vitro* activity is no guarantee of activity *in vivo;* also the degree of any activity *in vivo* is not necessarily related to the *in vitro* activity, and *in vivo* activity may require metabolism of the drug by the host, a feature which is excluded by an *in vitro* screen. With the target constraints indicated in the introductory discussion, we limit ourselves to *in vitro* screening against a variety of strains and species of *Candida* and assorted dermatophytes, and further evaluate compounds showing an interesting combination of *in vitro* activity and chemical structure in a series of animal models. Only if we had a compound which was a realistic candidate for development would we investigate its activity against the more exotic fungi. Although a primary *in vivo* screen might be preferred, the technical effort involved and the requirement for much larger samples of compound would result in a much smaller throughput of compounds than an *in vitro* screen, a very restricted spectrum of organisms would be covered, and any wide-ranging survey of a large compound collection precluded. It should be noted however that the antifungal activity of 5-FC would not have been discovered if Roche had relied entirely on their *in vitro* screen. The medium used for *in vitro* screening was complex, suppressing the activity of the drug, which was however revealed in the mouse screen which used a systemic infection with *C. albicans*. Similarly useful *in vivo* activity in imidazoles may be missed if the mycelial form of *C. albicans* is not included in the *in vitro* screen.

B. *In Vitro* Screening

1. *Basic Methods*

Although a wide range of techniques has been devised to measure the sensitivity of various fungi to specific antifungal agents, the methods used for large-scale screening programs have tended to be restricted to the traditional ones of broth-dilution, agar-diffusion, or agar-dilution (Ericsson and Sherris, 1971). Each of these methods is suitable for both yeasts and filamentous fungi. In any such test, the lowest concentration of compound which prevents growth is defined as the minimum inhibitory concentration (MIC).

The broth-dilution method consists of preparing tubes or flasks of drug-containing liquid medium, adding a specified fungal inoculum, incubating either stationary or shaken at the temperature of choice, and after a specific time comparing the growth in treated flasks or tubes with that in untreated drug-free controls. Normally each test unit consists of a single organism plus one concentration of the compound under investigation. If mixed inocula were to be used, the variations in growth rate for different organisms would make interpretation of such a system extremely complicated. The technique is cumbersome and becomes tedious when large numbers of samples are to be tested. The advent of microtitration equipment has enabled the magnitude of such operations to be reduced considerably. Such a system has been used for routine susceptibility testing of yeasts to 5-FC and amphotericin B (Mazens *et al.*, 1979).

The agar-diffusion method depends on the inhibition of growth of an assay organism seeded over the entire plate by drug diffusing radially from a reservoir (Holt, 1975). The reservoir contains a specified volume of test sample, and may be either a hole bored into the agar or a metal or porcelain cylinder placed on the surface. Alternatively, paper discs loaded with the agent can be prepared and used in place of the reservoir (Boyer, 1976; Saubolle and Hoeprich, 1978). Following incubation, the zones of inhibition of growth surrounding the reservoir may be measured to give an indication of activity.

Possibly the most suitable method for routine *in vitro* screening is that of agar-dilution. Here the drug is incorporated in an agar medium and dispensed into tubes (Shadomy, 1969) or petri plates. An inoculum is then applied to the surface of the agar, and following incubation, the plate is examined for growth of the test organism(s). The advantage of the method is that by using petri plates and some form of multipoint inoculator, numerous strains and/or species may be tested simultaneously.

In a study of the susceptibility of 70 yeast isolates to 5-FC, Marks and Eickhoff (1970) found that MICs by broth-dilution and agar-dilution methods were in close agreement, whereas assays using microtiter plates gave slightly lower values. By contrast, Brass *et al.* (1979), using nystatin and ketoconazole as representative drugs, observed poor agreement between the methods, the ratio of MICs determined by broth-dilution to agar-dilution varying from 2 to more than 10.

2. *Test Samples*

With the notable exception of 5-FC, antifungal agents are rarely soluble in water but are freely soluble in organic solvents. For an *in vitro* screen accepting a wide range of chemical types, it is preferable to use a solvent such as dimethyl sulfoxide (DMSO) or dimethyl formamide to prepare an initial solution of all samples. As such solvents are inhibitory for some fungi it is essential to reduce the final concentration in the test medium to a noninhibitory level. In practice we have found a final concentration of less than 1% DMSO to be satisfactory. It should be borne in mind that DMSO may enhance the susceptibility of some organisms by increasing their permeability to certain molecules. Other solvents commonly employed are acetone, ethanol, and polyethylene glycol. Solutions of certain chemicals in organic solvents when diluted in aqueous media frequently give a turbidity which precipitates on standing (e.g., imidazoles). However, provided the solutions are freshly mixed prior to further dilution, this does not appear to affect antifungal activity. Compounds which are insoluble may be treated mechanically by grinding, ball-milling, or sonication to produce a fine suspension. Whenever possible, compounds should be tested immediately after formulation to reduce any possible effects caused by compound instability.

The initial concentration at which compounds are tested is a matter for arbitrary decision. A search of the literature will reveal that for any given antifungal agent, a wide range of MIC values can be obtained depending upon the conditions of the test, and that activity *in vitro* does not necessarily imply a similar activity *in vivo*. Therefore in a primary screen accepting a wide variety of chemical types, one should test at a relatively high level—say 100 or 1000 μg/ml—to establish whether there is any basic interaction between the test organism and the compound. The concentration chosen should be such that 85–90% of samples tested are found to be inactive. The remaining 10–15% can then be further evaluated by serial dilution tests or secondary screens to assess their potential therapeutic value.

3. *Culture Media*

When choosing a test medium one has to consider the relative claims of both the test organism(s) and the compound being evaluated. The medium should be such that the organism is allowed to grow freely, but should not possess constituents which could antagonize the activity of the compound. It is known that the antifungal activity of 5-FC is antagonized by peptone and yeast and beef extracts—which contain purines and pyrimidines and are common constituents of many undefined culture media. Therefore when testing compounds of this nature, a defined medium free of such constituents must be used—e.g., yeast nitrogen base (YNB; Shadomy, 1969). YNB is poorly buffered and as such is not suitable for testing polyenes because of the low pH (<5.0) which results from the fermentation or assimilation of glucose (Shadomy and Espinell-Ingroff, 1974). This can be overcome by making up in 0.1 *M* phosphate buffer at pH 7 (Holt, 1975).

Hoeprich and Finn (1972) compared the ability of six undefined culture media to antagonize the activity of amphotericin B, 5-FC, and clotrimazole with that of a totally defined synthetic amino acid medium (SAAMF). The activity of both 5-FC and clotrimazole was reduced by the undefined media whereas that of amphotericin B was not markedly affected; Sabouraud's agar was the most unsuitable for clotrimazole. Similar observations were reported by Jevons *et al.* (1979) who compared four different agar media for their ability to antagonize the activities of miconazole and tioconazole; they selected diagnostic sensitivity test agar (Oxoid Ltd.) as the most suitable for assessing the activity of imidazoles. The inclusion of substances such as proteins and sterols which might bind antimicrobial agents and thus reduce their antifungal activity should in general be avoided, although the activity of ketoconazole was markedly enhanced by the addition of 10% inactivated bovine serum to Sabouraud's broth (Heeres *et al.*, 1979).

4. *Fungal Inoculum*

How many species should be used in a primary screen? Of the pathogenic yeasts, *C. albicans* is the obvious choice, and for the dermatophytes possibly *T. mentagrophytes* or *T. rubrum*. The number of species used depends on whether one wishes to test at an early stage for broad-spectrum activity, or limit the number of test organisms and simply establish whether there is any antifungal activity at all. Additionally one must decide how many strains of a particular species are to be used. Can a single strain be considered typical of a species? Should drug-resistant organisms be included in the battery of test organisms in order to provide an early indication of cross-resistance?

What morphological form of organism should be used? *C. albicans* and other pathogenic yeasts are normally prepared as suspensions of blastospores. Borgers *et al.* (1979) however advocated using the pseudomycelial form, as this is the prevailing one found in tissues infected with *C. albicans*. Since with some imidazoles (e.g., ketoconazole), activity against the blastospore form is poor considering their *in vivo* potential, but is outstanding—by a factor which may be 1000-fold greater—when determined against the pseudomycelial form, when screening imidazoles at least it is profitable to test them against both forms. With imidazoles, although growth in the mycelial form may be prevented by very low concentrations of drug, it proceeds nevertheless in the blastospore form, so that evaluation is preferable by microscopy rather than gross visual observation. Pseudomycelia predominate in the system described by Aerts *et al.* (1980) which consists of a mixed culture of human fibroblasts and fungi. Likewise for dermatophytes, rather than the usual inoculum of purified conidia or mixed mycelia and conidia, Granade and Artis (1980) prefer to use fragmented mycelia because this is the form present in infected stratum corneum. Yeast inocula are usually prepared by washing off the growth from a 24- to 48-hour old culture on agar medium with saline or buffer. The same procedure can be used for those dermatophytes which readily sporulate to produce conidia. To prepare suspensions of other fungi it may be necessary to scrape the surface of a mature culture (10–28 days, depending on the species), homogenize with a tissue grinder, separate out any large pieces of cellular material, and standardize the suspension of conidia and/or mycelial fragments produced. Granade and Artis (1980) favor growing dermatophytes in submerged culture for 3 to 5 days at 35°C to prevent sporulation, and then grinding the harvested mycelium to produce a standardized inoculum.

Inocula may be prepared at the start of each experiment from actively growing cultures or may be stored for short periods as spore suspensions in sterile distilled water at room temperature. Alternatively, fungal suspensions containing 5% DMSO may be stored frozen in liquid nitrogen to provide standardized inocula for successive assays or experiments (Georgopoulos, 1978). Another possibility is to prepare freeze-dried samples which are then reconstituted to a standard volume as required.

It is important that some effort be made to standardize the size of inoculum used. The most direct method is a microscopical count using a counting chamber or hemocytometer, while various photometric systems may be used to measure optical density or light scattering. Less exact methods involve comparison with barium chloride standards (Shadomy *et al.*, 1977a) or the "Wickerham card technique" (Shadomy and Espinell-Ingroff, 1974). Unfortunately although many authors have described the respective yardstick by which they have standardized their inoculum, they have failed to indicate how this relates to a direct count. Consequently it is extremely difficult, if not impossible, to correlate findings from different laboratories. None of the methods outlined above takes account of the viability of the inoculum. This may be confirmed by the traditional pour-plate or surface-dilution methods for viable counts, but a more attractive method, now available commercially, is to measure the ATP concentration of living cells using the firefly bioluminescence system. This could prove to be superior to the previous methods because it relates directly to the viable content of the inoculum.

With some chemical types, inoculum size is very important. Haller (1979a) using a broth-dilution method obtained MIC values for clotrimazole of 0.25 or 32 μg/ml when he used inocula of 10^3 or 10^5 cells/ml, respectively, whereas the activity of nystatin was unaffected by varying the inoculum size. Likewise Brass *et al.* (1979) using an agar-dilution method found that three strains of *C. albicans* were highly sensitive to ketoconazole (MIC 0.05 μg/ml) when 10^3 colony-forming units (CFU)/ml were used as inoculum, but highly resistant (MIC 100 μg/ml) when 10^4 CFU/ml were used; again no effect of inoculum size was apparent for nystatin. These results serve to highlight just one of the many variables which can affect *in vitro* assays for antifungal activity.

5. *Incubation Conditions*

As mentioned earlier, broth-dilution tests have traditionally been performed using test tubes or flasks, although microculture techniques are becoming more accepted. Since fungi are aerobes, the volume of medium used should always be such as to produce a shallow depth which will allow adequate aeration. If flask cultures are to be used, aeration can be improved by use of a gyratory shaker. Surface inoculation onto agar plates provides ideal aerobic conditions. In the majority of cases, sensitivity tests on fungi responsible for systemic mycoses would be performed at 37°C and for dermatophytes at 26–30°C, although Granade and Artis (1980) preferred an incubation temperature of 35°C for their antimycotic susceptibility testing of dermatophytes in microcultures. Marked variation in MIC values can occur by varying the incubation temperature. Thus Kitahara *et al.* (1976) found that MICs of amphotericin B, 5-FC, and rifampin for *Aspergillus* spp. were markedly lower at an incubation temperature of 25°C than at 37°C [ratios of MIC (37°C)/MIC (25°C) were 5/12.5, 8/20, and 2/40 for the respective agents]. The reverse situation was observed by Block *et al.* (1973) when testing the susceptibility of *Cryptococcus neoformans* isolates to 5-FC. Of eleven isolates tested, nine had identical MICs at 32 or 37°C, whereas two isolates were 5-FC resistant (MIC 320 μg/ml) at 32°C but markedly sensitive (MIC 2.5 μg/ml) at 37°C. Such variations in sensitivity may be attributed to differences in growth rate of the organisms at different temperatures.

Early researchers in antifungal chemotherapy were known to use incubation periods of up to 10 weeks (Bergman, 1955). In the context of modern screening and susceptibility testing, such extended periods of incubation are unthinkable. Time is at a premium, and due consideration must be given to the stability of the compound under test. For example amphotericin B is unstable in certain fungal culture media with a half-life of 18–24 hours (Cheung *et al.*, 1975). If a compound is fungistatic at the concentration tested, the longer the incubation period, the greater the potential for regrowth of the organism as the compound loses its activity; the shorter the incubation period, the more relevant the test. Such reasoning would not apply to stable fungicidal compounds where the possibility of regrowth on extended incubation does not exist.

If growth is to be assessed with the naked eye, then the time required to produce visible growth will be related to the size of the inoculum, the growth rate of the organism, and the growth capacity of the medium. In the context of susceptibility testing of a specific drug or compounds of the same chemical class and a single organism, ideal experimental conditions can be established by a series of exploratory experiments. However, for a screen involving a range of organisms and compounds of various chemical types, the incubation conditions can at best be a compromise.

6. *Estimation of Activity*

Provided there is a rapid transition from total inhibition of growth to totally uninhibited growth of the fungus, MIC determination with the naked eye is relatively simple. However, when testing imidazoles, quantitative assessment without any photometric aid is extremely difficult, because subinhibitory concentrations of imidazoles are able to reduce considerably the growth rate of yeasts. Odds (1979a) found that with miconazole, partial inhibitory effects were observed over a 128-fold range of concentrations for three strains of *C. albicans.* Such observations have been confirmed by Haller (1979b) for both broth-dilution and agar-dilution systems. Similar effects were not seen with nystatin (Haller, 1979b) or amphotericin B (Odds, 1979a) where the inhibitory effect ends almost immediately the concentration drops below the MIC. As imidazoles are able to reduce fungal growth at concentrations far below the MIC, they are able in association with host defense mechanisms to produce therapeutic effects *in vivo.* Thus for novel imidazoles it might be profitable to investigate the range of concentrations able to partially reduce fungal growth—rather than determine a straight MIC—when considering their potential for *in vivo* activity.

Visual determination of end-points is highly dependent on inoculum size, and wherever possible steps should be taken to reduce the risks of misinterpretation of "almost no growth." Fisher and Armstrong (1977) modified the broth-dilution system by incorporating bromothymol blue in the medium. Metabolizing cells caused a color change before growth could be assessed by turbidity, and thereby reduced the incubation time necessary for reading the test. From our own experience with this system, good correlation was obtained between MIC measured at 24 hours by color change and MIC measured at 48 hours by turbidity. Galgiani and Stevens (1976) advocated the use of a turbidimetric method, which is inoculum independent, is free from subjectivity and observer variability, and expresses inhibition as a function of control growth.

7. *Our Screen*

Each of the factors already discussed can influence the *in vitro* activity of a compound to a greater or less extent. In devising a high-throughput screen applicable to all types of synthetic chemicals and natural product samples in addition, compromise is essential. We agree with Haller (1979a) that "there are justifiable doubts whether test conditions equally appropriate for all antimycotics are feasible at all."

In our screen, compounds dissolved in DMSO are incorporated into yeast morphology agar (YMA) at 100 μg/ml and into Sabouraud's dextrose agar (SDA) at 25 μg/ml and poured into a two-compartment petri dish. By means of a Denley multipoint inoculator, the surface of the gelled YMA is inoculated with blastospores of a range of species and strains of *Candida* and the SDA with a variety of dermatophytes. The plates are examined for visible growth after 4 days incubation at 27°C. Such a system enables us to determine the breadth of the spectrum of activity at an early stage of the drug's evaluation. To enable us to detect (and eliminate) polyenes, we include an amphotericin B resistant strain of *C. albicans;* this is particularly valuable when testing unidentified samples of natural products. Because of the comparatively poor activity of the imidazoles against the blastospore form of *C. albicans* under these test conditions, we test compounds for activity against the mycelial phase of *C. albicans* in Eagle's minimum essential medium with fetal calf serum. Multiwell plates are incubated for 24 hours at 37°C in an atmosphere of 5% CO_2 : air, after which the degree of mycelial development is observed using an inverted microscope.

C. *In Vivo* Models

1. *Practical Considerations*

In view of the target orientation discussed in the introductory section, we shall only consider here infections with *C. albicans* and dermatophytes. Laboratory animal models are available for more exotic species such as *Histoplasma, Coccidioides, Cryptococcus,* etc., but we would not consider compound evaluation against such species worthwhile unless an encouraging degree of *in vivo* activity had already been established against vaginal candidosis and/or ringworm—a rare event indeed! Our own interest lies in the discovery of oral activity, and the models to be described are eminently suitable for this form of treatment. Some would consider that when looking for lead activity—rather than a final drug—then parenteral injection of the test compound might be preferable in the first instance in order to circumvent (hopefully!) the problem of absorption from the gut. Although we feel the needs and opportunities for further topical remedies are limited, the animal infections described can readily be treated in this way. When deciding on an animal model, due consideration needs to be given to the size of the animal used, since this influences considerably the requirement for compound—always a problem with research materials. Docility of the species too is a factor worth considering, especially in the case of ringworm infections.

2. *Vaginal Candidosis*

Vaginal infections with *C. albicans* for chemotherapeutic investigations have been described in both mice (Wildfeuer, 1974) and rats (Scholer, 1960). We are indebted to Dr. A. Polak for the outline of a screening method for topical activity based on that of Scholer (1960): Rats are ovariectomized, and 1–2 weeks later are injected subcutaneously with 1 mg microcrystalline estradiol benzoate (Ovocycline). Four days later they are inoculated in the vagina with 5×10^6 *C. albicans* suspended in 0.1 ml gum arabic (day 0). Groups of 6 animals are treated with test compounds formulated in a mixture of polyethylene glycols squirted into the vagina (0.1 ml/rat) twice daily on days 1, 2, and 3. Samples are taken by means of a wire loop between treatments on day 2, and again on days 4 and 7, and cultured on Sabouraud's agar. Colonies are counted, and the logarithm of the mean of the 3 counts determined. This is subtracted from the log of the control counts, and the results expressed as:

	log control − log treated
Maximum activity (MA)	>3.0
Active (A)	3.0–2.0
Slightly active (S)	2.0–0.7
Not active (NA)	<0.7

Table I indicates results obtained by Dr. Polak with some standard antifungals.

We have removed the ovaries and part of the uterine horns from female rats weighing 100–120 gm, and at weekly intervals thereafter administered 0.1 mg estradiol undecylate in sesame oil (Progynon: Schering) intramuscularly. Two weeks after operation, a suspension of an overnight culture of *C. albicans* at 10^8/ml in saline was introduced into the vagina until run-out using a blunt-ended Pasteur pipet. One week later, a vaginal sam-

TABLE I

TOPICAL TREATMENT OF RAT VAGINAL CANDIDOSIS

Treatment	MA	A	S
Gentian violet	1[a]	0.13	—
Clotrimazole	—	2	1
Miconazole	—	2	0.5
Econazole	—	2	1
5-FC	—	—	1–10
Nystatin	—	—	0.75–2
Amphotericin B	—	—	0.75–2
Candicidin	—	0.75	0.05
Rapamycin	0.025	0.003	—

[a] Figures are percentage concentration in polyethylene glycol giving the activity indicated.

ple was taken by means of a wire loop and plated on BiGGY agar, being incubated for 3 days at 37°C. If the cultures indicated an adequate degree of infection, treatment was started. Three days after the cessation of treatment, and again a week later if it seemed appropriate, further samples were taken with a wire loop and cultured. Cultures were scored on an arbitrary scale of 0–4; we have made no attempt to count colonies. Rats weighed 160–170 gm at the time of treatment. We have carried out tests in mice in an analogous manner except that the ovaries were not removed and estradiol benzoate ball-milled in 0.5% Tween 80 was given subcutaneously each week at the rate of 0.5 mg per mouse. Mice weighed around 33 gm at the time of treatment.

The infection in the mouse appears to be less stable than that in the rat—and possibly as a consequence, more amenable to chemotherapeutic treatment. We have had rats showing a good level of infection 5 months after inoculation, and it would appear that estradiol need only be given every 2 or even every 4 weeks rather than weekly; if estradiol treatment is not continued after inoculation, then the infection dies out after 1–2 months. With most mice however, the infection does not persist beyond about 2 months from inoculation. In neither rats nor mice are clinical symptoms of infection produced; there is no discharge, and no production of plaques. The animals do not improve with keeping, but symptoms—loss of hair in rats, enlarged vulvae in mice, and general malaise in both—would appear to be due to the operative, dosing and/or hormonal treatments rather than to the *Candida*. The infection in both species is confined to the lumen of the reproductive tract; we have found no evidence for tissue invasion. In both direct smears and in histological sections, fungal hyphae can be found in the keratinaceous debris of the lumen. Direct microscopical examination of vaginal samples however does not seem to be as reliable a method for monitoring infection as culture. The infection is not restricted to the vagina; in a large percentage of cases it penetrates the cervix and becomes established in the uterine horns. This means that if the model is to be used for evaluation of topical treatments, clearance of the vaginal infection may not be possible due to continual reinfection from the uterine reservoir.

Table II gives the results of a comparative trial on 7 commercially available antifungal creams applied topically in rats and mice. The creams were squirted into the vagina by means of a syringe and ball-ended metal canula twice daily for 5, 14, or 28 days. Cultures from treated animals made 3 days after the end of treatment were compared with controls, and results expressed as active (virtually no *Candida* recoverable from any animals), slightly active (an obvious reduction in score when compared with untreated controls), or inactive. From the table it will be seen that the results of topical treatment were not very impressive. With no preparation was it possible to eliminate the infection from rats, although three produced a reduction in infection after twice daily treatment for 28 days. The infection in mice was somewhat more susceptible, but even here elimination of the infection was achieved only with miconazole and clotrimazole, and only after prolonged treatment. Our results with some compounds are not as good as those of Dr. Polak (Table I) with a much shorter schedule of treatment, but in some cases she was using a higher concentration of drug. It should also be noted that she obtained maximal activity only with gentian violet and rapamycin. In further experiments we have found that some preparations gave better results when mice were inoculated the day before treatment was started rather than 10 days previously—possibly because less uterine infection was established before treatment started.

Total elimination of rather than reduction in the infection is desirable, and our experiences with oral treatments in rats and mice demonstrate that this is possible. Miconazole (prepared by ball-milling commercially available 250-mg tablets in 0.5% Tween 80) was active in the rat at 250 mg/kg when given twice daily for 5 days. Toxicity was evident at 1000 mg/kg or when treatment at 500 mg/kg was continued for a second week. Rather surprisingly, activity was not as marked in the mouse; some reduction in yeast burden was achieved—along with toxicity—at 1000 mg/kg, but little evidence of activity was noted at 500 mg/kg twice daily for 5 days. Ketoconazole in rats or mice would eliminate the infection in the majority of animals at a dose of 25–50 mg/kg for 5 days; there was little advantage in giving this dose twice instead of once daily. A single dose of 100 mg/kg or 2 doses of 50 mg/kg on succeeding days was also effective in eliminating the infection in mice.

TABLE II

TOPICAL TREATMENT OF VAGINAL INFECTIONS WITH *C. albicans* IN RATS AND MICE[a]

			Mice			Rats		
Preparation[b]	Manufacturer	Active ingredient	5 days	14 days	28 days	5 days	14 days	28 days
Canesten	Bayer	Clotrimazole 1%	S	S	A	NA	NA	S
Daktarin	Janssen	Miconazole 2%	S	A	A	NA	NA	NA
Pevaryl	Cilag-Chemie	Econazole 1%	NA	NA	S	NA	NA	NA
Fungilin	Squibb	Amphotericin B 3%	S	S	S	NA	NA	S
Candeptin	Pharmax	Candicidin 0.06%	NA	S	S	NA	NA	S
Nystan	Squibb	Nystatin 100,000 units/g (~2%)	NA	NA	S	NA	NA	NA
Pimafucin	Brocades	Natamycin 2%	NA	NA	NA	NA	NA	NA

[a] NA, not active; S, slight activity; A, active.

[b] Trademarks.

It can thus be seen that elimination of an experimental vaginal infection by oral treatment is possible, and that the techniques to demonstrate this are relatively simple. For testing large numbers of compounds, the infection in mice is preferable—since removal of the ovaries is not necessary, and only one-fifth the amount of compound needed for the rat is required for evaluation. For screening purposes, we feel a group of 5 mice is desirable. Once useful activity is discovered, then of course evaluation in alternative models is in order.

It should be remembered that the rat and mouse models are only models. Not only are the infections asymptomatic, but the conditions under which the yeasts are living are different from those in the human—where the vaginal pH is much lower and the normal flora is different. It may well be that indication of moderate activity in the rodent models foreshadows much more impressive activity in humans; certainly the results obtained with imidazoles (Tables I and II) are not as good as clinical trial results in women would lead us to expect.

3. *Dermatophyte Infections*

The classical dermatophyte model is *Trichophyton mentagrophytes* in guinea pigs—the infection used by Martin in our laboratories and later by Gentles (1958) to demonstrate the systemic activity of griseofulvin. Similar infections can be produced with *Microsporum canis* and *T. mentagrophytes* var. *quinkeanum* but we have been unable to infect guinea pigs with *T. rubrum,* which is probably the most prevalent dermatophyte affecting man. Dermatophyte infections in guinea pigs are self-limiting, animals showing spontaneous recovery in 3–6 weeks depending on the strain of fungus used. Fungal growth occurs in the surface layers of the skin during the first few days after inoculation, and during the latter part of the first week, fungal hyphae begin to invade hair follicles. During the second week, surface growth of the fungus is gradually eliminated, while penetration of the follicles and of the hair in the follicles increases, and sporulation takes place; some areas appear to be a mass of fungal spores with no signs of hyphae. No invasion of the follicle or hair shaft takes place below the level of keratinization. The intensity of infection declines during the third week; hyphae can be found in the follicles at 21 days, but in our infections have been eliminated by day 28. Macroscopically infection first shows around the fifth day as an area of reddening, soon accompanied by the production of a fine scale. The reddening increases over the next few days and the scale gradually gives way to a crust or scab. The lesions are raised and the skin thickened. Lesions appear to reach maximum severity by 10–12 days, but measurements on histological preparations indicate that maximal epidermal thickness does not occur until day 21—when recovery is setting in. As the animals recover, hair loss in heavy infections is pronounced; the bald patches in such animals are transformed by hair regrowth within a couple of weeks. If guinea pigs are reinoculated, erythema, scale, crust, and scab formation, skin thickening, etc. all take place, quite as severe as in the primary infection, but somewhat earlier in appearance. Examination of skin sections however reveals that fungal elements are absent, and the reaction is one of immunity.

Inoculation of experimental animals requires occlusion or scarification to be effective. Although occlusion may be relevant in view of the conditions leading to the establishment of many human infections—e.g., the increase in foot infections now that nylon socks and synthetic shoes are prevalent—it is far from simple to occlude with a wet dressing the inoculation site on a guinea pig in such a way that the animal will not remove the dressing. If large numbers of animals are to be used regularly on a routine basis, inoculation by this method is just not practicable. Scarification can be produced in many ways. If the animal is first clipped, adequate trauma can be produced by rubbing the skin with coarse sandpaper and then spreading on a spore suspension with a pipet. The most convenient method we have found however produces scarification and inoculation in one action. A small wire brush pad around 2 cm square, and with many short bristles (cut from a file-cleaning brush) is dipped in a spore suspension in a petri dish (4×10^6 CFU/ml) and scrubbed on the clipped area of the animal; we clip an area 10×6 cm on each side of the guinea pig. Little trace of scarification is evident by the time the fungal lesions begin to develop 5–6 days later. Lesions are scored on an arbitrary scale of 0–4 on a basis of erythema, scale/crust/scab formation, skin thickening, etc.; we discount hair loss in this reckoning, as there comes a time when the animal presents a smooth bald area, and has obviously eliminated its infection, although it will be a matter of weeks before hair regrowth takes place. In order to facilitate scoring during the course of the infection, we clip the hair on and around the lesions every 3–4 days. We do not measure skin thickness as such, and consider cultivating skin scrapings or hair fragments unnecessary, and sometimes indeed misleading. In the clinical situation, treatment will not be given until the lesion has become established and diagnosed. In the guinea pig model, with the complication of self-healing, drug activity would only be evident as an increase in the *rate* of healing, rather than an absolute heal/no heal situation, and may not reflect to any marked extent the antifungal activity of the drug. Treatment started at the time of inoculation will reflect the prophylactic potential of the test compound, and treatment started after inoculation the therapeutic potential. For compound testing it is convenient to start treatment 3 days after inoculation—i.e., at a time when the infection has become established, but before clinical signs are evident—and continue until 12–14 days after inoculation. In general a compound will show greater activity the earlier treatment is instituted. When treatment is started at day 3, very good control of the infection can be achieved with daily oral doses of 10–20 mg/kg griseofulvin, 100 mg/kg ambruticin, or 75 mg/kg ketoconazole. Figure 1 illustrates the effects of these doses of drug on an infection with *T. mentagrophytes* when dosing was started 0, 3, 5 or 7 days after inoculation. Topical preparations can be evaluated in this model, the preparation being applied to the lesion twice daily. We have had good control of experimental infections with creams containing tolnaftate or miconazole, and moderate control with creams containing clotrimazole or econazole. With topical preparations, it is desirable to have control groups treated with drug-free base—with experimental compounds we have used polyethylene glycol 400 as a solvent. Topical treatment of experimental infections is not as easy to evaluate as oral treatment. The base alone or the fact of just rubbing it into the lesion produces an effect; scale and crusts are modified, disguised, or rubbed off—hence affecting the scoring—and with rubbing the treatment into all parts of the lesions, lesions tend to spread.

We have inoculated cynomolgus monkeys (*Macaca irus*) with *T. mentagrophytes* and with *M. canis* and found that although similar infections were produced to those in guinea pigs, with eventual self-healing, the course of the infection was extended by several weeks, particularly with *M. canis*. Such infections could be of interest in evaluating a candidate drug—though of course monkeys are not too easy to handle, and twice daily topical treatment would be something of a problem! For initial testing of compounds, something smaller rather than larger than a guinea pig is wanted, primarily to reduce the requirement for compound.

T. mentagrophytes will not infect the mouse or rat unless inoculated during a very restricted part of the hair cycle, and for practical purposes is unsuitable. *T. mentagrophytes* var. *quinkeanum* on the other hand will readily produce a lesion, though the course of infection is only a couple of weeks. The wire brush pad used for scarifying and inoculating guinea pigs is too vicious for the mouse skin, and we find the easiest method of inoculation is to clip the hair on the back of the mouse (Oster clippers; No. 40 blade), produce mild scarification with five sideways strokes with a piercing saw fitted with a fine blade (No. 1), and then spread on a spore suspension (10^7/ml) by means of a soft brush. Erythema and fungal growth become apparent 3–4 days after inoculation, and by 6–7 days a solid, yellowish crust has formed. This is sloughed off during the second week, so that by day 14 few mice have any fungal crust left—though a large bald

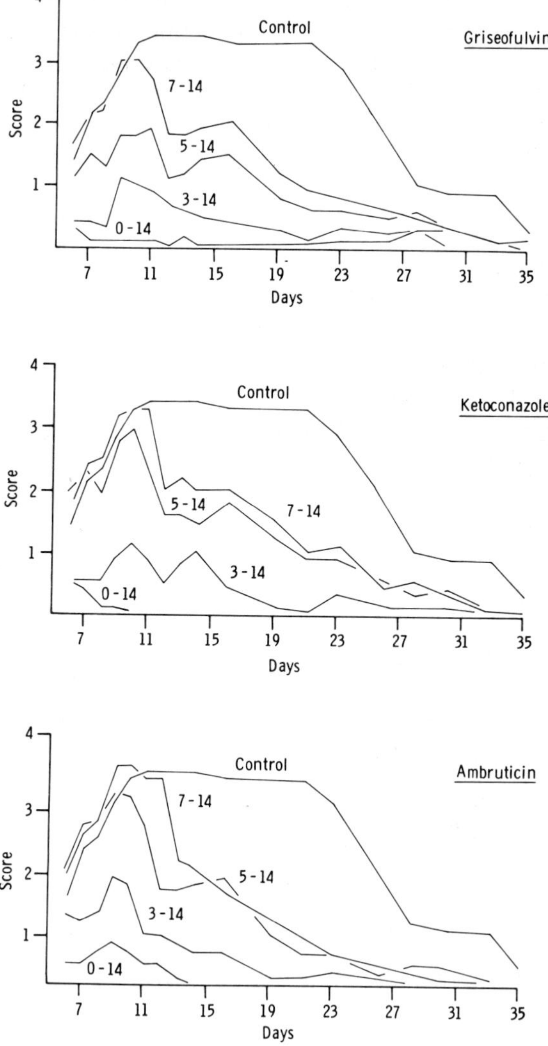

FIG. 1. Effect of griseofulvin (20 mg/kg), ketoconazole (75 mg/kg), and ambruticin (100 mg/kg) on the progress of an infection of *T. mentagrophytes* in guinea pigs. Dosing was by mouth, and was given daily starting on days 0, 3, 5, or 7 of the infection as indicated.

patch and a secondary scab are evident. This infection can be used for drug testing, but because the course of an untreated infection is so short, treatment needs to be started early. This infection can be readily controlled by oral ketoconazole, but is not very susceptible to ambruticin and particularly not to griseofulvin. Comparative tests have shown that *T. m.*

quinkeanum in the guinea pig is not as susceptible to griseofulvin or ambruticin as is *T. mentagrophytes,* but also that in the guinea pig it is more susceptible to ambruticin and griseofulvin than in the mouse. In choosing a model for drug screening one has to offset the marked saving of compound from testing in mice with the problem that a clinically effective drug, griseofulvin, is so much more effective in the guinea pig.

4. *An in Vivo Screen*

Given that vaginal candidosis and ringworm are the primary targets in the search for a new antifungal, and that amounts of compound for test are at a premium, we have combined the two mouse models such that an answer for both organisms can be obtained from one lot of compound in one lot of mice. Female mice around 30 gm are injected subcutaneously on a Friday with 0.5 mg estradiol benzoate. The following Monday (day 0) they are clipped and then dosed with the test compounds (orally or ip). They are then inoculated with *C. albicans* in the vagina and subsequently with *T. m. quinkeanum* on the back, and then given a second dose of compound. Dosing is repeated once daily on days 1–4. On day 7, skin lesions are scored and vaginal samples taken for culture on BiGGY agar. Table III indicates the doses of four antifungals necessary to give virtually complete control of the infections; partial control was evident at lower doses. For screening compounds we use groups of 5 mice and an initial dose level of 250 mg/kg; this means 250 mg of compound is required for test. The table also indicates that with three of the compounds—which are of course orally absorbed—the activity was no better when dosed ip; ambruticin was in fact toxic at 500 or 250 mg/kg ip, whereas oral doses at these levels were tolerated. Some speculative compounds might however show activity by the ip but not by the oral route, and provide a chemical

TABLE III

RESPONSE OF A MIXED INFECTION TO MEDICATION[a]

	C. albicans			*T. m. quinkeanum*		
Drug	Oral	ip	Food	Oral	ip	Food
Griseofulvin	NA 500	—	—	250	250	1000
Ambruticin	NA 500	—	—	250–100	100	Sl 1000–2000
Ketoconazole	25	25	500	25	25	500
Amphotericin B	Sl 100	—	—	25	—	—

[a] Figures are minimum effective doses for virtually complete control in mg/kg × 6 or in mg/kg of diet for 5 days; NA, not active, Sl, slightly active.

lead; experience with dosing compounds ip shows a much greater incidence of toxicity. Compounds can also be administered via the diet. An inclusion level of 1000 mg/kg of diet represents a daily intake of approximately 125 mg/kg. It will be noted that griseofulvin seems rather more active by this route and ambruticin and ketoconazole somewhat less active than by oral administration once daily.

III. Synthetic Chemicals

A survey has been made of various classes of synthetic chemicals for which antifungal activity has been claimed against human pathogens. The patent, medicinal chemical, and pharmacological literature have all been reviewed for the period 1970 through March 1980. This survey thus supplements and extends earlier reviews by Taylor and D'Arcy (1961), Cartwright (1975), Shadomy *et al.* (1977b), Kobayashi and Medoff (1977), and the regular updates in Annual Reports of Medicinal Chemistry (1966, 1967, 1968, 1969, 1970, 1972, 1973, 1974, 1975, 1976, 1978). These and other reviews have mostly focused on compounds which have advanced to some form of clinical trial. In the present report we have additionally attempted to assess patent claims and other publications of *in vitro* activity as a guide to possibly novel chemical types for future antifungal chemotherapy. The somewhat daunting nature of this task is illustrated by Odd's listing (1979b) of *some* compounds which have been reported as *in vitro* inhibitors of yeast pathogens alone.

The review is of necessity somewhat selective. Many patent claims do not satisfactorily distinguish between plant and human pathogens, while others describe compounds of potent chemical reactivity which would clearly be expected to interact widely with physiologically important thiol-mediated processes. Such types, although of possible interest as agricultural fungicides, are unlikely to be serious candidates for human usage in the light of today's drug toxicity/safety testing requirements, and have not therefore been considered. In general we have included only those classes of compound for which several publications have appeared, thus confirming the earlier observation of activity. Compounds have been classified rather arbitrarily in broad chemical types, and thus conform to our own prejudices concerning structure–activity relationships. References to the patent literature have been made directly in the text quoting the patentee, and the number and country of registration; dates are quoted as date of original application/date of publication of the complete specification. In the writing of cycloaliphatic or aliphatic structures, no stereochemistry is implied by the gross structures given.

A. Amines

Long chain and higher molecular weight aliphatic amines have been known for many decades to have fungicidal or fungistatic action, usually as their quaternary salts. Recent research has tended to concentrate on more detailed structure–activity relationships and the often subtle stereochemical factors involved. In a series of primary 2-amino alkanes examined for broad-spectrum antifungal action, 2-aminotridecane had the highest activity (Leiner *et al.*, 1970). In the same paper phenolic salts were described and the salt of 2-chloro-4-nitrophenol highlighted for its activity. A related study with other phenolic salts of this amine showed clear synergism between 2-aminotridecane and the phenols (Capek *et al.*, 1973). Thus the 2,4,5-trichlorophenol salt was active against *C. albicans* at 25 μg/ml, a potency five times that of the free base; the phenol itself was not inhibitory toward *C. albicans*.

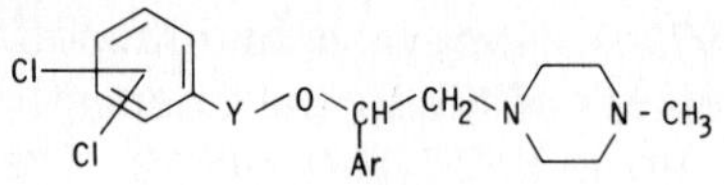

$Y = CH_2, CO, OCH_2CO$

(X)

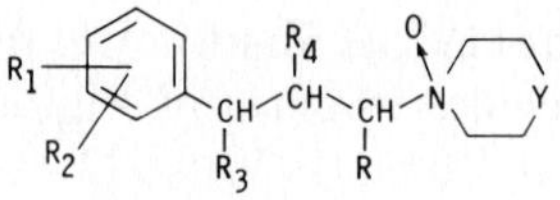

$Y = CH_2, O, C(R, R)$
$R_3 = H, R, OH,$
$R_1, R_2 =$ alkyl, cycloalkyl

(XI)

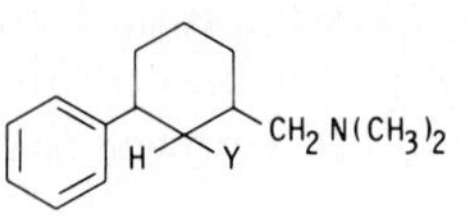

$Y = OH, OCOR$
R = aryl, alkyl

(XII)

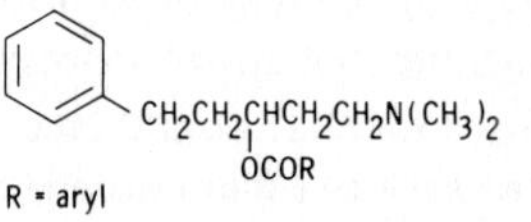

$CH_2CH_2CHCH_2CH_2N(CH_3)_2$ with OCOR
R = aryl

(XIII)

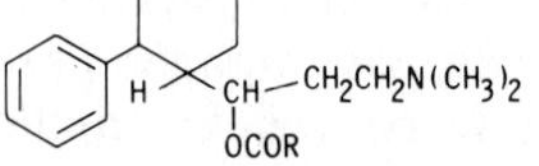

R = aryl

(XIV)

$R = (CH_2)_3-N\quad N-R_1$

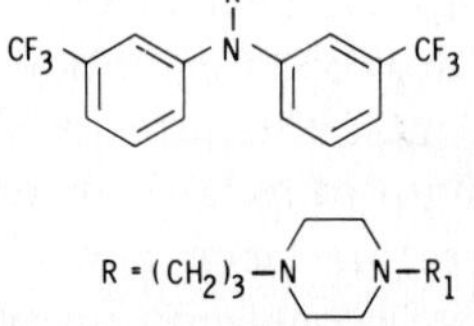

(XV)

Aliphatic tertiary amines form the other main class in this group. The early claims were for arylalkoxypiperazines of type X and their corresponding esters—for which widespread antibiotic action included antifungal and trichomonacidal activity (Pedrazzoli *et al.*, 1973). These compounds seem to have been the basis for later claims for arylalkylamines of type XI where piperidines and morpholines are exemplified (Roche: E.P. 5-541, 1978/1979; BE. 861003, 1977/1978). Widespread activity against plant mildews and yeasts is claimed in addition to activity against *C. albicans*, *T. mentagrophytes*, and *H. capsulatum*.

Interesting stereochemical specificity was noted in the activity of the phenyl cyclohexanol derivatives XII against *C. albicans* (Dimmock *et al.*, 1975). Axial and equatorial alcohols were produced by reduction of the corresponding ketone Mannich base. The axial alcohol (Y = OH) had activity against *C. albicans* at 3.2 μg/ml compared with 100 μg/ml for the epimer. Esters of the alcohols were in general not active except for the 10-undecenoyl derivatives where the equatorial alcohol ester was active against *C. albicans, M. gypseum,* and *Trichophyton granulosum*. This activity was apparently due to *in vivo* hydrolysis to give the parent acid. In a related study (Dimmock *et al.*, 1976) the conformationally "frozen" homolog XIV of the phenyl pentamines XIII was found to be active against the same three pathogenic fungi at approximately 10 μg/ml. Substituents in the benzoic acid function (R) of these esters were shown to influence activity directly and not via effects on rate of hydrolysis. The cyclic compounds had higher antimicrobial potency in general than the acyclic analogs, suggesting that a degree of rigidity between functional groups favored activity.

In a study aimed at establishing the possible role of the trifluoromethyltolyl residue in new drugs the diarylamines XV were found to have activity against *C. albicans* and *T. mentagrophytes* (Yale and Spitzmiller, 1977). Two compounds with $R_1 = CH_3$ and $R_1 = -(CH_2)_2OH$ were found to show activity at 25 and 12.5 μg/ml, respectively.

B. Amino Acids and Peptides

On the whole isolated amino acids or dipeptides have not shown activity as antifungal agents, and in some cases have been found to antagonize the uptake, and hence the activity, of other drugs. However *N-p*-phenoxyphenyl amino acids (XVI) and their *N*-nitroso derivatives were claimed to have broad spectrum antibacterial and antifungal activity (Searle: U.S. 3520922, 1967/1970). It is not known whether the potentially toxic *N*-nitroso function is an absolute requirement for activity.

R = H or NO

(XVI)

$CH_3(CH_2)_{14}CONH(Lys)_n OCH_2CH_2NH_2$

n = 1 - 3

(XVII)

$(CH_3)_2N-NH-CH(CH(CH_3)_2)-CONHCH_2COOC_2H_5$

(XVIII)

$R_1R_2CFCH(NH_2)COOH$

(XIX)

In a study of long chain fatty acid derivatives of amino acid esters, palmitoyl-lysine mono, di, and tripeptides (XVII) were found to have activity against several moulds and yeasts (Grye *et al.,* 1979). The ethanolamine ester function in these compounds presumably serves as a recognition feature for peptide transport systems in the fungi. In the case of some hydrazino dipeptides it is the additional basic function on the N-terminus of the peptide derivatives which acts as the transport recognition feature; American Home Products (U.S. 400013, 1973/1976) claim broad spectrum antibacterial, antifungal, and trichomonacidal activity for compounds typified by XVIII.

Various tripeptide derivatives were also studied for their effects on several fungi and pathogenic moulds (Eisele, 1975a,b). Seven tripeptides with the sequence L-arginine, DL-Y, L-phenylalanine were synthesized and tested against *Paecilomyces varioti* and *Mucor miehei.* Activity was found for three compounds with Y = DL-3-fluorophenylalanine, DL-4-chlorophenylalanine, or DL-phenylalanine. The terminal amino acids specified were found to be essential for activity. In the other study, tripeptides with Y = D-alanine, D-tryptophane, D-valine, D-leucine, or D-phenylalanine were found to have fungicidal activity at approximately 1 mg/ml. The activity of these tripeptides was antagonized *in vitro* by tripeptides containing the corresponding L-amino acid. Finally some 3-fluoroamino acids (XIX) were shown to have weak (10^{-2} to 10^{-4} *M*) activity against *A. niger, T. viride,* and *T. mentagrophytes* (Gershon *et al.,* 1973).

C. Azasteroids

Compounds of this class fall into two types, the 4-aza-androstanes (XX) and the 15-aza-D-homocholestadienes (XXII). Previous studies had shown that 4-aza-cholestanes had good activity against yeasts and gram-positive bacteria. The compound ND 502 [XX; R_1 = H; R_2 = $-CH(CH_3)(CH_2)_3$-$CH(CH_3)_2$] was reported to have activity against *S. cerevisiae, C. albicans,* and *A. niger* at 12.5, 0.75, and 0.75 μg/ml, respectively (Doorenbos and Bossle, 1970). Early studies had shown that 4-aza-androstanes and pregnanes were not active—apparently as a result of the polar C-17/20 hydroxy functions in these compounds, since the corresponding deoxy-4-aza-androstanes and pregnanes were approximately as active as the cholestane series. In order to test the hypothesis that hydrophilic residues attached to ring D were responsible for loss of activity, the alkoxy derivatives XX [R_1 = H; R_2 = $-CH(CH_3)O(CH_2)_2CH(CH_3)_2$] and XX [$R_1$ = H, CH_3; R_2 = $-O(CH_2)_2CH(CH_3)_2$] were prepared and tested (Doorenbos and Bossle, 1970; Doorenbos and Solomons, 1973). The high activities ob-

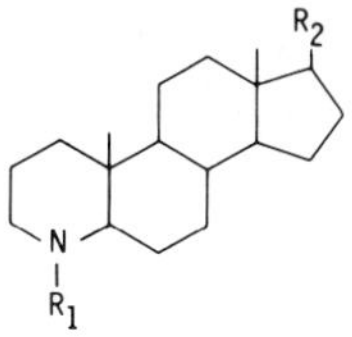

(XX) 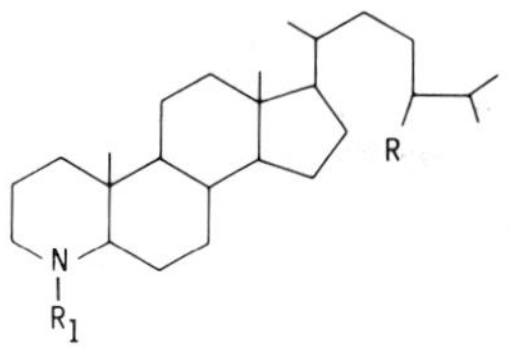 (XXI)

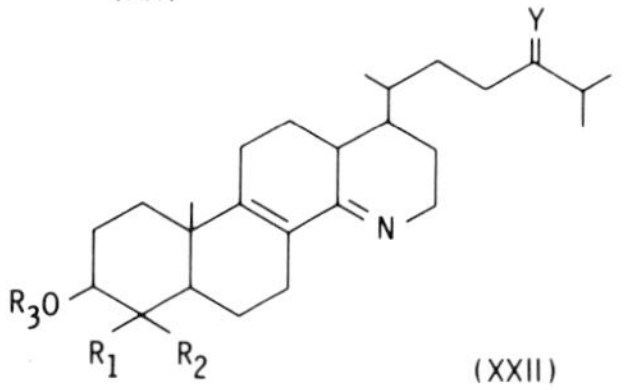

(XXII)

R_1, R_2, R_3, = H or alkyl
Y = O or OH, H

served for these compounds confirmed the hypothesis; the corresponding 17-amino derivatives were without activity (Doorenbos and Solomons, 1974). With confirmation of the positive effects of the C-17 lipophilic side chain on activity, other studies were undertaken to investigate the effects of substitution in the side chain (Doorenbos and Aboul-Enein, 1974a). The activity of the 4-aza-sitostane (XXI; R = Et) thus prepared was reduced compared with the parent tetracyclic series (Doorenbos and Aboul-Enein, 1974b).

Activity against *C. albicans, C. tropicalis,* and *T. mentagrophytes* has been claimed for the 15-aza-D-homocholestadienes XXII following topical application (Lilly: U.S. 3947453, 1974/1976; 3972884, 1974/1976; 4001246, 1976/1977; 4003238, 1976/1977). These compounds have two hydroxyl functions (optionally alkylated), and would be expected to be much more hydrophilic than the 4-aza types discussed above. The potential reactivity of these dienamines suggests a different mechanism of activity against *Candida* from the previous aza-steroids.

D. Guanyl Hydrazones, Guanidines

The most widely studied compounds in this class were the alkoxyacetophenone, alkoxybenzaldehyde, and alkoxycinnamaldehyde derivatives XXIII, XXIV, and XXV, respectively. Extensive investigations of the position and optimum chain length of alkyl substitution in the alkoxy function (Nishimura *et al.*, 1973a,b,c) of these derivatives drew the following conclusions: In the acetophenone series XXIII, *m*- or *p*-alkoxy substituted compounds showed optimum activity with R = C_6–C_7 and *o*-substituted compounds with R = C_8–C_{10}; ortho compounds had the best overall antibacterial and antifungal activity although meta derivatives were nearly as good. Alkylation of one of the terminal amine functions (as

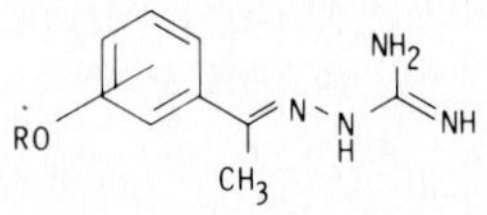

RO CH3 NH2 N N H NH

(XXIII)

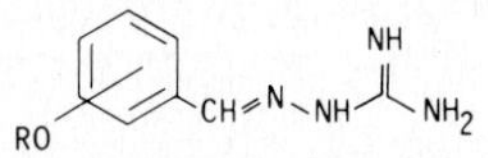

RO CH=N-NH NH NH2

(XXIV)

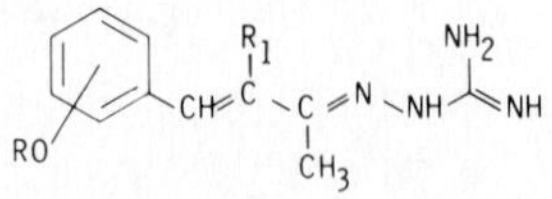

RO CH=C R1 C=N-NH NH2 NH CH3

R = C1 - C5 alkyl (XXV)

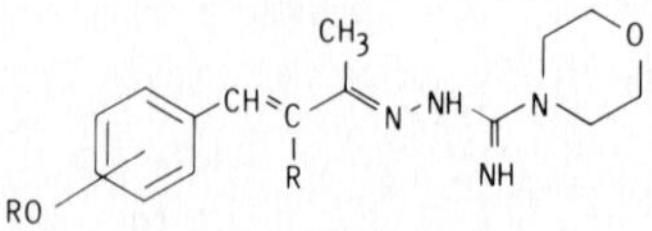

RO CH=C CH3 R N-NH N O NH

(XXVI)

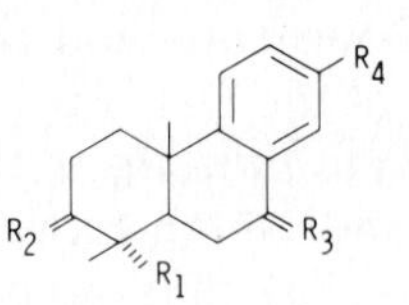

R4 R2 R1 R3

(XXVII)

OR N NH NH NH2

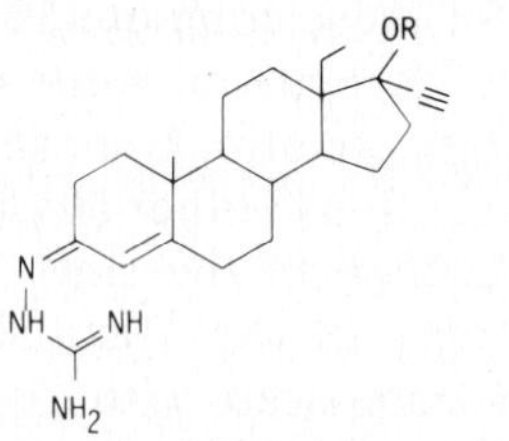

(XXVIII)

a pyrrolidine ring) generally lowered activity. For the benzaldehyde series XXIV rather different findings were obtained. With few exceptions *p*-alkoxy compounds showed maximum activity with R = C_6. Meta or *o*-alkoxy compounds were optimum with R = C_6 and C_{10}, respectively. Substitution of NH_2 by pyrrolidino in the amidine moiety of the ortho alkoxy series increased antifungal and gram-positive antibacterial activity. For the cinnamaldehyde/benzalacetone series XXV, maximum activity for *o*-, *m*-, and *p*-alkoxy substitution was at C_4–C_6. The position of the alkoxy residues and substitution in the alkylene chain by methyl seemed to have little effect; however, disubstitution with two alkoxy radicals almost abolished activity. Substitution of NH_2 by pyrrolidino generally decreased activity. All these compounds were tested against *C. albicans, S. cerevisiae, A. niger, M. gypseum, Penicillium chrysogeum,* and *Trichophyton interdigitale;* most potent activities were in the region of 6.3 μg/ml. A patent application addressed to morpholino guanyl hydrazones of the benzalacetone derivatives XXVI appeared claiming activity against *Candida,* but it apparently covers the active types described above (Gakuen, K.: JAP. 7105704, 1967/1971).

Based on the well-documented antibacterial activity of guanidine types in general, a Schering group undertook an extensive structure–activity study of some 100 amine and guanidine derivatives of the dehydroabietyl diterpene nucleus XXVII (Schroder, 1970). Guanidino methyl and ethyl substitution at C_4 (R_1) was explored together with guanyl hydrazones at C_3 (R_2) and C_7 (R_3). A guanidine residue at C_4 together with an isopropyl function at C_{13} (R_4) was found to give the best overall spectrum of activity against *C. albicans, M. gypseum, T. mentagrophytes,* and *Trichomonas vaginalis*. The C_3 [R_2 = =N.NH.C(NH_2)=NH] hydrazones were found to be particularly effective against *M. gypseum* and *T. vaginalis,* with activity at the 10–25 μg/ml level. A patent for steroid 3-ketoguanylhydrazones claimed compounds such as XXVIII to be fungicidal against *H. capsulatum* and also active against trichomonads (American Home Products: U.S. 3507857, 1967/1970).

E. *N*-Hydroxypyridones

The antibacterial activity of 2-pyridone-*N*-oxide (XXIX, X = O) has been known for many years (Newbold and Spring, 1948). Later development work showed that *N*-hydroxypyridin-2-thiones were even more potent, and *N*-hydroxypyridin-2-thione itself (XXIX, X = S) has been used extensively as an antifungal with agricultural and preservative applications. Compounds of the general type XXX, where R_1–R_4 were alkyl, cycloalkyl, etc., were claimed by Hoechst (NL. 6912934, 1969/1970) as antifungals. The cyclohexyl derivative HOE-296 (XXXI) soon emerged as the preferred compound (Dittmar and Lohaus, 1973). HOE-296 was shown to have antibacterial and trichomonacidal activity, and in particular very high potency and a wide spectrum of antifungal activity. Its MIC values are in the range 0.98–3.9 μg/ml, and average 2.0 for the more important human pathogens such as *C. albicans, T. mentagrophytes,* and *M. canis*. Topical activity against ringworm in guinea pigs was demonstrated. An extensive Hansch analysis of the various derivatives in the *M. canis*/guinea pig model revealed a remarkably linear relationship between

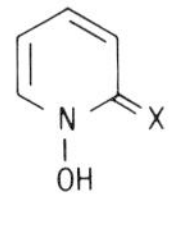

(XXIX) 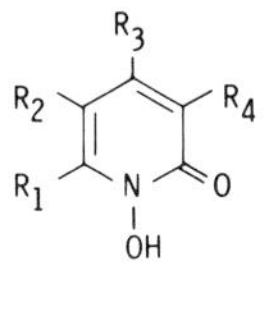 (XXX) 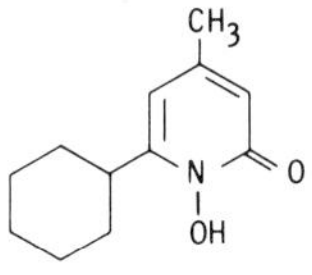 (XXXI)

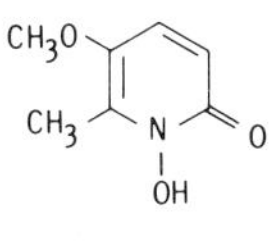

(XXXII) 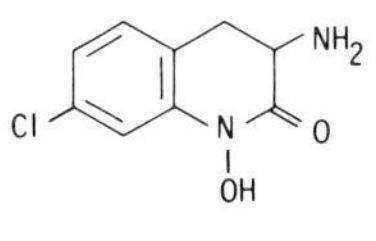 (XXXIII)

lipophilicity (extension of side-chain R_1 in XXX) and skin penetration/cure rate (Dittmar *et al.*, 1974). Thus the $C_{11}H_{23}$ derivative had an effect some 10^5 times better than the compound XXX ($R_1 = R_2 = R_4 = H$; $R_3 = CH_3$). Steric influences (Es) had no effect on activity in this assay even at the R_1 position. An unusual outcome was the finding that the ethanolamine salts of the series gave 50% higher activity than the free acids—presumably due to modification of the absorption properties of the skin at the site of penetration.

The closely related *N*-hydroxy pyridone XXXII has recently been isolated from two *Pseudomonas* species: BN227 (Itoh *et al.*, 1979) and *P. alcaligenes* (Barker *et al.*, 1979). The substance forms copper and iron complexes, has low toxicity, and is moderately active against gram-positive bacteria, fungi, and *T. vaginalis;* typical MIC values were in the region 8–125 μg/ml. The compound was obtained both as a tris ferric complex and a true ligand from BN227 and as the ligand alone from *P. alcaligenes.* Although formation of the ethanolamine salt or metal complexes increased activity against some species, notably yeasts, the effect was not general. It seems likely that the mode of action of these compounds is via metal chelation, e.g., magnesium or possibly iron. A related carbostyril derivative XXXIII has been reported active against gram-positive bacteria and *C. albicans* at 20 μg/ml (Davis *et al.*, 1977).

F. IMIDAZOLES

1. *Ring Fused Types*

The anthelmintic thiabendazole has long been known to have activity against a variety of dermatophytes, but not yeasts; it has been used topically in the treatment of ringworm and chromomycosis. A Merck study (Fisher and Lusi, 1972) on imidazo[1,2-*a*]pyridines (XXXIV) demon-

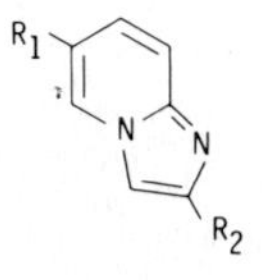

(XXXIV) 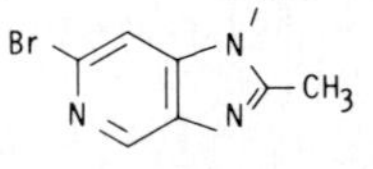 (XXXV) 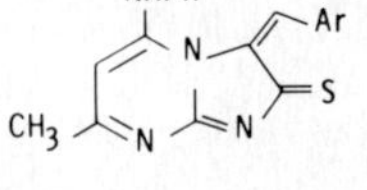 (XXXVI)

strated good *in vivo* anthelmintic activity for 6-substituted compounds (e.g., R_1 = EtOCONH, R_2 = 4-thiazolyl) which apparently were less susceptible to *in vivo* hydroxylation than derivatives where $R_1 = H$, which were only active *in vitro*. Broad spectrum antifungal activity was identified in these compounds, but did not correlate with anthelmintic activity and was generally rather weak, e.g., 100 μg/ml against *A. niger, P. luteum,* and *T. viride.* The isomeric imidazo[4,5-*c*]pyridines XXXV were reported in a Russian study to show strong activity against gram-positive bacteria and some fungi (Brantsevich *et al.,* 1975); the compounds where "sugar" was 1-β-D-glucopyranosyl or 1-β-D-ribopyranosyl for instance showed an MIC of 8 μg/ml against *T. rubrum.* Another Russian study (Mandrichenko *et al.,* 1978) examined a related ring system—the imidazopyrimidines XXXVI—but the compounds described probably owe their activity more to the unsaturated thioamide structure shown than to the imidazole part of the molecule.

2. *Mono-(N)-substituted*

This group of compounds represents the single largest class of synthetic antifungals, and has been the subject of extensive investigation by many companies and academic groups, resulting in several successful drugs already in clinical use, with probably more to follow. It is not the purpose of this article to give an exhaustive account of the development, clinical, pharmacological, and biochemical investigations of this large group of compounds, since these aspects have been well covered in many reports over the last few years (e.g., *Annu. Rep. Med. Chem.* 1969 *et seq.*). Instead, some of the more fundamental structure–activity relationships which have been discerned for members of various series will be discussed, and the resulting direction of present research on mechanisms of action and further synthetic effort will be highlighted. Patent applications have not been included for this group in view of the large numbers involved and the wealth of pharmacological papers otherwise available.

The first reports of activity in N-substituted imidazoles were by the Bayer and Janssen groups (Plempel *et al.,* 1969; Godefroi *et al.,* 1969) for 1-triphenylmethane and 1-phenethyl derivatives of imidazole, respectively (XXXVII and XXXVIII). The tritylimidazoles were synthesized on the hypothesis that substances producing reactive carbonium ions *in vivo* might be biologically active—such as the known antifungal tropylium derivatives. Substantial structure–activity work however demonstrated that the rate of hydrolysis of these compounds to the trityl carbonium ion did not correlate with *in vivo* activity (Buchel *et al.,* 1972). There was also no marked effect of lipophilicity on activity. The best compounds—e.g., clotrimazole (VI; XXXVII X = Y = H, Z = *o*-Cl)—were in the group showing a moderate rate of hydrolysis. A marked correlation *did* emerge with steric effects of ortho-substituents (e.g., clotrimazole), and it was concluded that the preferred molecular conformation for activity involved a "propeller" form with the aryl rings out of plane. Clotrimazole has wide

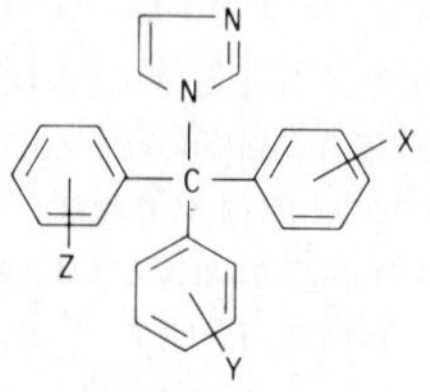

(XXXVII) 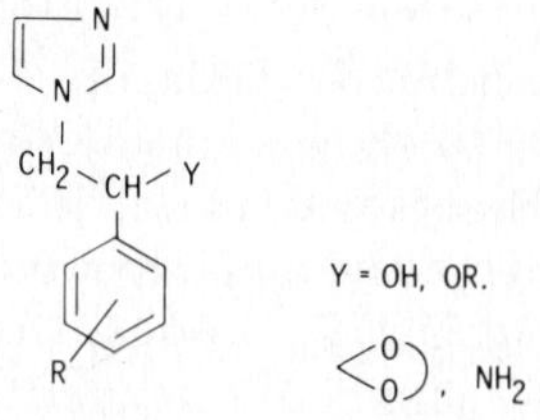 (XXXVIII)

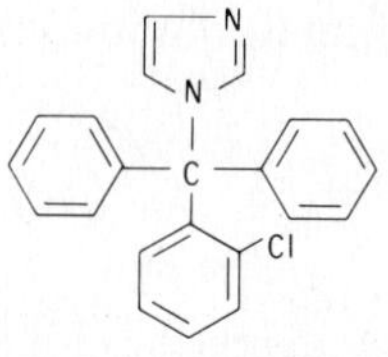

Y = OH, OR, $\langle^{O}_{O}\rangle$, NH_2

(VI) clotrimazole 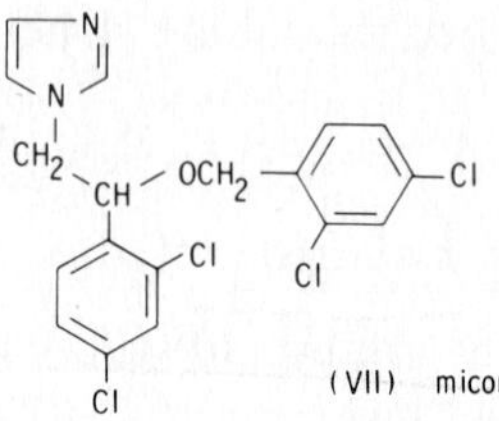 (VII) miconazole

spectrum activity against many dermatophytes and yeasts—a property which generally characterizes this class of compound; most *Candida* isolates are inhibited in the 0.02–4 μg/ml range.

The Janssen phenethyl compounds XXXVIII were also found active against dermatophytes, yeasts, and gram-positive bacteria when Y = OR, although the amines (Y = NH_2) were active only against dermatophytes, and that at a lower level. Ketals and the alcohols [Y = $O(CH_2)_nO$ and OH] were intermediate in activity. The best compounds in the series were ethers (Y = OR) with antidermatophyte activity from 0.01 μg/ml. The first drug of this type with clinical utility was miconazole (VII). This compound inhibits most yeasts at 3–15 μg/ml, and has broad spectrum antifungal activity. Both miconazole and clotrimazole are poorly absorbed from the digestive tract and are similar in their mode of action; they appear to affect the membrane permeability of susceptible organisms and cause visible damage to the structure and function of intracellular organelles. At very low concentrations (1.04×10^{-9} *M*) miconazole has selective effects on the uptake of various nutrients by *C. albicans* (Van den Bossche, 1974). De Nollin and Borgers (1974, 1976) found that miconazole produced ultrastructural changes in *C. albicans*. Low concentrations caused changes in the cell periphery with thickening of the wall and proliferation of the plasmalemma, while higher concentrations caused progressively more severe changes, with an increase in cell volume, proliferation of peroxisomes, and eventually complete necrosis. De Nollin *et al.* (1977) followed this with enzyme studies which showed that at low concentrations (fungistatic) of miconazole there was decreased cytochrome c oxidase and peroxidase activity and an increase in catalase, while at higher concentrations (fungicidal), all three enzymes disappeared; cell death could be caused by hydrogen peroxide accumulation. Yamaguchi (1977, 1978) believed that the plasma membrane is the primary target for imidazoles, and found that activity could be antagonized by lipids containing fatty acids; his results are supported by observations of Sud *et al.* (1979) on liposome model membranes. Although differences in liposome phospholipid fatty acid unsaturation did not correlate with susceptibility to imidazoles, the presence of free fatty acids had marked effects on susceptibility to clotrimazole and miconazole, and the degree of unsaturation was the key factor. It is interesting to note that lipids of fungi and gram-positive bacteria susceptible to imidazoles contain substantial quantities of free fatty acids whereas mammalian cells and gram-negative bacteria have little or none. Ergosterol is the key sterol in the fungal plasma membrane, playing an analogous role to cholesterol in the mammal. Van den Bossche *et al.* (1978) found that 10^{-7} *M* miconazole would inhibit ergosterol biosynthesis in *C. albicans* by blocking demethylation at C_{14}, the penultimate stage in ergosterol formation. Cope (1980) has studied the rapid release of K^+ ions from *C. albicans* following exposure to miconazole and the immediate effects on growth. She feels that her observations suggest that the damage is more likely due to a direct interaction of the plasma membrane with miconazole than to an effect on ergosterol synthesis. Her observations are supported by those of Dufour *et al.* (1980), who observed that miconazole is a powerful competitive inhibitor of the plasma membrane ATPase of *Schizosaccharomyces pombe,* inducing a rapid efflux of K^+ accompanied by the stoichiometric influx of H^+.

In studies designed to explore structure–activity relationships in the miconazole series, the Janssen group explored compounds of types XXXIX, XL, and XLI (Heeres *et al.*, 1976, 1977). In the alkyl substituted

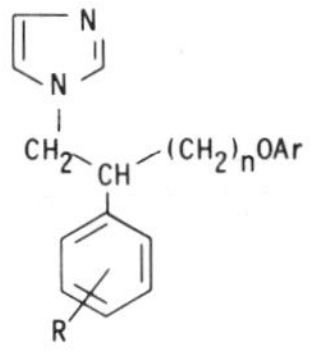

(XXXIX) 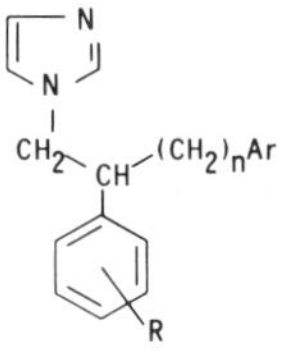 (XL) 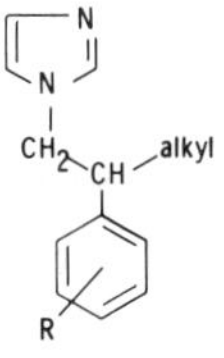 (XLI)

series XLI, most were active against dermatophytes at 1 μg/ml and also against yeasts; alkyl groups of at least four carbon atoms were required for significant activity, and substitution in the phenyl ring was optimum in the ortho/para positions. In general, *in vitro* activity was predictive of *in vivo* activity in a cutaneous candidosis/guinea pig model following oral administration. For the phenoxy and phenalkyl series XXXIX and XL the same biological profile was found, but chain length was not important; *in vitro* potency *did not* correlate with *in vivo* activity following oral administration.

The problem of poor correlation between *in vitro* and *in vivo* results was also found for a series of 1-imidazolyl phenol ethers and 1-imidazolylmethyl phenyl ethers synthesized by a Schering group (XLII and XLIII; Strehlke and Kessler, 1979). Among allylic, propargylic, and

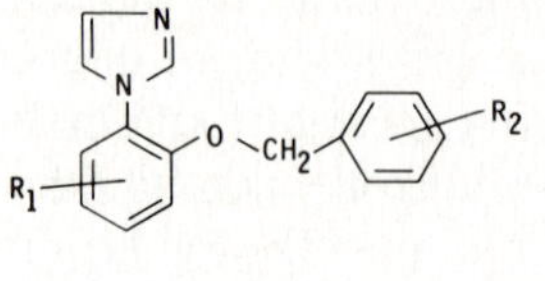

(XLII) 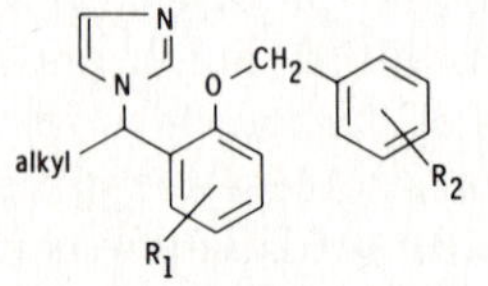 (XLIII)

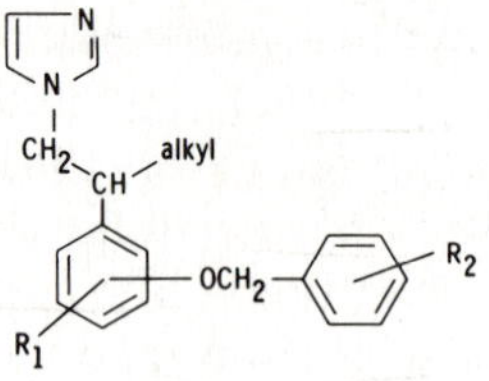

(XLIV) 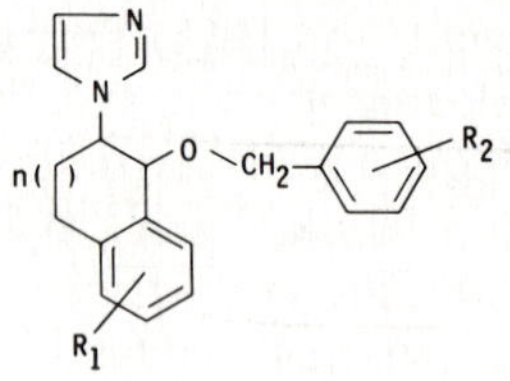 (XLV)

benzylic ethers of 1-imidazoyl phenol, the benzylic compounds (XLII) were superior (Strehlke, 1979) and 3,4-dichloro substitution (R_2) gave optimum potency. The compounds were active against *T. mentagrophytes, T. rubrum,* and *M. gypseum* at 1.6–12.5 μg/ml; activity against *C. albicans* was generally poor (>100 μg/ml). The corresponding methylphenyl ether homologs XLIII were similar in potency and spectrum of activity, with optimum alkyl substitution being *n*-propyl (R_1 = H; R_2 = 2,4–Cl_2). Compounds with other alkyl substituents were active *in vitro* but not *in vivo*. Compounds in this and the homologous series XLIV were examined for activity in a rat vaginal candidosis model; structure–activity relationships were studied using the animal model rather than *in vitro* data. The related ring fused alkyl chain series XLV (n = 0 and 1) was also examined and somewhat better *in vitro* activities obtained (0.8–1.6 μg/ml; Strehlke *et al.*, 1975).

Much Janssen work seems to have been directed at the problem of oral absorption, and several compounds from their dioxolane series have reached the stage of clinical evaluation. Parconazole (R 39,500; XLVI) and doconazole (R 34,000; XLVII) were found to be more active against *Coccidioides immitis* than miconazole but to have less activity in other systemic fungal infections (Dixon *et al.,* 1978a); doconazole has been described as the drug of choice for oral treatment of murine coccidioidomycosis (Levine, 1977), but was dropped because it produced glaucoma in dogs. Other compounds in the series such as ketoconazole (R 41,000; IX) have much improved water solubility, and in general, broad-spectrum activity (Dixon *et al.,* 1978b). Ketoconazole appears to hold considerable promise as an orally absorbed antifungal agent, e.g., Levine and Cobb (1978), Botter *et al.* (1979).

Many other compounds which have reached some stage of clinical trial represent only minor variations in the parent miconazole structure. Thus sulconazole (XLVIII) and butoconazole (RS 35,887; IL) are thioether analogs of miconazole with similar *in vitro* profiles. The *in vivo* profile of butoconazole is claimed to be markedly superior, with consistently higher cure rates and less recurrence of infection (Walker *et al.,* 1978a). Other variations on the miconazole theme are oxiconazole (L), democonazole (LI), tioconazole (LII), isoconazole (LIII), and REC 15/1476 (LIV). Other studies have investigated the replacement of the ether group in miconazole by oxy and thioester functions (LV; Walker *et al.,* 1978b). Activity in this series was markedly influenced by lipophilicity, significant activity against *C. albicans* only being associated with compounds with properties similar to miconazole itself. Another series with potent activity contains *N*-ketomethylimidazoles typified by structure LVI (Ueno *et al.,* 1973) and the Bayer compound climazole (LVII). In the LVI type the optimum chain length for the alkyl residue was eight carbon atoms, and these compounds were active against *C. albicans, T. mentagrophytes, T. rubrum,* and *C. neoformans* at 0.2–2 μg/ml; topical activity against *Trichophyton* infections in animals was also good (3% concentration). A recent trend in this area is to replace the imidazole residue itself with the related 1,2,4-triazole

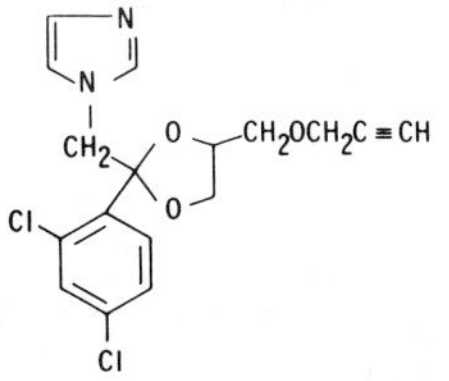

(XLVI) parconazole

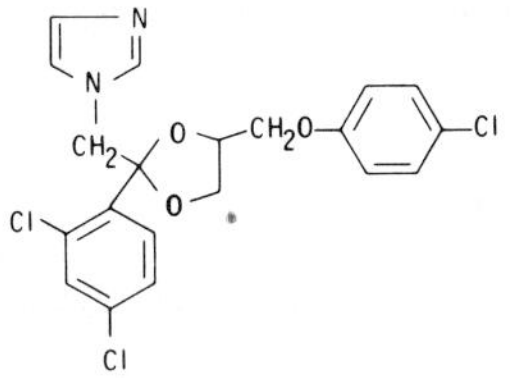

(XLVII) doconazole

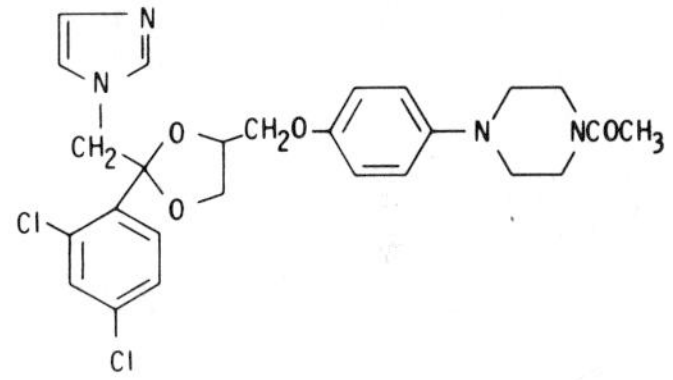

(IX) ketoconazole

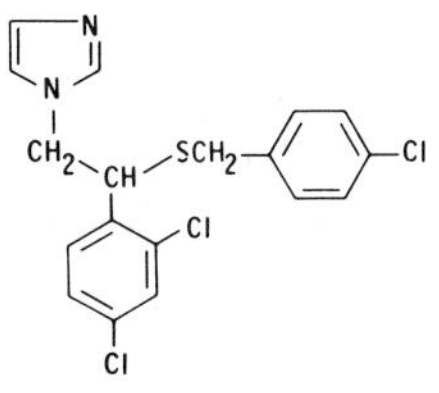

(XLVIII) sulconazole

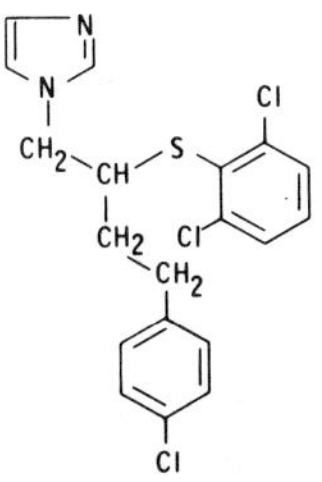

(IL) butoconazole

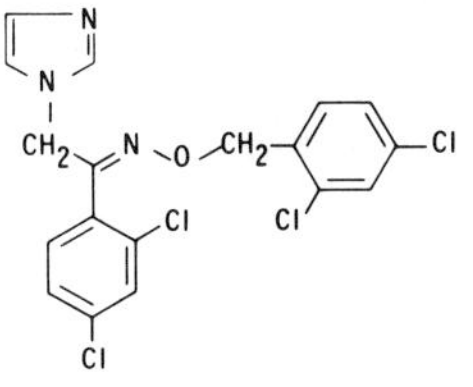

(L) oxiconazole

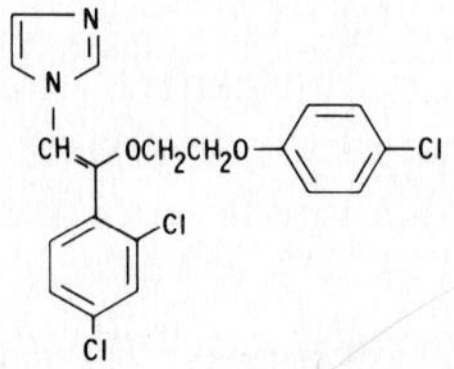

(LI) democonazole 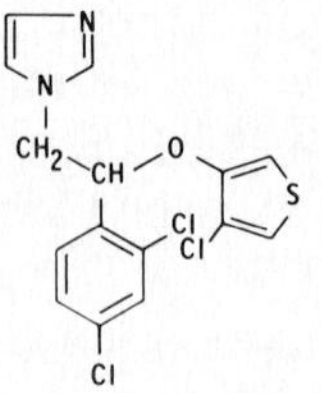 (LII) tioconazole 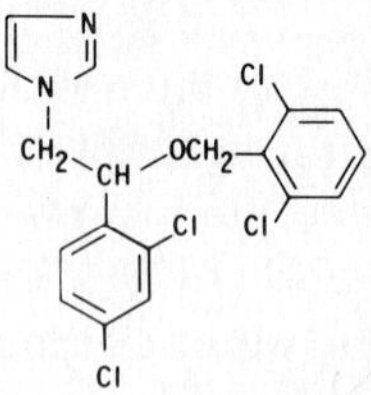 (LIII) isoconazole

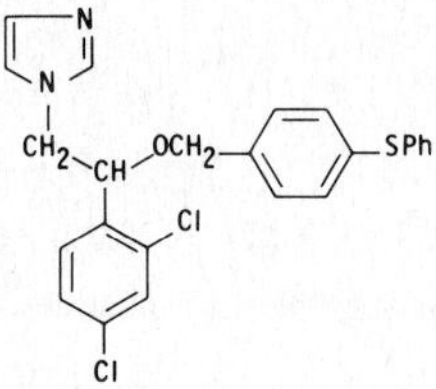

(LIV) 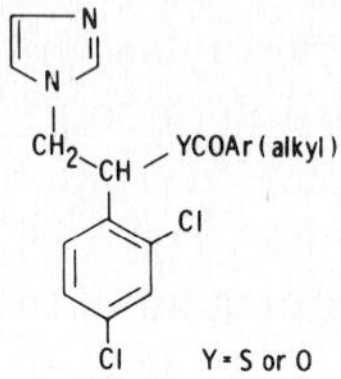 (LV) 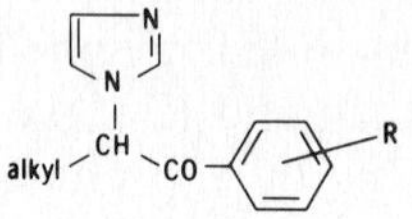 (LVI)

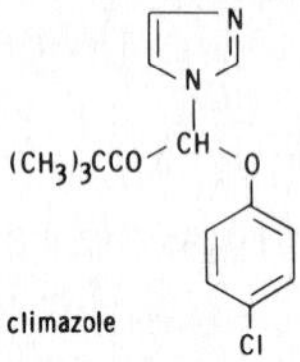

Y = S or O

(LVII) climazole 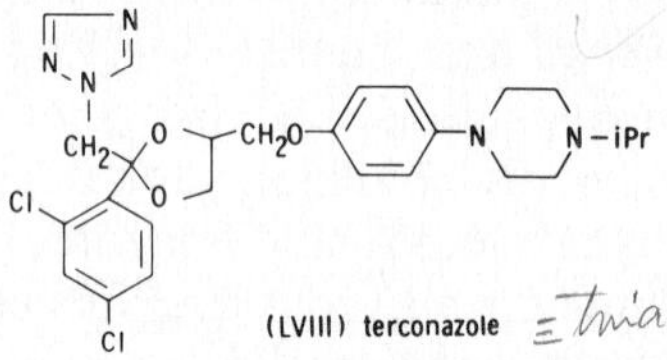 (LVIII) terconazole

moiety. Thus the water-soluble terconazole (LVIII) seems to be showing considerable promise at present as a topical agent; experimentally, terconazole also has oral activity but is more toxic than ketoconazole.

G. Indoles

Indole produced by *E. coli* was found by Oimomi *et al.* (1974) to have widespread but feeble activity (e.g., 100–400 μg/ml for *Candida*). In a large scale investigation of some 400 simple indole derivatives against 51 microbial species, Whitehead and Whitesitt (1974) found that 54% of the compounds inhibited one or more species, 36% inhibited two or more, and 8% inhibited fifteen or more; 5-bromoindole was assessed as having the best overall antifungal activity (against six species). Substitution of the 2- and 3-positions by diarylmethyl residues surprisingly produced compounds of considerable antibacterial but no antifungal interest; thus 5-bromo-3-diphenylmethylindole had a spectrum comparable to current clinically important antibacterials. More highly substituted indoles have also been examined: 2-amino or aminomethyl derivatives (LIX) have been described with activity against unspecified organisms at 4–8 μg/ml (Grinev *et al.*, 1977); the phenylthioureido derivatives (R_2 = PhNHCS)

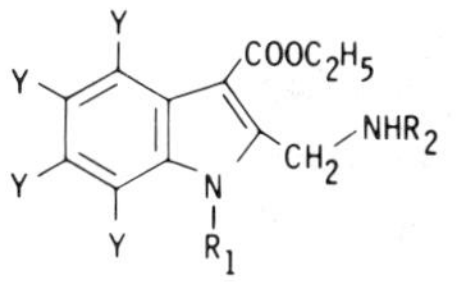

(LIX) 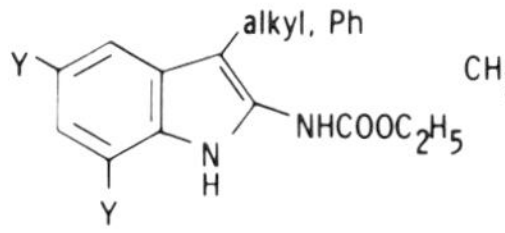 (LX) 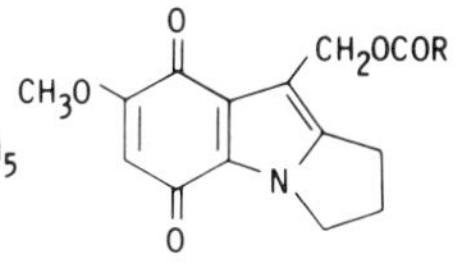 (LXI) 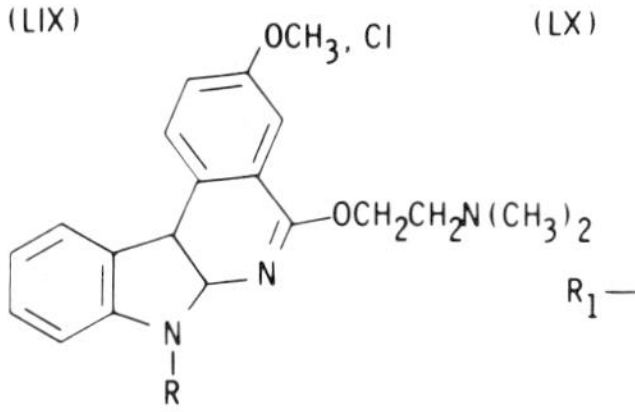 (LXII) 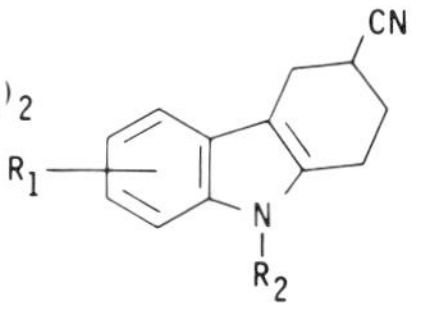 (LXIII)

were particularly interesting. In a similar study the polyhaloindoles (LX) were also investigated (Hiremath *et al.,* 1978).

Three fused indole ring systems are of some interest; pyrrolo[1,2-*a*]indoloquinones of type LXI were investigated for antimicrobial activity on a basis of their similarity to mitomycin (Yamada *et al.,* 1974). Compounds where R = alkyl were active against *C. albicans* at 1.25–12.5 μg/ml, but the corresponding carbamoyloxy derivatives (R = NHR′) were less active against fungi and more active against bacteria. A series of indolo[2,3-*c*]isoquinolines (LXII) were shown to have wide spectrum activity against fungi at 5–20 μg/ml (Winters *et al.,* 1979). The activity was consistently reduced by the presence of serum, and there was no activity at 250 mg/kg in mice. Schering patents have appeared claiming topical activity in a related series of tetrahydrocarbazoles (LXIII; Schering: DT. 2240880, 1974/1976; DT. 2438022, 1974/1976; U.S. 3835152, 1972/1974); a specifically claimed compound was R_1 = H, R_2 = benzoyl in LXIII. The first carbazole antibiotics, carbazomycins A and B, have recently been isolated from an unidentified *Streptomyces* species (Sakano *et al.,* 1980). Carbazomycin B (hydroxy-methoxy-dimethylcarbazole) was slightly active against dermatophytes, yeasts, and some phytopathogens.

H. Nucleoside Derivatives

The literature in this area seems to be confined to patent claims. There are two main types of interest: compounds featuring variations in the base attached to ribofuranose sugars of natural configuration, and natural pyrimidine bases with modified sugar residues. The first type is represented by three classes (LXIV, LXV, and LXVI). The 1,2,3-triazole nucleosides (LXV) are claimed in an ICN patent (U.S. 3968103, 1972/1976) to be active against a variety of bacteria and fungi including *C.*

albicans and *A. niger;* R_1 in these compounds is an electron-withdrawing function, e.g., NO_2, $CONH_2$, CN, $COOCH_3$. The related pyrazole nucleosides (LXIV)—which are formally derivatives of the antibiotic pyrazofurin—have antiviral, antifungal, and antitumor properties (Lilly: NL. 7508706, 1975/1976); R_1, R_2, and R_3 in these compounds may be alkyl or alkanoyl. The cytosine derivatives (LXVI) appear to be attempts to modify the transport characteristics of the natural nucleoside, R_1 being a long chain fatty acid residue such as margaroyl (C_{17}); cytostatic activity is emphasized in this claim (Asaki Chem. Co.: DT. 2461862, 1974/1976). In

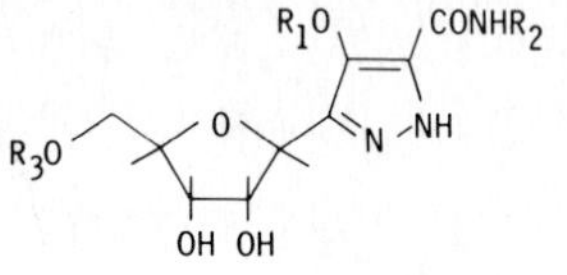

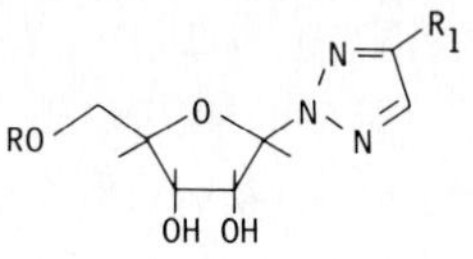

(LXIV) (LXV)

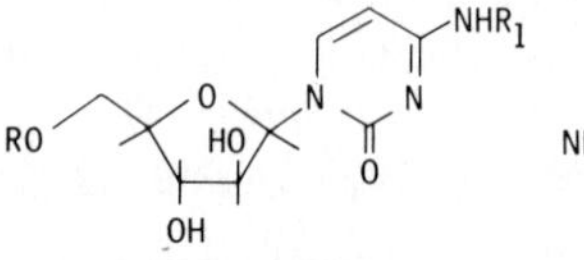

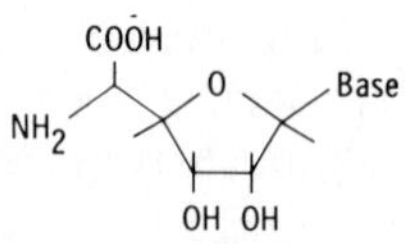

(LXVI) (LXVII)

the second type the sugar residue in purine and pyrimidine nucleosides was converted to a 5′-uronic acid as found in the polyoxin C type nucleosides (Syntex: U.S. 3936184, 1972/1976). Widespread antibiotic and antifungal activity was claimed for these products (LXVII), but no specific examples are given.

I. Isoxazoles, Oxadiazoles, and Oxazoles

This heterogeneous group has been assembled on grounds of rather superficial resemblance; it is possible that the oxadiazoles in fact have more in common with the thiadiazoles discussed later. Significantly the 1,3,4-oxadiazoles of type LXVIII have thioamide residues as a probably vital toxophore. Both Mazzone and Bonina (1979) and Singh and Yadav (1977) described activity for the Mannich bases LXVIII where R_3 is optimally a substituted benzamido (e.g., with *o*-Cl, *m*-Cl, *p*-Cl, or *p*-F) or a phthalimido residue. Both electron-withdrawing and electron-releasing substituents R_1 and R_2 gave activities against *C. albicans, C. tropicalis, C. triadis, T. glabrata, T. rubrum,* and *M. gypseum* at 6.25–50 μg/ml. Singh and Yadav (1976) examined the related 2-aryl-5-amino compounds LXIX and

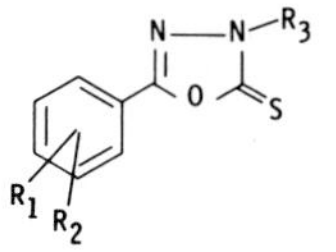

(LXVIII) 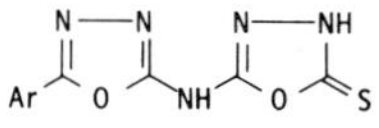 (LXIX)

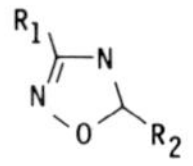

(LXX) 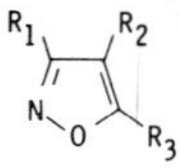 (LXXI) 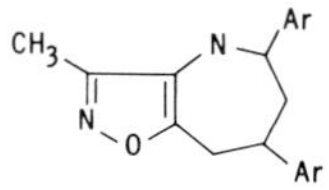 (LXXII)

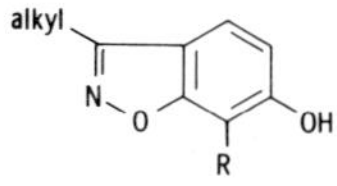

(LXXIII) 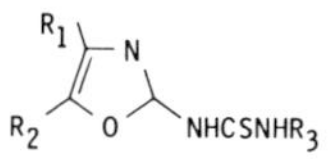 (LXXIV)

found activity against *A. niger* and *A. flavus*. The corresponding 5-substituted thioethers (LXIX; S for NH) have also been described as having activity against these pathogens (Suman and Bahel, 1979), i.e., $\geq 50\%$ inhibition at 10 ppm for Ar = *o, m,* or *p*-nitrophenyl. The isomeric 1,2,4-oxadiazoles LXX have been claimed in an Abbot patent (U.S. 3651054, 1967/1972) to have antibacterial, antifungal, and trichomonacidal activity following topical application; one of the substituents in these compounds is 5-NO_2-2-furyl, the other being a basic group.

Isoxazoles are represented by the ring-fused and free heterocyclic examples LXXI, LXXII, and LXXIII. Claims of antifungal activity were made for LXXI with R_1 and R_3 = aryl, R_2 = H (Murthy *et al.*, 1973), and with $R_1 = CH_3$, R_2 = NHCOR, R_3 = CH═CHR (Murthy *et al.*, 1976), but no details are recorded. The pyrazyl-isoxazole LXXI with R_1 = 3-methyl-4-nitrosopyraz-5-yl, R_2 = H, $R_3 = CH_3$—which was an intermediate in a pyrazolopyridine synthesis—was found active against *M. canis* at 6.25 μg/ml (Ajello, 1971). In the benzisoxazole series LXXIII, a range of antibacterial and antifungal properties were found. The compounds with R = H or CHO and alkyl = ethyl in particular were active against *C. albicans* at 40–200 μg/ml (Thakar and Ghawal, 1977). For the ring expanded and reduced series LXXII the general examples shown were active against *C. albicans* and *C. neoformans,* but were not antibacterial (*E. coli* or *S. aureus*).

Finally the oxazoles LXXIV—which may be regarded as the parent ring system for the oxadiazoles above—were investigated for antifungal activity as part of a general study of the biological activities of this group (Crank *et al.*, 1973). The compounds were active against plant and human fungal pathogens, the best compound for the latter having $R_1 = R_2$ = H,

R_3 = Et; MICs were: *T. mentagrophytes* 4–128 μg/ml; *C. neoformans* 32–500 μg/ml; and *S. cerevisiae* 32–64 μg/ml.

J. Phenylacetic Acid Derivatives

Only two similar types of derivative have been described, but patent activity in the area suggests the interest to be sustained. Ciba-Geigy have produced a number of claims for tertiary (aminophenyl) acetic acids (U.S. 3868391, U.S. 3936467, U.S. 3997609, U.S. 4126691, U.S. 4163788, 1972/1979) which are all based on derivatives of type LXXV, including the amine oxides; R_1 and R_2 are drawn widely as alkyl, aryl, or cycloalkyl. The compounds are claimed to be analgesic and antiinflammatory as well as active against dermatophytes. The 2-arylaminophenylacetyl amides LXXVI have been recently described to have antibacterial and antifungal properties; no biological details are available (Mehta *et al.*, 1978).

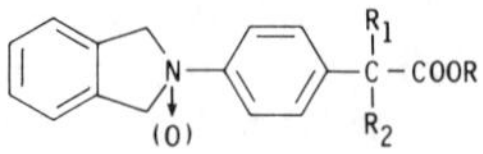

(LXXV) 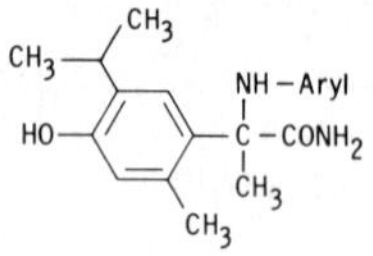 LXXVI)

K. Pyridine Derivatives

This group includes saturated pyridines, but not the *N*-hydroxypyridones described in Section III,E. In a systematic study of pyridoxal analogs (Korytnyk and Paul, 1970; Korytnyk and Ahrens, 1971; Korytnyk *et al.*, 1972) various homologs of the aldehyde or alcohol functions at C_4 (R_1) and C_5 (R_2) in LXXVII were prepared. It was found that homologation of the C_4 function in LXXVII [R_1 = $(CH_2)_3OH$, R_2 = CH_2OH] gave weak antagonists of *S. cerevisiae* $IC_{50} = 5 \times 10^{-4}$ *M*). However the corresponding isomer homologated at C_5 [R_1 = CH_2OH, R_2 = $(CH_2)_2OH$] inhibited this yeast with an IC_{50} of 5×10^{-8} *M*. The closer analog of pyridoxal itself with R = CHO was less active ($IC_{50} = 5 \times 10^{-5}$ *M*). Although these compounds were inhibitors of pyridoxyl phosphokinase and acted as substrates for pyridoxine dehydrogenase, these properties could not be correlated with their *in vivo* activity; their activity was however consistent with antagonism of vitamin B_6 uptake.

A Merck study of some 4-phenyl tetrahydropyridinium salts (based on the known antimicrobial effectiveness of quaternary compounds in general) showed that compounds of the type LXXVIII were active against

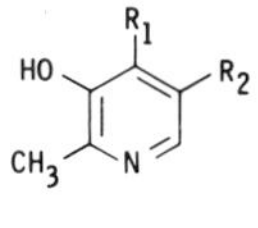

(LXXVII) 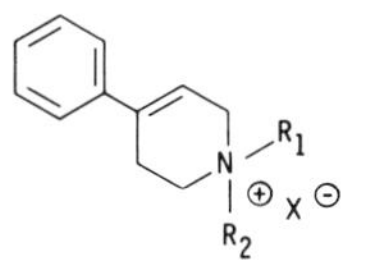 (LXXVIII) 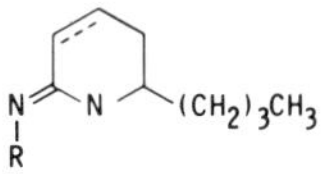 (LXXIX)

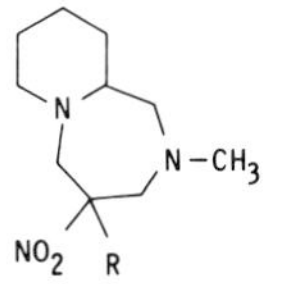

(LXXX) 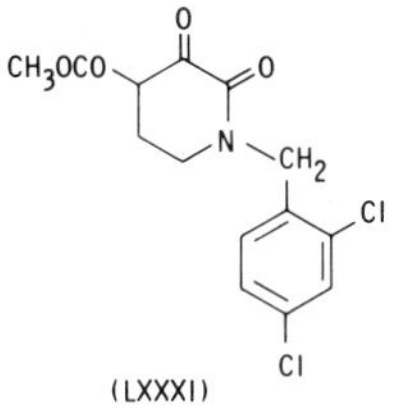 (LXXXI)

gram-positive and gram-negative bacteria and also fungi (Grier, 1979); the optimum chain length for R_1 was nonyl through dodecyl for both types of activity. The best MIC values against *Aspergillus niger* and *Aureobasidium pullulans* were 10 μg/ml for the latter compounds ($R_2 = CH_3$). Piperidines (and tetrahydropyridines) of type LXXIX were active against *B. subtilis, T. mentagrophytes,* and *M. gypseum* when R was an electron-withdrawing function such as CN or *p*-NH_2–$C_6H_4SO_2$ (Ondrus and Kraus, 1979). Nitroperhydropyridodiazepines of type LXXX showed broad spectrum antifungal and antibacterial properties (Biere and Redmann, 1976); optimum substitution was found when R was in the C_2–C_7 range, with a sharp drop in activity at higher chain lengths, e.g., C_{11}. Typical compounds had MIC values of 4 μg/ml for *M. gypseum,* 0.5 μg/ml for *T. mentagrophytes,* 1 μg/ml for *T. rubrum,* and 8 μg/ml for *A. niger*. These compounds are probably analogous to the well-known "bromopol" type of NO_2 alkane diol antimicrobials. An isolated report (Schwan *et al.*, 1979) describes activity against pathogenic fungi for the dioxopyridine LXXXI. Various *Candida* species were inhibited at 20 μg/ml and *A. niger* at 100 μg/ml, but no synthetic rationale was given for this compound.

L. Pyrimidine Derivatives

An ICN group—as part of a systematic study of heterocyclic systems resembling nucleosides—investigated the antimicrobial properties of imidazo[1,2-*a*]pyrimidines (LXXXII) and pyrazolo[1,5-*a*]pyrimidines (LXXXIII; Revankar *et al.*, 1975; Novinson *et al.*, 1977). In each case the substituted amino derivatives corresponding to adenosine were examined. In the imidazopyrimidine series LXXXII only the 5-*n*-octylamino ($R = C_8H_{17}$) derivative showed "significant" activity against all the organisms tested (bacterial and fungal): MICs were *C. albicans* 0.08, *E. floccosum* 0.08, *M. canis* 0.04, *T. mentagrophytes* 0.08, and *S. aureus* 0.16

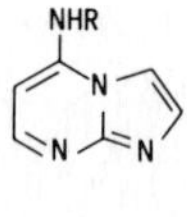

(LXXXII)

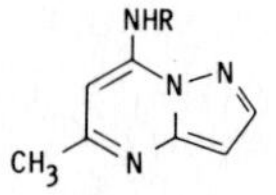

(LXXXIII)

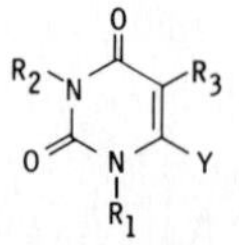

(LXXXIV)

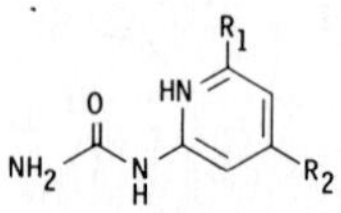

(LXXXV)

μg/ml; activity against gram-negative bacteria was not detected. By contrast the pyrazolopyrimidines LXXXIII showed a clear structure–activity relationship between chain length R and fungicidal properties. Thus antifungal efficacy of saturated nonbranched units increased to a maximum with the octylamino compound (see above), but in this series maximum overall potency was achieved with the oleylamino derivative [R = CH_3-$(CH_2)_7CH{=}CH(CH_2)_8$—], the corresponding derivative being uninteresting in the imidazopyrimidine series. This compound gave an average MIC value of 0.005 μg/ml for the above species. Topical testing against *T. mentagrophytes* in guinea pigs was unfortunately abortive because of skin irritation.

Two groups of free pyrimidines were included in another investigation. Structure–activity relationships were studied in a series of alkylated uracils (LXXXIV) using *T. rubrum, M. gypseum, T. mentagrophytes,* and *E. floccosum* (Gauri and Meyer-Rohn, 1974). Compounds with Y = H or alkyl were inactive, but when Y = Cl, activity was found at low (0.005 *M*) concentrations. Optimum potency was found with $R_1 + R_2 + R_3 = 7$ or 8 carbon atoms, but no clear optimum in positional substitution emerged. This finding paralleled earlier studies on yeast alcohol dehydrogenase with alkylated uracils (Gauri, 1970), but the mechanism for the compounds' antifungal activity was not clear.

2-Ureidopyrimidines (LXXXV) were prepared by Kreutzberger and Schimmelpfennig (1980) and claimed to show marked antifungal activity; R_1 and R_2 were simple alkyl residues, and the best compound had $R_1 = CH_3$. "Simple" pyrimidines as a class are widely represented in the field of plant antifungal agents.

M. Pyridazines, Pyrazoles

Although sparsely represented here, many pyrazole and pyridazine types have found agricultural applications. The 5-aminopyrazoles

LXXXVI were prepared and studied by Giori *et al.* (1979); the 4-thiocyanato or 5-amino compounds were found active against *C. albicans* and *T. mentagrophytes* at 5–10 μg/ml. In general there was no correlation of potency between species, compound R_1 = Ph, R_2 = CH_3, R_3 = *o*-$MeOC_6H_4CO$, R_4 = H being best against *Candida* and compound R_1 = CH_3, R_2 = Ph, R_3 = H, R_4 = SCN being optimum for *Trichophyton*.

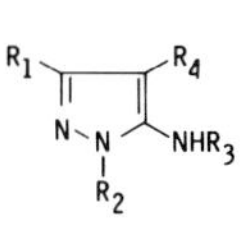

(LXXXVI) 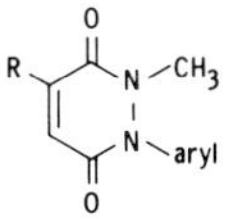 (LXXXVII) 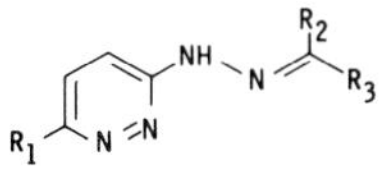 (LXXXVIII)

Two types of pyridazines have been examined. Of the pyridazinediones LXXXVII studied for inhibitory activity against bacteria and fungi, compounds with R = EtNH were found to be best with "moderate" activity (Baloniak *et al.*, 1975). The hydrazinopyridazines (LXXXVIII) were prepared as a series of alkylidene, cycloalkylidene, and arylidene derivatives, and activity against various pathogenic fungi noted (Schauer *et al.*, 1972); the best compound (R_1 = Cl, R_2 = R_3 = CH_3) was "effective" against *N. asteroides, C. neoformans, T. rubrum,* and *T. mentagrophytes*.

N. Quinazolines

The major interest in compounds of this type has been in the 2,4-diaminoquinazolines LXXXIX and XC which are structural analogs of known antagonists of the folic acid pathway. In a systematic study of selected 2,4-diaminoquinazolines against *C. albicans in vitro,* Hynes *et al.* (1976) explored the effects of various linking residues in the structure LXXXIX. While both NHCO and $NHCOCH_2$ functions were best, the elongated or reversed compounds CH_2NHCO and $CH_2NHCOCH_2$ were of no value; the most potent compounds had Y = H. The two most effective compounds in the series (R = 3,4-dichloro, with the linking groups mentioned above) had IC_{50} values of 0.6–4 μg/ml, and were selected for *in vivo* study. Although the amide (Z = NHCO) was more toxic than the homolog (Z = $NHCOCH_2$), both compounds were nontoxic to mice at 100 mg/kg. There was no correlation between activity or toxicity and inhibitory effects on rat liver dihydrofolate reductase. A parallel study of the amide (Z = NHCO; Hairi and Larsh, 1976) against *C. neoformans* showed activity *in vitro* at 6–8.25 μg/ml; partial inhibition of RNA and protein synthesis was observed at concentrations below the MIC. Oral treatment of infected mice failed to cure, but ip injection resulted in complete recovery; lack of absorption was thus suspected.

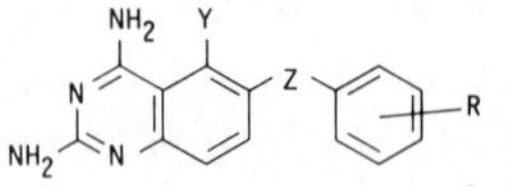

NH2 Y N Z R NH2 N (LXXXIX)

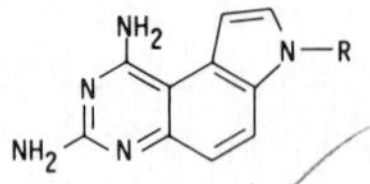

NH2 N—R N NH2 N (XC)

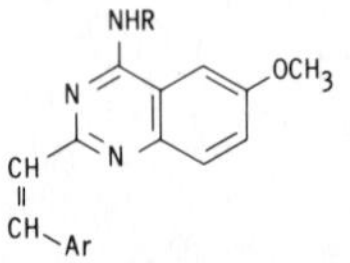

NHR OCH3 N CH N CH Ar (XCI)

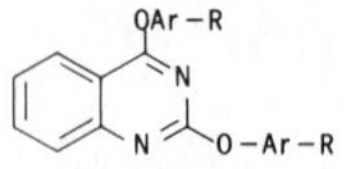

OAr—R N N O—Ar—R (XCII)

OCH3 Cl N N OH (XCIII)

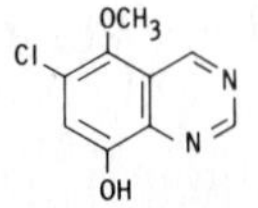

A further study involving some 40 clinical isolates of *Candida* has been undertaken to compare diaminoquinazolines (DAQ) with the pyrrolo-[3,2-*f*]quinazolines XC (Castaldo *et al.*, 1979). For compounds LXXXIX where Z = CH_2NH or $NHCH_2$, activity was very marginal or nonexistent. However the ring fused series XC yielded two compounds [R = benzyl (DAQA); R = cyclopropylmethyl (DAQB)] which were as potent as 5-FC and amphotericin B (AMB); geometric means of MICs were DAQA 0.64 μg/ml, DAQB 1.39 μg/ml, AMB 1.03 μg/ml, and 5-FC 0.72 μg/ml. Synergism was demonstrated between AMB and the DAQs, but *antagonism* between the DAQs and 5-FC. In addition, synergism between the DAQs and sulfamethoxazole—a folic acid synthesis inhibitor—was observed (Castaldo *et al.*, 1978). Since these particular DAQs are dihydrofolate reductase inhibitors, such sequential synergism would be expected. The observed antagonism of 5-FC can be explained by suppression of 5,10-methylenetetrahydrofolate formation due to DAQ inhibition of dihydrofolate reductase; 5,10-methylenetetrahydrofolate is the substrate for thymidylate synthetase, the enzyme sensitive to 5-FUdRMP (produced from 5-FC). Interestingly enough, other dihydrofolate reductase inhibitors—trimethoprim, pyrimethamine, and methotrexate—showed no antifungal activity at 50 μg/ml in this study. It would thus appear that the fungal enzyme is much less sensitive to these particular inhibitors than the enzyme from other eukaryotic (mammalian) cells.

Other quinazolines reported to have antifungal activity would appear to be acting by different mechanisms. The 2-styryl-4-amino-6-methoxyquinazolines (XCI) were active against gram-positive bacteria but were less active against fungi ($>$30 μg/ml; Zhikhareva *et al.*, 1976). The diaryloxy compounds (XCII) seemed to be effective only as pentachloro derivatives (R = Cl_5), and had an MIC against *C. albicans* and *C. tropicalis* of 20 μg/ml (Serafin *et al.*, 1977). The 5-methoxy-8-hydroxy-6-chloroquinazoline (XCIII) was active against gram-positive organisms in the presence of Fe^{2+} and against *C. albicans* in the presence of Cu^{2+}; it would thus appear to be operating by its undoubted chelating potential.

O. Quinolines, Isoquinolines

A substantial amount of interest in this group has centered on the well known chelating properties of the 8-substituted quinolines and the antifungal toxicity of their metal derivatives. Gershon *et al.* (1972a,b,c; Gershon, 1974) in particular have undertaken systematic studies on the effects of various substituents on the activity of the copper chelates of these compounds. In the 8-quinolinols (XCIV) the effects of substitution at Z showed that I = Br > Cl > F > H; these compounds were fungicidal to *T. mentagrophytes* at 0.003–0.01 μM/ml. Other studies showed that these compounds have antifungal mechanisms in addition to chelation. Thus the 8-methoxy compounds were active, but at a much lower level than the parent phenol. The 8-amino compounds were active at 0.1–8 μM/ml. These studies on structure–activity relationships were used to estimate the pore dimensions in the spore wall of five fungal species. Taking an ellipse as the model for the pore opening, the long and short axes were determined as 15/10.8 Å for *A. niger* and 16.6/10.7 Å for *T. mentagrophytes*. A series of 7-nitro-8-quinolol esters (XCV) were prepared and tested for toxicity/potency relative to the parent phenol (Massarani *et al.*, 1974). The esters were in general less active against *C. albicans* but also less toxic *in vivo*.

In the nitroalcohol series XCVI, the only active compounds were those where R = H, the 4-substituted derivatives being best (MIC against *C. albicans* <50 μg/ml; Osumi, 1972). In the trichloroalcohol series XCVII,

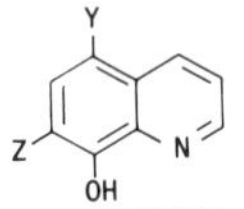

(XCIV) 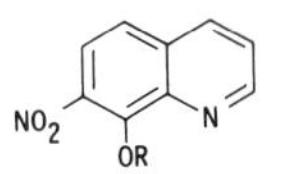 (XCV) 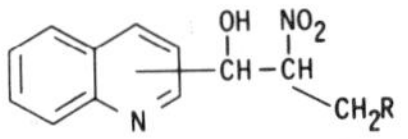 (XCVI)

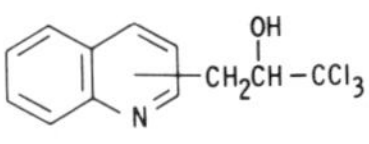

(XCVII) 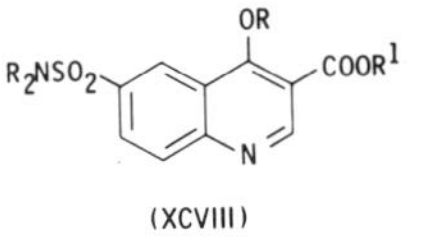 (XCVIII) 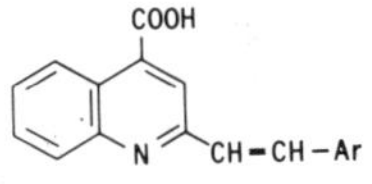 (IC)

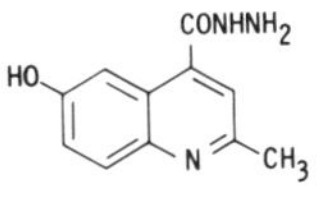

(C) 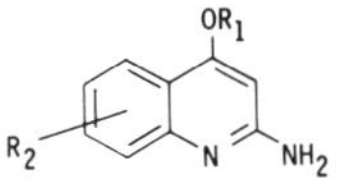 (CI) 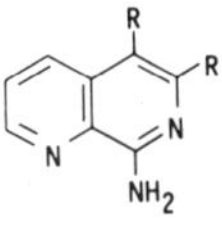 (CII)

activity against *C. albicans* and *G. candidum* was recorded at 12.5 μg/ml, but not against gram-negative bacteria. Carboxy-substituted quinolines were considered in three papers. The sulfonamido quinoline acid esters XCVIII were active against a wide range of species but activity was of a very low order (200 μg/ml on average; Parrini *et al.*, 1973). A Russian paper described the 4-quinoline carboxylic acids (IC) with the best compound (Ar = phenyl) being "active" against *C. albicans* (Lipkin and Bespalova, 1970). A series of quinolinic hydrazides were active against *C. albicans* with the best compound *in vitro* being C; it was not active *in vivo* (Anghel and Silberg, 1971).

An extensive study by an SKF group (Actor *et al.*, 1974) of 2-amino-4-alkoxyquinolines (CI) led to the conclusion that optimum potency was associated with longer alkyl side chains (R_1), and that acylation/alkylation on the amino group reduced activity. The compounds were active against *C. albicans, C. neoformans, H. capsulatum*, and *B. dermatitidis* at 12.5 μg/ml or less. These compounds, although somewhat analogous to known quinazoline antimalarials, were not folic acid antagonists. Unfortunately the compounds were inactive *in vivo*. Patent claims of antibacterial and antifungal activity opposite the 1,7-naphthyridines have been made; these compounds (CII) may be seen as combined quinolines/isoquinolines (Schering: U.S. 3928367, 1973/1975; U.S. 4017500, 1975/1977). Antiobesity properties seem to be the major interest in the series.

P. Thiazolidinones, Rhodanines, Thiazoles

This large and rather ill-defined group includes many compounds of agricultural importance, particularly ones with thiocarbonyl functions where interference with fungal primary thiol metabolism must be suspected. With the 5-substituted rhodanines (CIII; Y = S) and thiazolidines (Y = O) information on the degree of activity is scanty. The bis compounds (linked by $-CH_2-$ at R_2; R_1 = PhCH) of a Russian study "inhibited" *C. albicans* (Zdorenko *et al.*, 1978). The corresponding polynitrodiaryl compounds [R_1 = aryl-CH, $R_2 = (NO_2)_n$-aryl] were active against a range of agricultural pathogens including *A. niger* (Gupta and Sarita, 1978). Both these series could well be Michael acceptors for fungal thiol

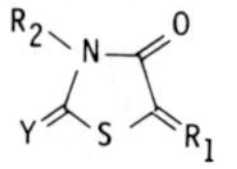

(CIII) 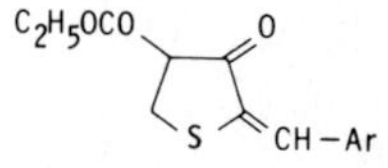 (CIV) 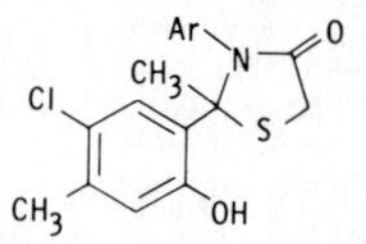 (CV)

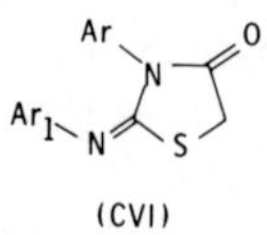

(CVI) 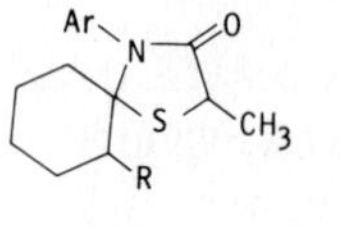 (CVII) 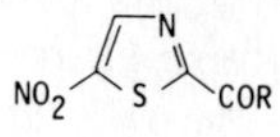 (CVIII)

groups when compared with the corresponding tetrahydrothiophenes (CIV) in which antifungal properties and sulfhydryl inhibition have been studied (Rees and Sugden, 1973). Unsaturation at C_5 does not appear however to be essential for activity, since the saturated rhodanine series (CIII; R_2 = aryl, R_1 = H, $-CH_2COOR$) were active against *C. albicans* at 30–60 μg/ml (Harefield and Hinz, 1980).

The other group of thiazolidines represented are those bearing alkyl, aryl, or arylimino residues at C_2. The hydroxyphenyl compound CV was the best of a series of phenyl/methyl substituted examples tested and found active against unspecified species at 100 μg/ml (Jadhav *et al.*, 1978). The corresponding imino compounds CVI had "amebicidal" and "fungicidal" activity, the best one having Ar_1 = *p*-tolyl, Ar_2 = 3-pyridyl (Gupta *et al.*, 1978). The spiro derivatives CVII were active against *A. niger* and *S. aureus*, the best compounds having R = H or CH_3, Ar = *o*-$NO_2C_6H_4$, *o*-$CH_3C_6H_4$, or C_6H_5 (Mehta and Parikh, 1978).

Thiazoles represented by the 5-nitro substituted example CVIII, where R was an aryl residue such as hydroxyphenyl or furyl, were active against *T. rubrum* at 0.8–3 μg/ml (Strehlke and Schroeder, 1974). Compounds with R = NHR′, piperidino, morpholino, etc. were additionally active against *C. albicans* and *Trichophyton* spp. at 6.3–12.5 μg/ml.

Q. Thiadiazoles, Dithiazoles, Isothiazoles

The thiadiazoles are probably more similar to the thiazoles in overall properties, but are included in this group as those possessing two adjacent hetero atoms (see also isoxazoles in Section III,I). Thus the 2-nitrothiadiazoles CIX are almost certainly very similar in action to the 5-nitrothiazoles. The most potent compounds were those where X is 5-aryl, having activities of 0.4–1.6 μg/ml against *T. rubrum, T. mentagrophytes,* and *C. albicans;* compounds where X = NR were active at 25–50 μg/ml and where X = CH_2OR at 12.5–25 μg/ml (Heindl *et al.*, 1975a). The 2-arylidenamino compounds CX were weakly active against *A. niger* (100

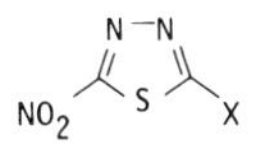

(CIX) 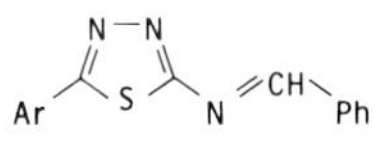 (CX) 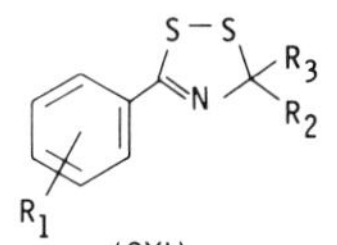 (CXI)

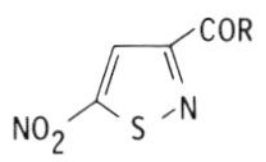

(CXII) 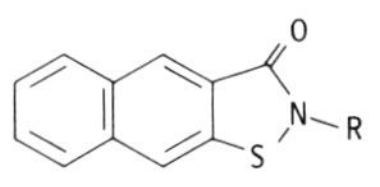 (CXIII) 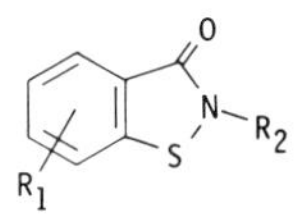 (CXIV)

μg/ml), the ones of interest having a dihydroxyaryl substituent (Singh *et al.*, 1975).

In the dithiazole series, the 5-aryl compounds CXI were tested against a range of fungi and were particularly active against *Trichophyton, Candida,* and *Aspergillus* species (Böhme and Ahrens, 1974). The compound with $R_1 = R_2 = R_3 = H$ was the most potent overall, although some substituted examples with R_2 = Cl, Me, iPr, etc. approached it in activity.

Unfused isothiazoles are represented only by the 5-nitro examples CXII which were found active against *C. albicans, T. mentagrophytes,* and *T. rubrum* down to 0.8–1.6 μg/ml. In general the esters (R = OR′) were superior to the corresponding amides (R = NHR′; Heindl *et al.*, 1975b). Two series of fused isothiazolones were reported to have antifungal activity. The naphtho[3,2-*d*]isothiazolin-2-ones CXIII were active against *C. albicans* and *T. mentagrophytes* at 2–20 and 0.5–20 μg/ml, respectively. Surprisingly the R = benzyl and phenethyl compounds were active against *Trichophyton* spp. but not (>100 μg/ml) against *Candida* (Vitali *et al.*, 1974). For the benzisothiazolin-3-ones CXIV most examples investigated had activities against *C. albicans, T. mentagrophytes,* and *C. torulopsis* in the 1–20 μg/ml range. The reduction potentials in a polarographic investigation were shown to correlate with antifungal activity, the compound with lowest reduction potential having greatest potency (R_1 = 7-Cl, R_2 = H; Riganti and Spini, 1973).

R. Triazines (Ring Fused)

The main interest in this type has been with the Norwich triazino [5,6-*c*]quinolines CXV and the corresponding pyrido[3,4-*c*]triazines CXVI. A study of CXV types against pathogenic yeasts including *C. albicans, C. krusei, C. tropicalis, C. guilliermondii,* and *T. glabrata* showed that for compounds where R = NHR, MIC values were 20–50 μg/ml. However, when R = Cl, activities of ≤10 μg/ml against all species were recorded (Wright *et al.*, 1974). The compound CXVI has undergone some development under the USAN of oxifungin.

In a study on azapteridines, the thiazalumizines (CXVII; Y = CHR, Z = N with R = aryl or pyridyl) were investigated for activity against *T.*

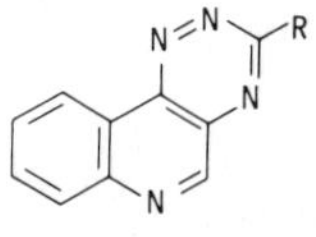

(CXV) 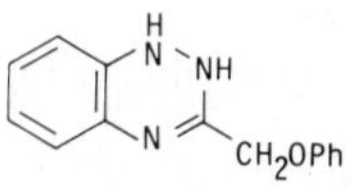 (CXVI) oxifungin 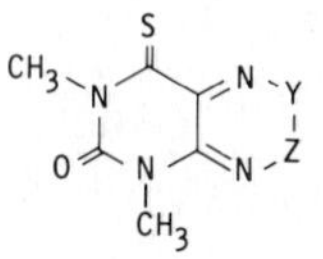 (CXVII)

mentagrophytes and found effective at 6.25–50 μg/ml; the isomeric series (Y = N, Z = CHR) were in general somewhat less active (Yoneda *et al.*, 1973).

IV. Antifungal Antibiotics

Natural sources have been particularly fruitful in providing antibacterial agents of novel structure and varied spectrum of activity—β-lactams, aminoglycosides, tetracyclines, etc. Some of these agents—possibly as many as 2% (Perlman, 1978)—find use in human chemotherapy as such or after chemical modification. In the case of antifungal antibiotics, however, success has been much more limited; the grisans and polyenes are the only types which have so far found a place in the treatment of mycoses in man, and are all far from ideal. In the present section, emphasis will be placed on those antibiotics with claimed antifungal activity which have appeared in the scientific and patent literature between 1970 and mid-1980. Classification will be into families distinguished by structural type, as knowledge of mode(s) of action is often limited for newer agents. Where possible, however, these will be discussed, together with some indication of biological profile and relative toxicity. Unless they present some feature of particular interest, generally toxic compounds will not be included.

Various aspects of antifungal antibiotics have been treated in reviews and articles, usually side by side with their synthetic counterparts. D'Arcy and Scott (1978) give a good general review, although the structures of all but four natural products are omitted. The mechanisms of action of a wide range of antibiotics have received detailed treatment by Gottlieb and Shaw (1970), and more recently by Arai (1974). Cartwright (1978a,b) has summarized this aspect in addition to the therapeutic applications of clinically useful drugs, a subject also covered by Medoff and Kobayashi (1980a). For a description of the human mycoses and dosage regimes of available treatments, the reader is referred to the chapter by Shadomy *et al.* (1977b) and the book edited by Speller (1980). Progress in the field of antifungal agents has been concisely reported in the series of articles in *Annual Reviews in Medicinal Chemistry* previously mentioned, which include references to the latest antibiotics to be isolated.

A. Polyenes

This family of poorly absorbed polyhydroxylated macrolides with characteristic conjugated olefinic chromophores has provided the majority of antifungal antibiotics of clinical importance. In particular amphotericin B (IV) and candicidin (CXVIII) which are both heptaenes, nystatin (V) a pseudo-heptaene/tetraene, and pimaricin (CXIX) a tetraene, have all found use in the topical treatment of superficial infections.

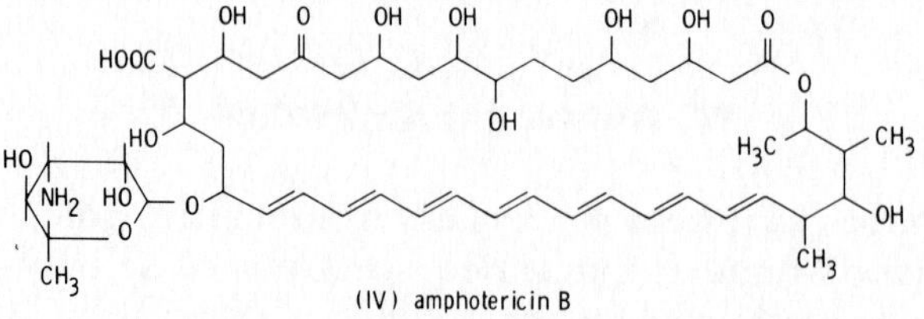

(IV) amphotericin B

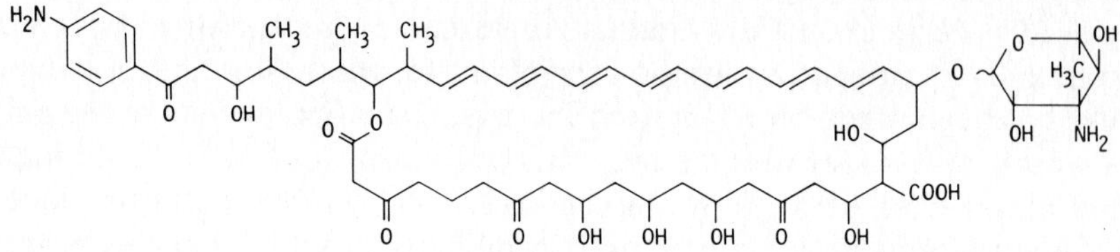

(CXVIII) candicidin D

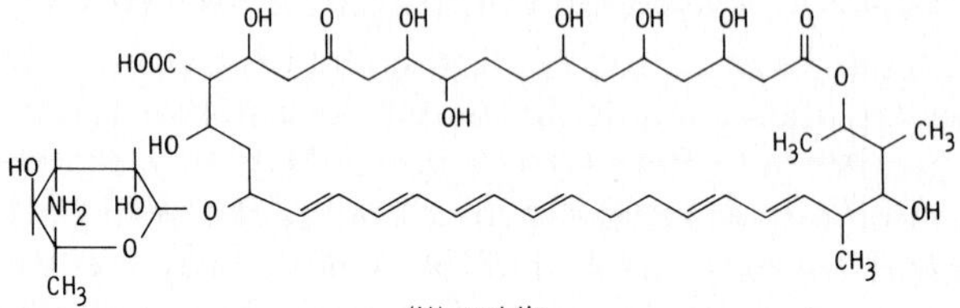

(V) nystatin

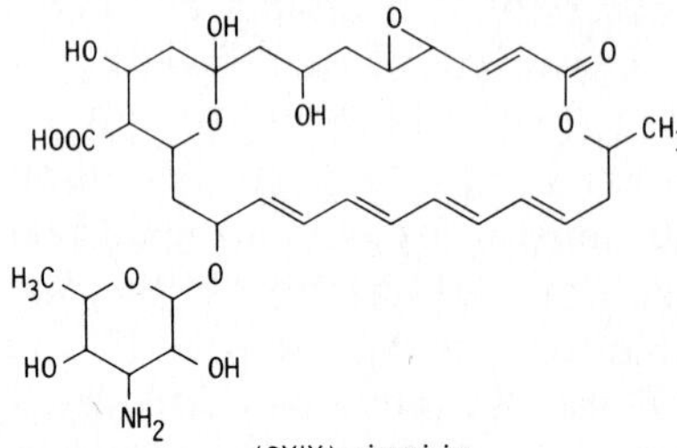

(CXIX) pimaricin

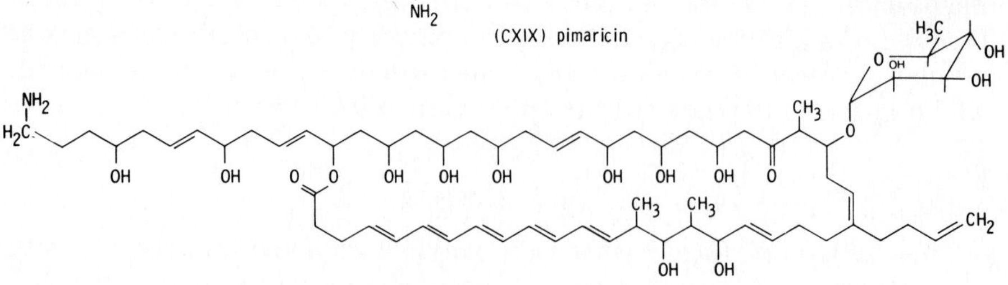

(CXX) lienomycin

The somewhat more favorable therapeutic ratio of amphotericin B has allowed it to find wider application following parenteral administration. For detailed accounts, reference should be made to any of the reviews mentioned in the introduction to this section. In addition, Hammond (1977) and Martín (1979) have devoted wide-ranging reviews exclusively to the polyenes. The former can be particularly recommended for its account of the mechanism of action of the polyenes, and the latter for fermentation and biosynthetic aspects.

1. *Origin, Structure, and Properties*

The overwhelming majority of polyenes is produced by *Streptomyces* species. *Chainia,* another genus of the family *Streptomycetaceae,* and the genera *Actinoplanes, Streptoverticillium,* and *Actinosporangium* of the family *Actinoplanaceae* have species which are also capable of polyene production. It is postulated that polyenes are components of the sheath of the aerial mycelium. The mold *Epicoccum nigrum* has been shown to contain a red photosensitive antifungal pigment with a typical polyene mode of action. The compound—which has been named epirodin—appears to be a polyhydroxylated carbonyl-conjugated octaene, though its macrolide nature has still to be established (Ikawa *et al.,* 1978).

Chemically the polyenes possess a very large lactone ring [44 atoms in the pentaene lienomycin (CXX; Pawlak *et al.,* 1979)] consisting of a rigid lipophilic chain of from three to seven conjugated double bonds, and a flexible hydrophilic region bearing a number of hydroxyl groups. The length of the chromophore gives rise to the characteristic UV spectrum, enabling ready recognition and classification into subgroups. The instability of some polyenes to heat, light, and pH can also be attributed to this part of the molecule. Most polyenes contain a sugar unit, the majority having the aminosugar mycosamine (3-amino-3,6-dideoxy-D-mannose) linked by a glycosidic bond to the carbon atom α to the chromophore. The aminosugar perosamine (4-amino-4,6-dideoxy-D-mannose) from perimycin, and the sugar L-digitoxose (2,6-dideoxy-L-ribohexopyranose) from nystatin A_3 and others, have also been reported (Martín and Gil, 1979; Zieliński *et al.,* 1979). α-L-Rhamnopyranose is present in lienomycin at a site nonadjacent to the conjugated system (Pawlak *et al.,* 1979). However this polyene from *Actinomyces diastatochromogenes* var. *lienomycini* is atypical structurally in several ways, and exhibits antibacterial and antitumor properties in addition to antifungal activity. Working with the candihexin-complex producer *Streptomyces viridoflavus* IMRU 3961, Martín and Gil (1979) have suggested that the sugar unit (mycosamine) is added to the molecule during passage through the cell membrane. One further feature worthy of mention is the occurrence in some heptaenes of a side chain terminating in a *p*-amino- or *p*-*N*-methylaminobenzoyl group.

2. *Mode of Action, Toxicity, and Derivatives*

It is now well established that polyenes owe their antifungal properties to interaction with membrane sterols, resulting in cells being rendered selectively permeable to small vital constituents, especially potassium ions. Exogenous sterol antagonizes this effect. The presence of appropriate sterols in the cell membrane is therefore a necessary requirement for susceptibility to polyenes. Thus bacteria (including bacterial protoplasts) are insensitive, whereas mammalian red blood cells are lysed, a fact which is at the root of the problem of polyene toxicity. Kotler-Brajtburg *et al.* (1979) have divided the polyenes into two groups, those provoking potassium leakage/cell death in *Saccharomyces cerevisiae* and hemolysis in mouse erythrocytes at comparable concentrations, and a second group in which hemolysis occurs at much higher concentrations than yeast potassium leakage. With the exception of the topically active pimaricin (natamycin), the useful polyenes are all of the second type and are all heptaenes: amphotericin B, candicidin, aureofungins A and B, hamycins A and B, nystatin (a pseudo-heptaene), and certain of their methyl esters and *N*-acetyl derivatives. Amphotericin B, candicidin, and nystatin are also reputed to have immunoadjuvant properties. Rapamycin (CXXI), a triene, has been shown to be an immunosuppressant (Martel *et al.,* 1977).

The affinities of polyenes for various sterols and the nature of this interaction have received much attention. Patterson *et al.* (1979) have shown that filipin (CXXII) has a higher affinity for cholesterol (or stigmas-

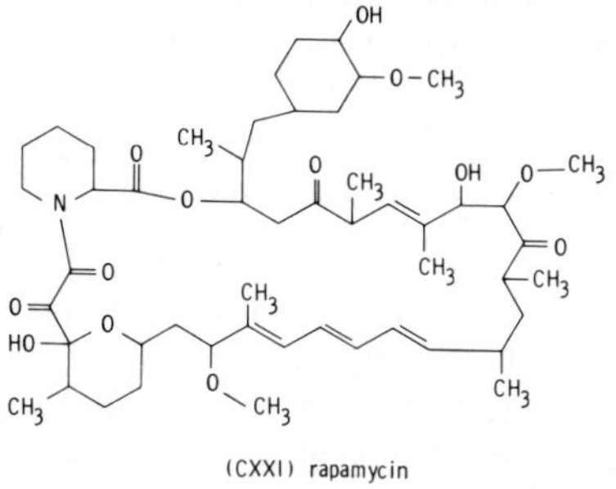

(CXXI) rapamycin

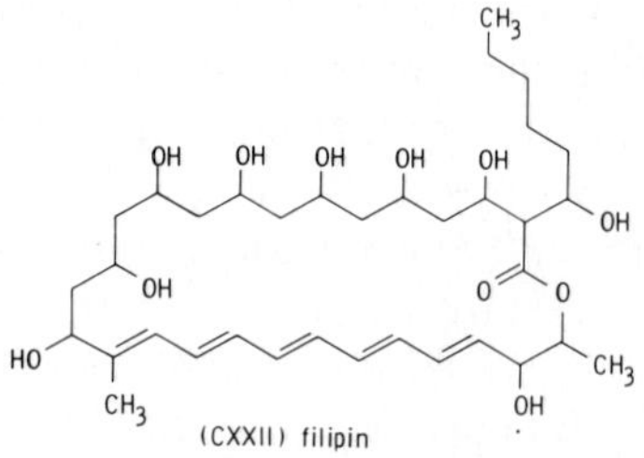

(CXXII) filipin

terol) than does amphotericin B, pimaricin, or nystatin, whereas it has less affinity for ergosterol. Filipin is particularly toxic to mammalian cells, the membranes of which contain cholesterol, and the resulting complex has been used to demonstrate the inhomogeneous distribution of cholesterol in the membrane (Montesano, 1979). Ergosterol is the predominant fungal sterol, and it is the interaction of heptaenes with this sterol which results in the formation of lethal membrane "pores."

In a search for more favorable therapeutic ratios and for compounds which lend themselves to more stable or more suitable formulation, a variety of water-soluble derivatives has been made. *N*-Acetylheptaenes exhibit less than a fifth of the activity of the parent amines. Similarly amide derivatives are reported to be both less toxic and less potent (Falkowski *et al.*, 1980). In contrast, the methyl ester hydrochloride salts of heptaenes retain full activity, but are much less toxic (Hammond, 1977). Some indications of reduced nephrotoxicity have been observed for amphotericin B methyl ester in a limited number of patients (Medoff and Kobayashi, 1980a). A significant advance may have been achieved with the highly water-soluble acid salt of D-ornithyl amphotericin B methyl ester (Wright *et al.*, 1980; Loebenberg *et al.*, 1980); this derivative in mice has an 8-fold larger therapeutic ratio than amphotericin B itself and a 5-fold better ratio than amphotericin B methyl ester. Another favorable example is methyl partricin, which is four times more potent against *C. albicans* and 400 times less toxic ip to mice than partricin. It also renders *C. guilliermondii* more susceptible to human polymorphonuclear leukocytes *in vitro* (Sacchi *et al.*, 1979). Recently patents have appeared disclosing the preparation of *N,N,N*-trimethyl derivatives of amphoteric polyenes (Vainshtein, V. A. *et al.*: DT. 2706156, 1977/1978). These zwitterions are 7–10 times less toxic than the parent compounds. Falkowski *et al.* (1979) have found that if this reaction is continued, the carboxylic acid group becomes methylated, and where an aromatic amine is also present, the mono- and dimethyl-derivatives are formed. Compounds such as the methosulfate salt of *N,N,N*-trimethylamphotericin B methyl ester are readily soluble in water, are equipotent with the parent antibiotic, and are several times less toxic. Another approach has been to prepare sugar derivatives of polyenes containing a free amino group. *N*-Glycosylamphotericin B is unchanged in potency and forms water-soluble salts. Furthermore, Plociennik *et al.* (1978) have shown that the *N*-methylglucamine salt of *N*-glycosylpolifungin could be stored for 2 years at 4°C without loss of biological activity. In contrast a series of polyenes was shown to be more effective as inhibitors of *C. guilliermondii* intact cells or protoplasts than the corresponding perhydro derivatives (Haupt *et al.*, 1979). Finally, a strain of *Streptomyces chartreusis* IMRU 3962 produces chartreusin and a nonaromatic mycosamine-containing heptaene, hydroheptin, unique in being water-soluble at pH 7. Its activity against yeasts and other fungi is comparable to that of *N*-acylated heptaenes, and its parenteral toxicity is less than that of the parent compounds (Tunac *et al.*, 1979).

3. *Resistance*

Polyene resistance can be produced in the laboratory, particularly with the help of UV light or mutagenic agents (Medoff and Kobayashi, 1980b). In some cases it is associated with a decreased level of membrane ergosterol, although in other instances an *increased* content of total ergosterol has been noted; at all events one of the major changes would seem to concern sterol metabolism. Resistant strains grow more slowly than parent strains, and are less pathogenic in mice; cross resistance among the polyenes is observed. Fortunately genotypic resistance has been rarely observed in the clinical situation, presumably due to the characteristics of resistant strains which mitigate against survival in a competitive situation.

Phenotypic resistance however is readily observed, and may have clinical significance; Gale and associates have conducted a long series of studies on this phenomenon (e.g., Cassone *et al.*, 1979). *C. albicans* during exponential growth is highly sensitive to amphotericin B methyl ester as measured by its ability to provoke K^+ leakage from cells. Cessation of growth however is marked by a pronounced change in antibiotic sensitivity, which in late stationary phase may be 100-fold less. This change in sensitivity is associated with modifications of the wall, since isolated protoplasts prepared from resistant organisms display a normal sensitivity. The change initially involves a loss of the layered appearance seen in sensitive cells at the electron microscope level, and eventually is associated in a marked increase in wall thickness due to glucan deposition. Normal sensitivity returns as growth restarts following subculture into fresh medium. These observations suggest that in the clinical situation, actively growing organisms should be eliminated during polyene treatment, but quiescent organisms—such as may be associated with plaques in lesions—will not be affected, and will be a potential source of relapse infection following cessation of treatment.

4. *Recent Polyenes*

There is some contention in the literature concerning the classification of trienes as true polyene antibiotics. Certainly rapamycin (CXXI; Swindells *et al.*, 1978), isolated from an Easter Island strain of *Streptomyces hygroscopicus* NRRL 5491, does not affect cell permeability nor is its potent candicidal action reversed by sterols (MIC versus *C. albicans* 0.02 μg/ml). It is rather an inhibitor of nucleic acid synthesis (Singh *et al.*, 1979). Although devoid of antibacterial properties it has shown sufficient antitumor activity to be of interest to the National Cancer Institute as a potential anticancer agent, and it will shortly undergo clinical trials. Rapamycin is effective orally against systemic candidosis in mice (PD_{50} 11 mg/kg) and against vaginal infection in rats (91% cure rate), while showing low acute toxicity by a number of routes (Baker *et al.*, 1978). However amphotericin B is orally absorbed in mice, but not in man. It is encouraging therefore that rapamycin is also absorbed orally in the dog. It is worth mentioning that in the solid state at least, the triene chromophore of the 32-membered ring of rapamycin is significantly nonplanar (Swindells *et al.*, 1978), resulting in a reduction in intensity of absorption in the UV spectrum and possibly influencing the biological properties.

In addition to lienomycin and rapamycin, the structures of several other polyenes have recently been published. Falkowski *et al.* (1978) used the *N*-acetyldimethoxime methyl ester of the tetraene rimocidin (from *Streptomyces rimosus*) as a key derivative. Tetramycin, produced by a strain of *Streptomyces noursei*, is related structurally to pimaricin (26-membered macrolide ring; Dornberger *et al.*, 1979). A close relative of amphotericin B, mycoheptin, is a metabolite of *Actinomyces netropsis* for which Borowski *et al.* (1978) have proposed a complete structure. Chakrabarti and Chandra (1979) have described antibiotic A-7 from *Streptomyces aureus*. Three species of *Streptoverticillium* have furnished the pentaenes mycopenten-1, mycopenten-2, and kokandomycin, and the heptaene O-185 I (Severinets *et al.*, 1977; Konev *et al.*, 1977, 1978); kokandomycin is antibacterial as well as antifungal. Kulalaeva *et al.* (1978) have found two new members of the carbonyl-conjugated pentaene group: flavopentin and brunefungin. A method has been developed to enable the aromatic heptaenes to be readily characterized using HPLC (Mechlinski and Schaffner, 1980).

5. *Synergy/Potentiation*

It is an attractive approach to reduce the dosage of polyenes by seeking synergists or potentiators. In the treatment of disseminated infection with dimorphic fungi for example, combination therapy with 5-FC is now common. The rifamycins, which are inhibitors of nucleic acid polymerases, have also been reported to behave synergistically with amphotericin B (Hammond, 1977). Recently Lew *et al.* (1978) have shown that the lipid-soluble minocycline is the best of several tetracyclines in combination with amphotericin B against strains of several species of *Candida, T. glabrata,* and *C. neoformans in vitro.*

Similarly potentiators have been found in nature. Two basic metabolites of unknown structure, enactin (H-646-SY3) from *Streptomyces roseoviridis* (Otani *et al.*, 1977) and neo-enactin (H-829-MY10) from *Streptoverticillium olivoreticuli* subsp. *neoenacticus* (Kondo *et al.*, 1979; Banyu: Japan Kokai 79117401, 1978), have been isolated using a test system capable of distinguishing between polyenes, nonpolyenes, synergists for polyenes, and antagonists of cholesterol. Enactin is weakly active against *Candida* (25–50 μg/ml) and neo-enactin is some 100 times more active. They are of particular interest however, because they potentiate the antifungal properties of the polyenes, trichomycin in the former case and an unidentified tetraene cometabolite in the latter. Neo-enactin is relatively nontoxic and furnishes L-serine on acid hydrolysis; further details of structure and mode of potentiation are awaited with interest. It is worth mentioning that the most important group of synthetic antifungals, the imidazoles, act antagonistically to the polyenes. They are believed to work by inhibition of the 14-demethylase enzyme in steroid biosynthesis, presumably lowering the ergosterol content of the cell membrane and hence reducing the effectiveness of the polyenes.

6. *Nonpolyene Membrane Active Agents*

Several other families of antibiotics which affect the cytoplasmic membrane have been the subject of a useful review (Lambert, 1978). Some such as the cyclic peptides tyrocidins and polymixins have a cationic detergent-like effect; others, for example the ionophores, inhibit processes involving electron transport or oxidative phosphorylation. Frequently the antifungal properties described for such compounds are part of a much wider, poorly selective biological profile with little real practical potential. This is the case for the quinone methides citrinin and ascochitine which cause leakage of cell contents and are active against a range of bacteria, fungi, yeasts, and plants (Gottlieb and Shaw, 1970). Antifungal compounds with this mode of action will be discussed in the section relevant to the structural type (e.g., the nonactins, the polyethers, and echinocandins).

B. Other Macrolides

1. *"Small" Ring Macrolides*

The smaller ring lactone antibiotics are generally antibacterial rather than antifungal and are typified by erythromycin. Brefeldin A (CXXIII), for which Bartlett and Green (1978) have published a further total synthesis, is nonspecific, being active against fungi, viruses, and tumors. By contrast oligomycins A, B, and C, rutamycin, ossamycin, and venturicidins A, B, and X are principally antifungals, with some toxicity to animal cells. They act by inhibiting in a related manner the mitochondrial energy transfer system. The venturicidins are active against fungi—including plant pathogens such as *Venturia inequalis* (apple scab)—venturicidin X (the aglycone of CXXIV) being three times as potent as the 2-deoxy-D-rhamnosyl glycosides A and B (CXXIVa and b; Brufani *et al.*, 1972). Venturicidin A has recently been isolated as a cometabolite of polyether Ro 21-6150 from *Streptomyces hygroscopicus* X-14563 (Liu *et al.*, 1976).

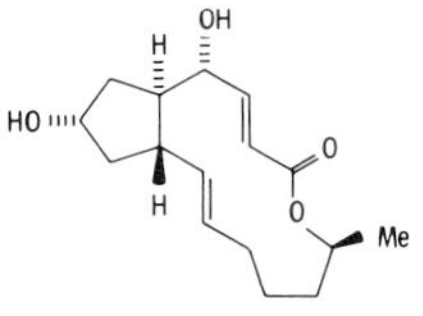

(CXXIII) brefeldin A

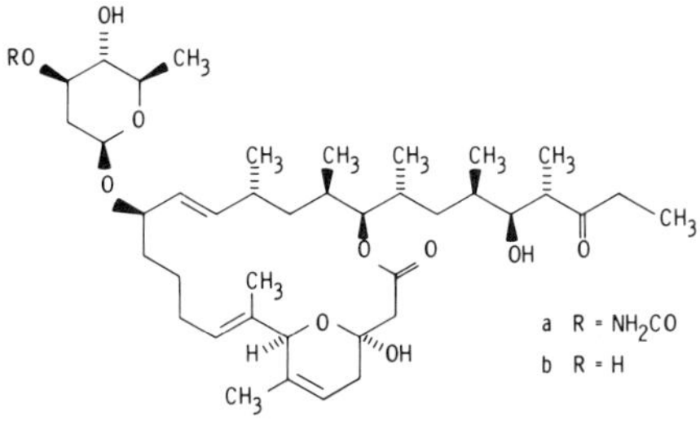

a R = NH_2CO
b R = H

(CXXIV) venturicidin

A species of *Aspergillus* has furnished two polyhydroxylated macrolides, niphimycins A_1 and A_2 (Blinov *et al.*, 1974), and the related memomycin (L1A-0775) containing no amino acids or sugars has been obtained from *Actinomyces memokrassinus* (Shenin *et al.*, 1978). They show activity against gram-positive bacteria, yeasts, and other fungi, but the structures and modes of action have not as yet been determined. The niphimycins appear to be 18-ring macrolides of molecular weight around 1200.

2. *Large Ring, Nonpolyene Macrolides*

Although most of the membrane-active large ring macrolides are polyenes, there are a few exceptions. Primycin was originally isolated from *Streptomyces primycini* from the intestinal tract of the wax moth *Galeria melonella* and later from *Micromonospora galeriensis*. The "saturated polyene-like" structure CXXV has been deduced for it in which a D-arabinose unit and two side chains, one ending in a guanidinium sulfate group, are attached to a 36-membered ring (Aberhart *et al.*, 1970). Some analogy with the polyene lienomycin (CXX) can be drawn, and both compounds act as ionophores rendering the inner membrane of energized mitochondria permeable to K^+, Na^+, and $Tris^+$. At higher concentrations primycin causes additional H^+ and Cl^- permeability changes, possibly via Mg^{2+} depletion of the inner membrane (Mészáros *et al.*, 1979, 1980). It is toxic to mammals. In addition to its activity against gram-positive bacteria and viruses, antifungal properties of primycin have only recently been recognized. Using crystalline material, Uri and Actor (1979) have deter-

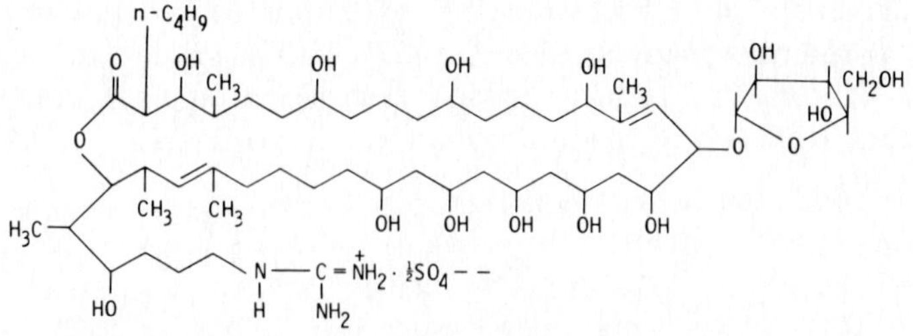

(CXXV) primycin

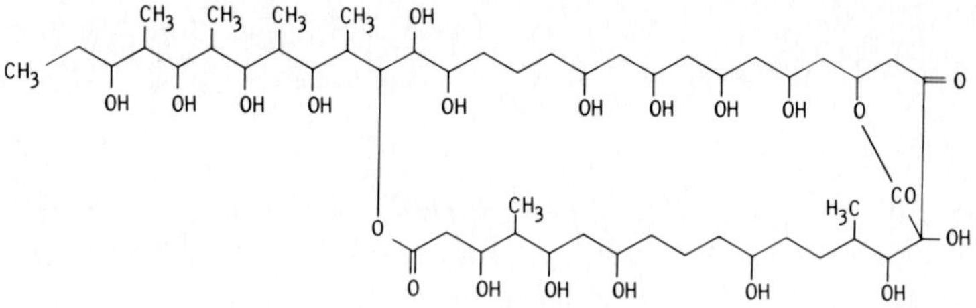

(CXXVI) axenolide

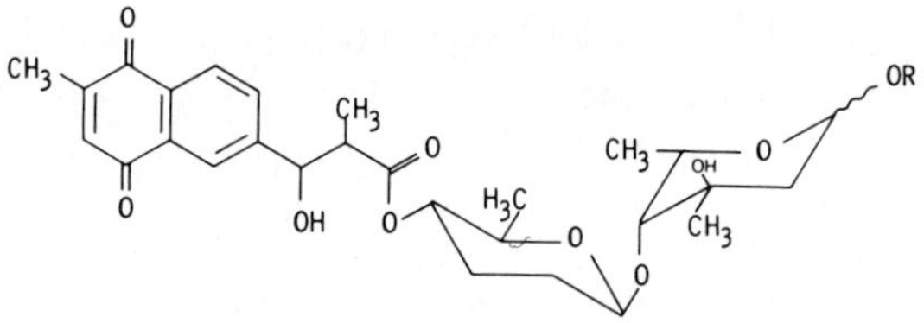

(CXXVII)

mined MICs in peptone-glucose broth buffered at pH 7.4 against species of *Candida* (2–10 μg/ml) and against *T. mentagrophytes* (1 μg/ml).

Of the "saturated polyene" axenomycins A, B, and D produced by *Streptomyces lysandri* (Bianchi *et al.*, 1974), axenomycin B is the most potent against yeasts. It appears to have a polyene-like mode of action although it does not have the usual olefinic chromophore. The 34-membered ring aglycone axenolide (CXXVI) and the 2-methylnaphthoquinone disaccharide derivatives CXXVII can be obtained from axenomycin B by methanolysis (Arcamone *et al.*, 1972). The amphoteric antibiotic desertomycin from *Streptomyces flavofungini* contains D-fructose, is membrane-active, antibacterial, antifungal, and cytotoxic, and may also be of this saturated polyene type (Betina *et al.*, 1969). From the foregoing it is clear that division of the macrolides according to the size of the lactone ring is very artificial and does not necessarily reflect biological properties.

3. *"Ansa" Macrolides*

This class of antibiotic is characterized by a large lactam ring bridging two nonadjacent positions of a benzenoid or naphthalenoid system. Rinehart and Shield (1976) have reviewed the chemistry of the various subgroups. Biological activities range from mainly antibacterial to antitumor together with antifungal and other properties in many cases. However the compounds are often too toxic to be of any real interest in the management of fungal infections. Modes of action involve inhibition of DNA-dependent RNA polymerase and of reverse transcriptases. By way of example from the recent literature, *Streptomyces spectabilis* is reported to produce damavaricin D (CXXVIII) which has both gram-positive and gram-negative antibacterial, and antifungal properties (Rinehart *et al.*, 1976; Deshmukh *et al.*, 1976). It is a member of the streptovaricin family of 2,5-bridged 1,4-naphthoquinones and occurs at an early stage of the biosynthetic sequence to streptovaricin A.

Herbimycins A (CXXIX) and B contain a benzoquinone nucleus and are related to geldanamycin; they were isolated by Omura *et al.* (1979a,b, 1980a; Furusaki *et al.*, 1980) from *Streptomyces hygroscopicus* AM-3672.

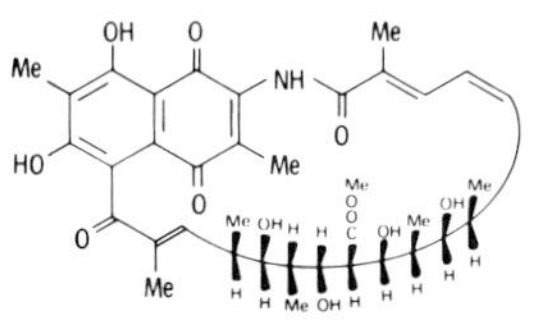

(CXXVIII) damavaricin D 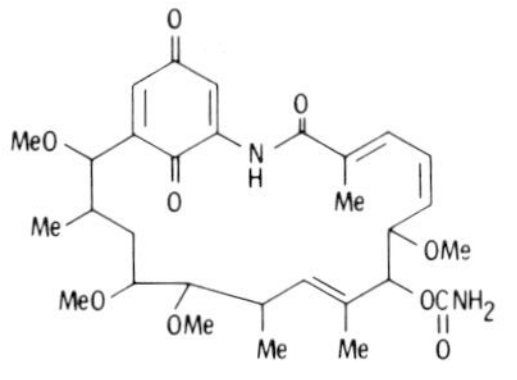 (CXXIX) herbimycin 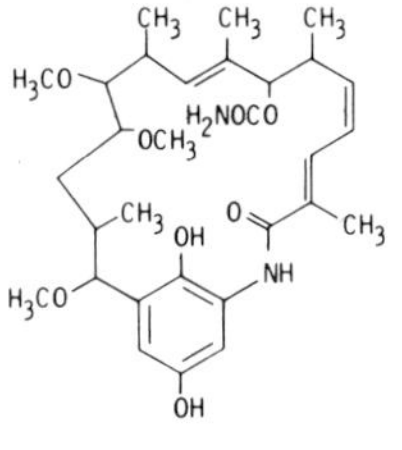 (CXXX) macbecin II

As their name implies they are herbicidal—to mono- and dicotyledonous plants—but they also possess weak activity against yeasts and other fungi and protozoa.

Nocardia sp. C-14919 has furnished macbecin I and macbecin II (CXXX; Muroi *et al.*, 1980a,b). The former is another example of a benzoquinone, whereas macbecin II is the first reported hydroquinone ansamycin isolated from a broth. Biological activity includes *in vitro* activity against gram-positive bacteria, fungi, and protozoa and *in vivo* inhibition of murine leukemia P388 with relatively low toxicity (Tanida *et al.*, 1980b).

The ansamycins are generally yellow to orange. The only exceptions are macbecin II and the potent antitumor maytansinoids, which are colorless. The discovery of minute amounts of maytansine and homologous amido-esters (CXXXIa–d) from species of the plant families *Maytenus* and *Putterlickia* (*Celestraceae*) and the recognition of their possible clinical potential prompted a flurry of effort toward their chemical synthesis. Another plant *Colubrina texensis* (*Rhamnaceae*) furnished the related colubrinol (CXXXIe) and its acetate (CXXXIf). However a most significant advance was the report of the discovery of ansamitocins P1, 2, 3, 3′, and 4

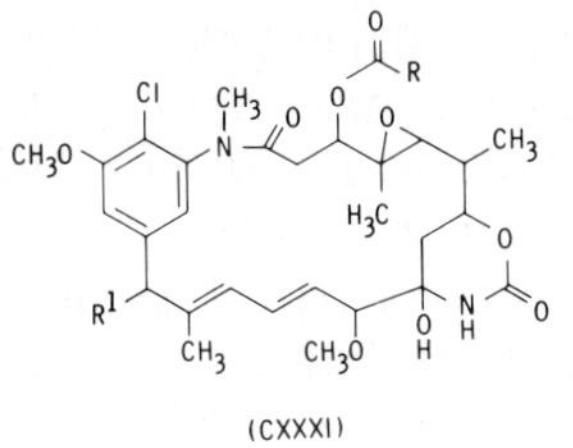

(CXXXI)

	R	R^1		R	R^1
a	$CHMeNMe\underset{\overset{\|}{O}}{C}Me$	H	g	Me	H
b	$CHMeNMe\underset{\overset{\|}{O}}{C}CHMe_2$	H	h	Et	H
c	$CHMeNMe\underset{\overset{\|}{O}}{C}Et$	H	i	$CHMe_2$	H
d	$CHMeNMe\underset{\overset{\|}{O}}{C}CH_2CHMe_2$	H	j	CH_2CH_2Me	H
e	$CHMeNMe\underset{\overset{\|}{O}}{C}CHMe_2$	OH	k	CH_2CHMe_2	H
f	$CHMeNMe\underset{\overset{\|}{O}}{C}CHMe_2$	OAc			

(CXXXIg–k) in *Actinomyces* C-15003(N-1), several of which had previously been found in plants (Higashide *et al.,* 1977; Tanida *et al.,* 1980a; Takeda: DT. 2849696, 1977/1979 and JAP. 77139384, 1977). This not only raised the question of their origin as possible metabolites of microorganisms on the plant, but also furnished sufficient material to permit semisynthetic work around these important compounds (Takeda: U.S. 4137230, 1977/1979). In this way it is hoped that an improvement in their therapeutic ratio will allow not only their use in human cancer treatment, but also the exploitation of their antifungal properties.

4. *Nonactins*

Very common among metabolites from streptomyces are the nonactins: nonactin, monactin, dinactin (CXXXII), trinactin, peliomycin, etc. These homologous macrotetralides are neutral ionophores which alter membrane permeability (microbial or mammalian) toward small inorganic ions

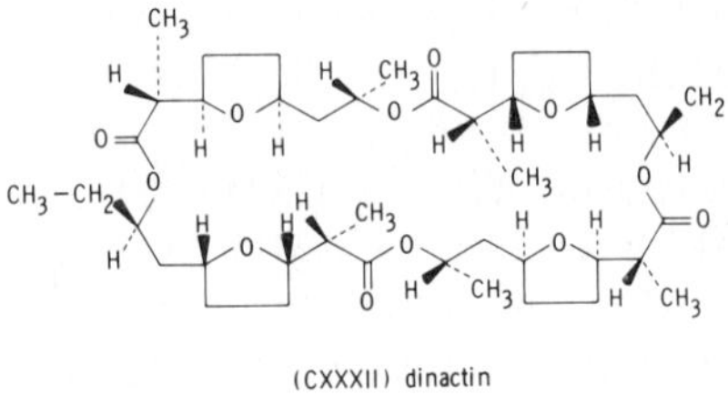

(CXXXII) dinactin

such as K^+. They form lipid-soluble complexes, probably akin to those formed by the cyclic depsipeptides valinomycin and enniatin B, in which the hydrophilic groups of the molecule are oriented toward the interior of the macrolide by coordination to the cation. The monomeric hydroxylated tetrahydrofuranylpropionic acids can also be found in the broths, and both (+) and (−) forms go to make up the tetramer. Nonactin contains two molecules of each antipode of nonactinic acid, whereas dinactin has the (+)-isomers replaced by (+)-homononactinic acid (Keller-Schierlein and Gerlach, 1968). Apart from their moderate candidicidal and antidermatophyte properties, there is some evidence that the nonactins permit antimicrobial activity in small toxic molecules which do not normally enter the cells.

C. Polyethers

The polyethers are ionophorous antibiotics produced by *Streptomyces*. Typically they are linear long-chain monocarboxylic acids, consisting of pyran or furan rings bearing alkyl and oxygen functional groups. In a metal salt, a hydroxyl group near the end of the chain forms a hydrogen bond to the carboxylate moiety, with other oxygen atoms acting as ligands to the cation. This results in the cation being encircled by the polyether, the exposed alkyl groups rendering the salt very lipophilic. The polyethers have potent gram-positive antibacterial activity and are antiprotozoal. Some have found use in the animal health area as growth promoters and anticoccidials, in particular monensin and lasalocid. This is possible because, although the polyethers are very toxic when given parenterally, they are not absorbed orally. Activity against yeasts and other fungi is reported or claimed for many of the polyethers: antibiotics 38986, A-6016, A-28695B, alborixin, carriomycin, etheromycin, grisorixin, lasalocid, lonomycins A, B, and C, mutalomycin, narasin, and nigericin. In the case of antibiotic 5057 and leuseramycin, activity is limited to phytopathogenic fungi. It is unlikely however that these observations will lead to therapeutic application in human medicine, although derivatives such as bromolasalocid and bromoisolasalocid are claimed to have useful antihypertensive effects when administered orally to warm-blooded animals (Roche: U.S. 4161520, 1976/1979).

D. Long-Chain Unsaturated Carboxylic Acids and Related Compounds

There are many antifungal natural products which bear some resemblance to the olefinic part of the polyenes, though lacking to a greater or lesser extent their amphophilic character, and which may thus act by different mechanisms. Furthermore it is by no means uncommon for antifungal antibiotics to occur as the esters of long-chain unsaturated carboxylic acids: the nucleosides (MM19290 and tunicamycin), the C-glycosides (papulacandins) and the peptides [antibiotics 20561/2 (W10 complex), bacillomycin-L, griseoviridin, iturin A, lipopeptin A, MSD-A43F, mycosubtilin, pantomycin, and stendomycin]. Some of these examples will be discussed in other sections.

1. *Cerulenin, Conocandin, Variotin, and Wyerone*

The antimicrobial activity of undec-10-enoic acid and the use of its zinc salt as a topical treatment for dermatophyte infections such as athlete's foot are well known. Of the examples which follow, pecilocin (Variotin) is also active against dermatophytes, whereas cerulenin and conocandin are effective against *Candida*.

Cephalosporium caerulens produces an antibacterial and antifungal C_{12}-acid derivative (+)-cerulenin which is particularly active against *Candida* (Matsumae *et al.,* 1972), as is tetrahydrocerulenin. The structure originally proposed was revised to CXXXIII by Arison and Omura (1974). In protic solvents however, the 4-keto-2,3-epoxy amide undergoes a tautomerism favoring the cyclic lactam form CXXXIV. Three syntheses of racemic cerulenin have appeared (Boeckman and Thomas, 1977; Jakubowski *et al.,* 1977; Corey and Williams, 1977). More recently both (+) and (−) tetrahydrocerulenin have been synthesized from D-glucose—confirming the absolute stereochemistry of CXXXIII (Ohrui

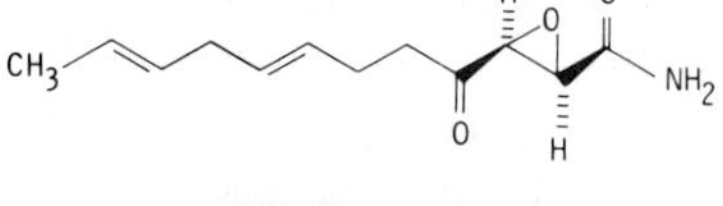

(CXXXIII) cerulenin

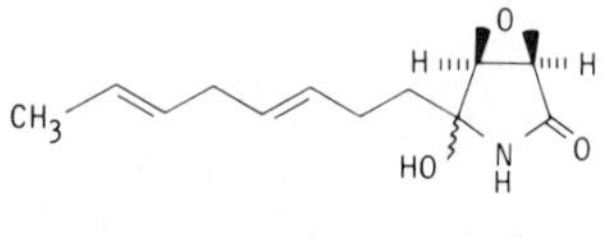

(CXXXIV)

and Emoto, 1978)—D-xylose (Pougny and Sinaÿ, 1978), and from optically active butenolides (Vigneron and Blanchard, 1980). D-Glucose has also served as a chiral template for the total synthesis of the natural parent antibiotic (Sueda *et al.,* 1979; Pietraszkiewicz and Sinaÿ, 1979). The number of research groups involved in these synthetic efforts is a reflection of the interest in the biological properties of this compound, which outweighs the moderate structural challenge. (+)-Cerulenin has been shown to interfere with lipid biosynthesis in *Escherichia coli* by binding irreversibly—possibly via opening of the epoxide by an active site amino acid group?—to the β-ketoacyl-acyl carrier protein synthetase concerned in chain-lengthening in fatty acid biosynthesis. It therefore specifically inhibits fatty acid and polyketide synthesis and promises to be a useful biochemical tool with potential medical application in obesity or mycoses (Kitao *et al.,* 1979). Screening for antagonists of lipids has recently detected the macrolide oligomycin A, a known inhibitor of energy metabolism, in *Streptomyces* sp. No. 178 (Nakakita *et al.,* 1980).

Conocandin (CXXXV) is a longer chain α-methylenic β,γ-epoxy acid which powerfully inhibits the growth of *C. albicans* (MIC 0.1 μg/ml). It is an oil, and was isolated as antibiotic A32,287 from *Hormococcus conorum* by the Ciba-Geigy group (Muller *et al.,* 1976). It has a fungistatic action, and is equipotent to but shows no cross-resistance with another Ciba-Geigy anti-*Candida* agent papulacandin B. The latter compound has two esterified unsaturated acid chains and is an inhibitor of cell wall glucan synthetase. Although conocandin shows only medium cytotoxicity, and is nontoxic in mice when given subcutaneously at 300 mg/kg, it is unfortunately inactive *in vivo.*

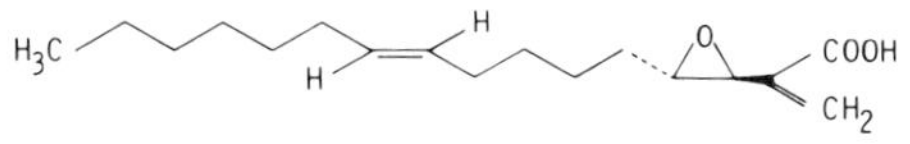

H_3C H H O COOH CH_2

(CXXXV) conocandin

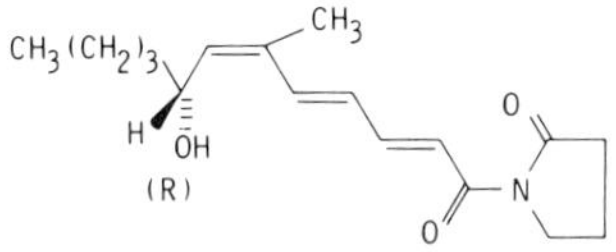

$CH_3(CH_2)_3$ CH_3 H OH (R) O N O

(CXXXVI) pecilocin

Another amidic fungal metabolite is pecilocin (CXXXVI) obtained from *Paecilomyces variotus* var. *antibioticus* as a fragrant oil which can be crystallized as a monohydrate (Takeuchi *et al.,* 1964). It is relatively unstable and of low toxicity and shows good *in vitro* control of *Trichophyton, Cryptococcus,* and some phytopathogens, but not of bacteria or yeasts; its activity is greatly reduced in the presence of serum. This has not prevented investigation of its topical utility (as Variotin) in patients with dermatophyte infections, where some success has been achieved.

Three related phytoalexins, wyeronic acid, wyerone, and wyerone 11,12-epoxide (CXXXVIIa, b, and c) are produced by the broad bean *Vicia faba* when infected with *Botrytis* species (Hargreaves *et al.,* 1976). These C_{14}-unsaturated acid derivatives are more fungitoxic to *B. cinerea* than to *B. fabae.* That the latter is the more efficient detoxifier is certainly a contributing factor to this observation, and is of relevance concerning the relative pathogenicity of these species. Whether wyerone and the other furanoylacetylenes offer any scope for the treatment of human

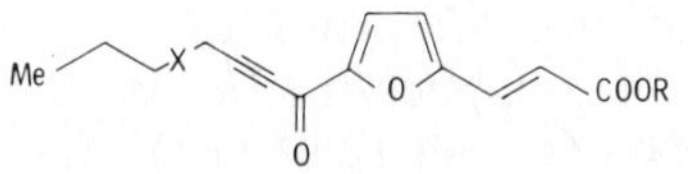

a R = H ; X = $\Delta^{11,12}$–
b R = Me ; X = $\Delta^{11,12}$–
c R = Me ; X = 11, 12–epoxide

(CXXXVII) wyerone (b)

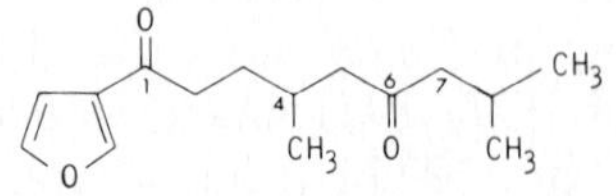

(CXXXVIII) myoporone

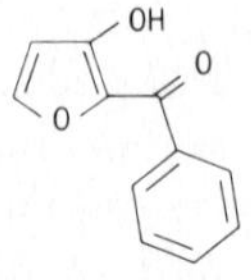

(CXXXIX) adustin

pathogens will be better appreciated in the light of discussion of other phytoalexins (Section IV,G) and of polyacetylenes (Section IV,F). It is worth noting here in passing two other furanoyl compounds: the phytoalexin furanosesquiterpenes, for example myoporone (CXXXVIII) from the sweet potato *Ipomoea batatas* (*Convolvulaceae;* Burka and Iles, 1979), and 2-benzoyl-3-hydroxyfuran, isolated by Chinese workers from *Steccherinum adustur* (*Basidiomycetes*) and named adustin (CXXXIX; Fang *et al.,* 1979). A patent (Deutsche Gold und Silber: BE. 869140, 1977/1979) has appeared claiming fungicidal activity for a series of synthetic fatty α-ketocarboxamides, which are also intermediates for preparing α-amino acids.

2. *Arylalkenes*

The *alkyl* trienoic acid carboxamide pecilocin has useful topical activity against dermatophyte infections. Several fungal metabolites with an *aryl*-triene structure have also been described, for one of which, mucidin, similar claims have been made. Crystalline dextrorotatory mucidin, $C_{16}H_{18}O_3$, can be extracted from submerged cultures of *Oudemansiella mucida* (Vondráček *et al.*; Czech 136495, 1967/1970). It is active against fungi but not bacteria, and is relatively nontoxic. Mucidin is a specific inhibitor of ubiquinol–cytochrome c reductase and therefore of respiration. From its physical characteristics it would appear to be different from the oily achiral strobilurin A, $C_{16}H_{18}O_3$ (CXL: $R_1 = H = R_2$; Anke *et al.,* 1977; Schramm *et al.,* 1978) which has been obtained together with strobilurin B (CXL: R_1 = OMe, R_2 = Cl) from *Strobilurius tenecellus,* and from other sources—*Cyphellopsis* species, *Mycena zephira,* and *M. fagetorum.* The Czechoslovak group (M. Nadrchalova and J. Capkova: Czech 172754, 1974/1978) have also claimed methods of detection of CXL ($R_1 = H = R_2$). Anke *et al.* (1979) have described another crystalline

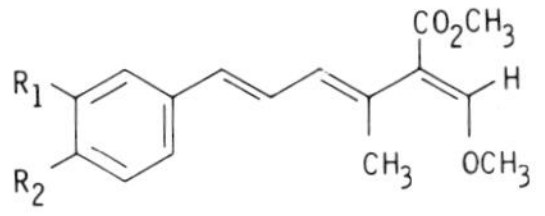

(CXL) strobilurin

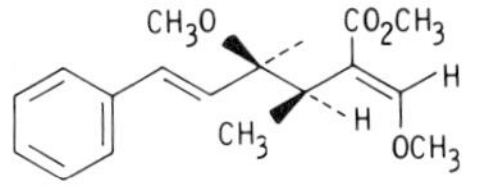

(CXLI) oudemansin

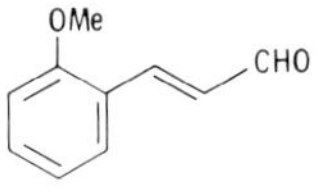

(CXLII)

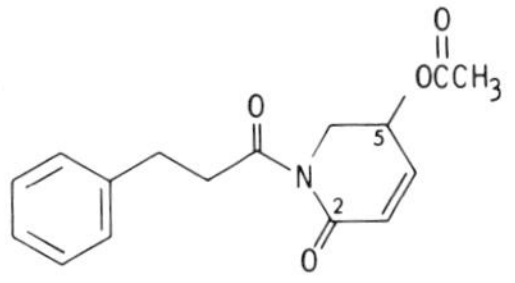

(CXLIII) pipermethystine

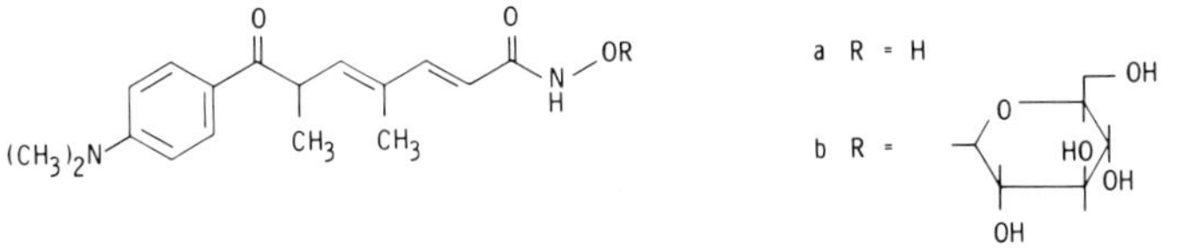

a R = H

b R =

(CXLIV) trichostatin

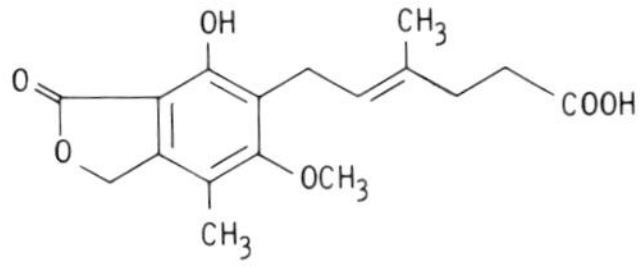

(CXLV) mycophenolic acid

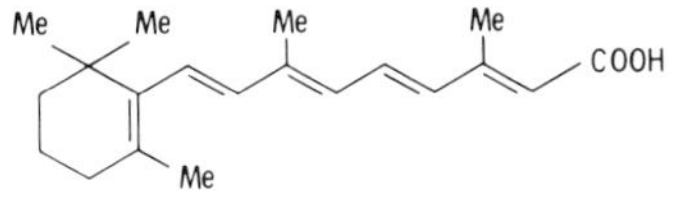

(CXLVI) retinoic acid

metabolite of *O. mucida,* the laevorotatory oudemansin, for which X-ray studies have established the relative configuration shown in CXLI. It has analogous properties to the other members of this series and the inhibition of respiration can be reversed by added glucose. Presumably the biological effects arise from a depletion of the intracellular ATP pool. All these compounds possess a β-methoxymethacrylate moiety, and it is possible to speculate that nucleophilic displacement of the methoxy group may be involved. A generally applicable 5-step synthesis of strobilurin A from cinnamaldehyde has been achieved (Schramm and Steglich, 1980), and has established the importance of the geometry of the β-methoxymethacrylate group. The penultimate product of the synthesis differs only in this respect from strobilurin A, and is inactive.

Three other types of aromatic natural products deserve mention in this section since they bear a distant relationship to the above. *o-*

Methoxycinnamaldehyde (CXLII) has been isolated from cinnamon powder and has MICs of 3.12–6.25 μg/ml against dermatophytes (Morozumi, 1978). Two *N*-cinnamoylpyrrolidines and the related 5,6-dihydropyridone, piperlongumine (piplartine) have been reported from species of *Piperaceae*. Smith (1979) isolated pipermethystine (CXLIII) from the leaves of the tropical shrub *Piper methysticum*. This is widely cultivated in the South Pacific for its roots and stems which are used in folk medicine and for preparing the drink "kawa." The plant also contains a series of α-pyrones which have antifungal as well as several other pharmacological effects.

The aroyl unsaturated hydroxamic acid trichostatin A and its glucopyranoside trichostatin C (CXLIV) are elaborated by *Streptomyces hygroscopicus* Y-50 (Tsuji and Kobayashi, 1978); activity is again confined to dermatophytes. As would be expected, trichostatin A forms a Fe^{2+} chelate, which has also been isolated under the name trichostatin B.

A great deal of interest has been aroused by the biological properties of mycophenolic acid (CXLV), a metabolite of several *Penicillium* species. The phthalide moiety is derived biosynthetically from acetate and the alkenoic acid from mevalonate by cleavage of a farnesyl side-chain (Doerfler *et al.*, 1980). Mycophenolic acid is cytostatic and has been tested in the clinic against cancer and psoriasis, and it is active against viruses and staphylococci. It exhibits good *in vitro* antifungal effects against *C. albicans* and some other *Candida* species (MICs 6.25–12.5 μg/ml at pH 5.2), *Cryptococcus neoformans* and *Trichophyton* species (6.25 μg/ml), and it is effective against *T. asteroides* in the guinea pig. The activity is fungistatic rather than fungicidal. No blood levels in mice were detectable microbiologically after oral, ip, or im administration, although some excretion in the urine was observed (Noto *et al.*, 1969). Acute toxicity was low, although cytotoxic damage to the intestinal mucosa was observed (Carter *et al.*, 1969). Interest continues in finding derivatives with improved characteristics, and efficient glucosylation for example has now been achieved microbiologically using *Streptomyces aureofaciens* (Abbott *et al.*, 1980). Finally, structural analogy with another series of naturally occurring cell growth inhibitors, retinoic acids (CXLVI), should be pointed out.

3. *Ambruticin and Other C-Glycosides*

W7783, 5,6-dihydroxypolyangioic acid or ambruticin, one of the most interesting antifungal antibiotics to emerge for some time, was discovered by Ringel and colleagues at Warner-Lambert during systematic screening of slime bacteria (*Myxobacteriales;* Ringel *et al.*, 1977; Ringel, 1978). Isolated as an amber gum from *Polyangium cellulosum* var. *fulvum*, it has a

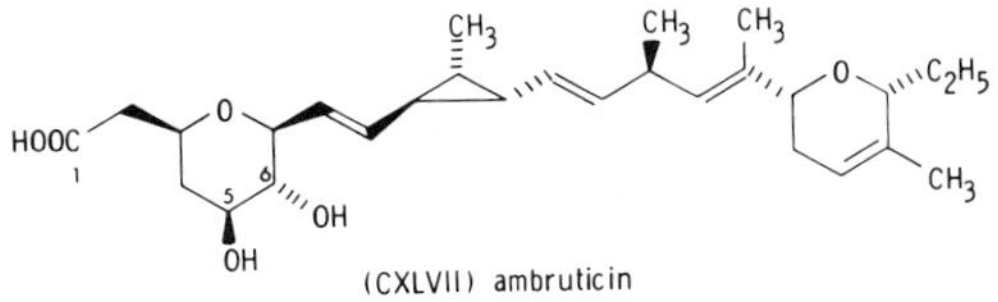

(CXLVII) ambruticin

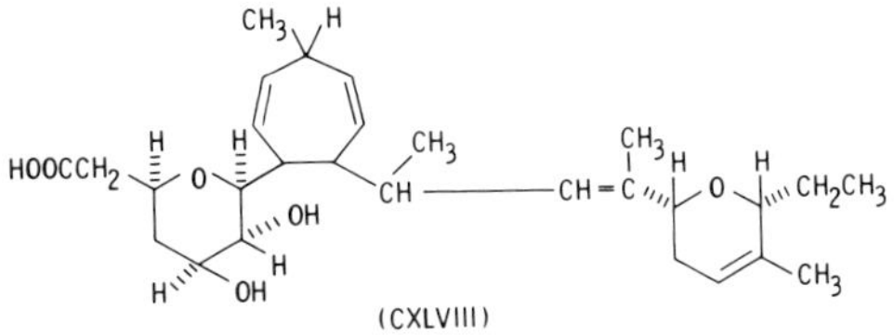

(CXLVIII)

highly unusual structure containing a cyclopropyl and two pyran rings in an unsaturated acid chain; it has since been obtained in our laboratories in the form of white crystals. The relative configuration of ambruticin as determined by X-ray crystallographic studies of the triformate derivative of the corresponding alcohol is shown in CXLVII. Ambruticin is produced together with small amounts of the less polar 5-epimer (Connor and von Strandtmann, 1978). Ambruticin possesses modest antibacterial activity, but is very active *in vitro* against a variety of dermatophytes and more serious fungal pathogens. It is however inactive against most strains of *C. albicans,* although some strains of *C. parapsilosis* are very sensitive. *In vivo,* ambruticin is active by mouth against ringworm in the mouse and guinea pig, but in the latter its activity is only about one-fifth that of griseofulvin (p. 70). It has activity against coccidioidomycosis in the mouse (Levine *et al.,* 1978) and against histoplasmosis in the mouse (Shadomy *et al.,* 1978). Acute toxicity is low—LD_{50} 315 mg/kg iv and >1000 mg/kg orally in the mouse—but the compound is unlikely to be developed due to its lack of activity against *C. albicans,* its poor showing (compared with griseofulvin) against dermatophytes, and low and variable yields in fermentation. Ambruticin is 95% serum-bound and has a half-life of 3.1 hours in the mouse, excretion being principally biliary. With 10 asymmetric centers it represents a formidable synthetic challenge, and has excited the interest of several groups. The synthesis of the C_{1-8} fragment in protected form from L-arabinose and comparison with material obtained from the antibiotic itself has confirmed the absolute configuration shown in CXLVII (Just and Potvin, 1981). A variety of ester, amide, alcohol, ketone, aldehyde, and oxime analogs has been made (Connor and Strandtmann, 1979). No improvement in the spectrum of activity was achieved, although molecules with unhindered polar substituents on carbons 1, 5, and 6 retained comparable antifungal properties. By virtue of its divinylcyclopropane moiety, ambruticin undergoes a thermal Cope rearrangement to the cycloheptadiene (CXLVIII), which is biologically inactive (Connor *et al.*, 1979); the chain length or steric bulk in this region is therefore of some significance. Little is known concerning the biosynthesis and mode of action of ambruticin. Although there is a superficial resemblance to the amphophilic polyenes, it is unlikely that they share a common mechanism. There are some indications that ambruticin inhibits the uptake of leucine and may be an inhibitor of protein synthesis.

Of the few recently discovered antibiotics to rival ambruticin in potential interest, papulacandin B (CILb) probably heads the list (Traxler *et al.*, 1977a). Papulacandins A–E are metabolites of *Papularia sphaerosperma* extracted at pH 8.4–8.6 (Traxler *et al.*, 1977b; Ciba-Geigy: G.B. 1543986, 1976/1979). Papulacandins A, B, and C have very high activity confined almost specifically to yeasts, and differ structurally only in one of the two unsaturated fatty acid ester chains attached to the spiro-dihydrobenzofuranyl disaccharide nucleus. *In vitro,* papulacandin B has a lower MIC against *Candida* than amphotericin B, nystatin, or clotrimazole (0.1, 0.8, 3.1, and 0.8 μg/ml, respectively) with the exception of *C. guilliermondii* K 334, against which only clotrimazole (0.8 μg/ml) is active. In mice, papulacandins A and B both combine low acute toxicity ($LD_{50} > 1000$ mg/kg) with effective control of systemic *C. albicans* infection (ED_{50} 180 and 80 mg/kg, respectively) when given subcutaneously; no protection was achieved orally even at 1000 mg/kg. Ethers of papulacan-

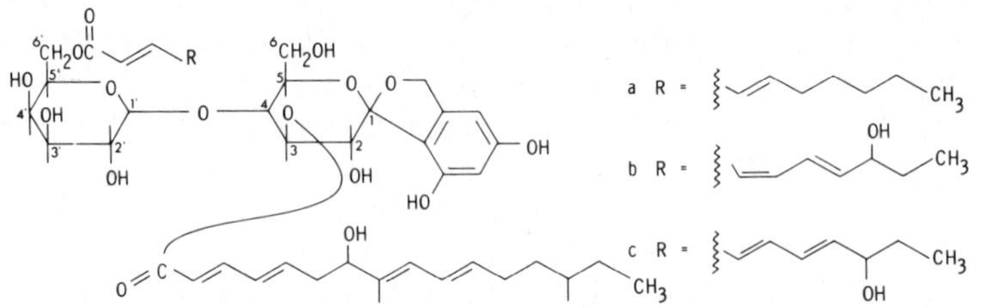

(CIL) papulacandin

dins A and B in which one or both phenolic hydroxyl groups are etherified are the subject of a patent (Ciba-Geigy: Swiss 613993, 1975/1979). Although the papulacandins are highly amphophilic, as are the polyenes, there is no cross-resistance between them, nor is there any with miconazole or clotrimazole, and a different mode of action is indicated. They do not cause release of potassium ions from yeast cells. Using spheroplasts of *Saccharomyces cerevisiae* and *C. albicans,* papulacandin B has IC_{50}s of 0.16 and 0.03 μg/ml, respectively, for glucan synthesis. As glucans form an important component of the yeast cell wall, it is probably through ensuing osmotic instability that these antibiotics have their effect.

Echinocandin B, a cyclic polypeptide bearing a linoleic acid chain, and aculeacin A (Section IV,J,2) also inhibit the synthesis of cell wall glucan; echinocandin B shows some cross-resistance with papulacandin B as determined with a strain of *C. albicans* made resistant to papulacandin (Baguley *et al.*, 1979). Although nothing has been published by way of structure–activity relationships, papulacandin D which has the 3-hydroxy group esterified as usual, but which lacks the 6′-esterified β-D-1′ → 4-galactopyranose in the 4-position of the β-D-glucopyranoside, is without significant antifungal properties. Since this mode of action is very selective for yeasts, it offers attractive therapeutic possibilities for the future, and search for similar agents will certainly intensify.

Another C-glycoside, which has been isolated independently from two thermophilic microorganisms *Myriococcum albomyces* (*Ascomycetaceae*) (Kluepfel *et al.*, 1972) and a eumycete *Albomyces* ATCC 20349 (Craveri *et al.*, 1972), is the amino acid (+)-myriocin (thermozymocidin; CL). An X-ray crystallographic study has been carried out on the *N*-acetyl-γ-lactone derivative CLI (Destro and Colombo, 1979). Biosynthetically (+)-myriocin appears to be formed from L-serine and an acetate-derived linear C_{18} carboxylic acid. (+)-Myriocin and anhydromyriocin have comparable *in vitro* activity against *C. albicans* (MIC 0.32–25 μg/ml), whereas only the latter inhibited the growth of dermatophytes. The compounds are probably too toxic to be taken further. A synthesis of the (−)-enantiomer of (+)-anhydromyriocin from L-arabinose has now been achieved, proving (+)-anhydromyriocin to have the absolute configura-

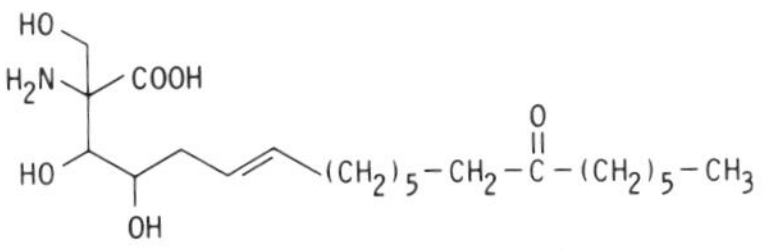

(CL) myriocin

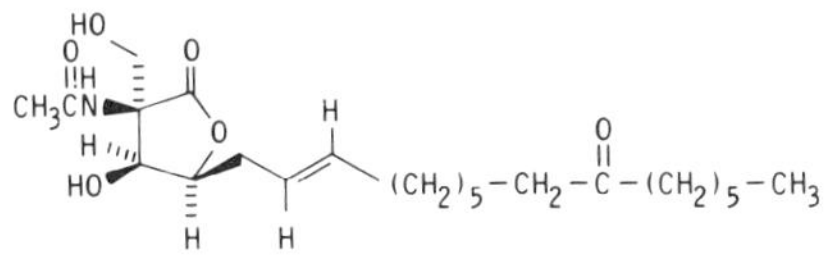

(CLI)

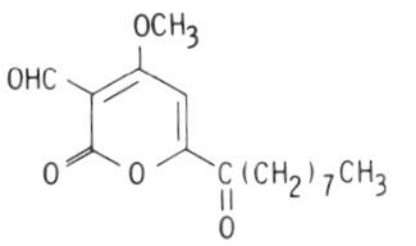

	R	R^1
a	Me	H
b	H	OH

(CLII) phacidin

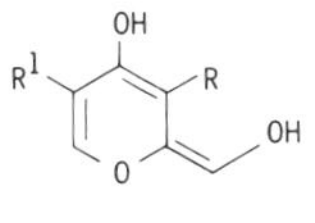

(CLIII) versicolin (a)
kojic acid (b)

tion shown in CLI (Just and Payette, 1980). The mode of action has also received some attention (Manachini and Aragozzini, 1972). Growth inhibition of *S. cerevisiae* is obtained at a concentration of 0.5 μg/ml. No effect on anaerobic or aerobic glucose metabolism was observed nor on the synthesis of RNA or protein; by contrast the DNA content was found to increase at the expense of nonprotein nitrogen.

γ-Pyrones such as phacidin obtained from *Potebniamyces balsamicola* (responsible for a bark disease in *Abies grandis*) can be considered as unusual C-glycosides. Phacidin (CLII) has the revised structure shown (Poulton and Cyr, 1980) and has broad-spectrum antifungal properties (Sekhon and Funk, 1977). Other examples of γ-pyrones include aureothin, colletotrichitin, spectinabilin, tridachione, and versicolin. The latter, which is produced by *Aspergillus versicolor,* has the structure CLIIIa (Rickards, 1971) and is closely related to kojic acid (CLIIIb), one of four compounds occurring in fungi which are derived directly from D-glucose. Versicolin may in fact prove to be a useful agent for the oral treatment of *T. rubrum,* the organism responsible for 90% of dermatophyte infections in eastern India (Nandi and Bose, 1976). The MIC against *T. rubrum* is 1.2–1.5 μg/ml and effective control of infection in guinea pigs can be obtained with as little as 15 daily doses of 2.5 mg/kg. In mice LD_{50}s are 33, 61, 80, and 330 mg/kg by the iv, ip, subcutaneous, and oral routes, respectively. Although inactivated by serum, blood levels 15–20 times the MIC can be sustained for more than 4 hours after 25 mg/kg iv (the maximum tolerated dose); no subacute toxicity was apparent, and excretion was principally via the urine (65%).

4. *Miscellaneous Compounds*

A marine tunicate of the *Aplidium* family has been found to contain a C_{22} aminoalcohol aplidiasphingosine (CLIV; Carter and Rinehart, 1978). It is mainly of interest as an antibacterial, antitumor, and cytotoxic agent (monkey kidney cells and *Herpes* virus type I), but shows slight activity against *C. albicans* and *Penicillium oxalicum.* It may function in this organism in the way that sphingosine does in higher animals and plants, and thus act by interference with the latter. Synthetic 11-aminoundecanol derivatives have been patented as fungicides and plant growth regulators (Ciba-Geigy: DT. 2831299, 1977/1979).

Another series of compounds, structurally related to the arylhexatrienes, are the triprenyl(chloro)phenols. These are active against *Candida* as well as against tumors and viruses, but are not cytotoxic to cultures of chick embryo fibroblasts. Members of this group have a sesquiterpene unit attached to a polyketide-derived aromatic nucleus. They include an-

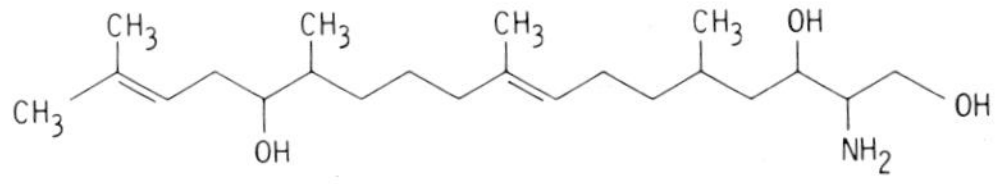

(CLIV) aplidiasphingosine

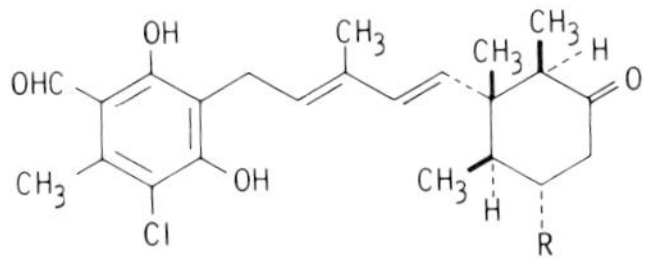

a R = H
b R = OAc

(CLV)

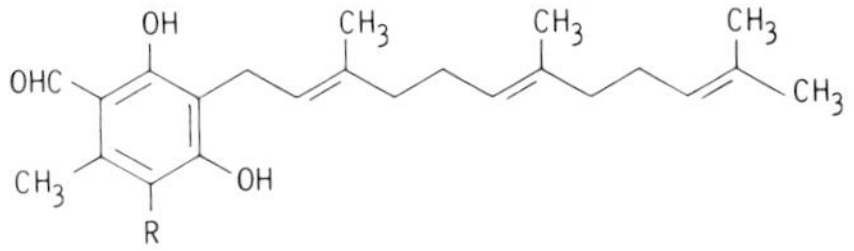

a R = Cl
b R = H

(CLVI)

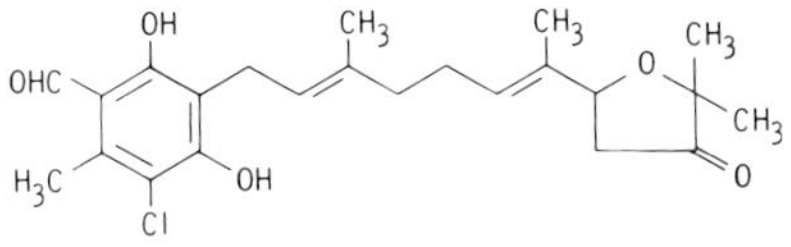

(CLVII) ascofuranone

tibiotics LL-Z 1272 α (ilicicolin A; CLVIa), β (ilicicolin B; CLVIb), δ (ilicicolin C), ϵ, ξ (ilicicolin F), and γ (ilicicolin D; CLVa) from a *Fusarium* species and cylindrochlorin (ilicicolin E). Ascochlorin, produced by *Ascochyta viciae* (Nawata *et al.,* 1969), is also identical to ilicicolin D, which together with ilicicolins A–G were isolated from *Cylindrocladium ilicicola* (Minato *et al.,* 1972). It is significant that the related ascofuranone (CLVII) retains activity against viruses and some tumors, but is without effect on bacteria, fungi, and yeasts. A series of synthetic arylmethylethylenes, halogenated on the double bond, have been patented as fungicides and plant growth regulators (ICI: G.B. 2033380A, 1978/1980).

E. Pyridone Olefins

Pipermethystine (CXLIII), an *N*-phenylpropionyldihydropyridone alkaloid, has already been mentioned. The literature contains several other examples of pyridones with antifungal properties arising from quite different modes of action. Takahashi *et al.* (1965) have described the isolation from *Streptomyces mobaraensis* of the insecticidal 4-pyridone piericidin A

(CLVIIIa) and the corresponding methyl ether piericidin B (CLVIIIe) which show a structural resemblance to coenzyme Q. At low concentrations, piericidin A inhibits the oxidation of $NADH_2$ and reduction of coenzyme Q in mitochondria; at higher concentrations it blocks the succinate–coenzyme Q pathway. A total of 16 piericidins (A_1–A_4, B_1–B_4, C_1–C_4, D_1–D_4) has now been reported from *Streptomyces pactum* (Yoshida *et al.*, 1977). These are pale yellow viscous oils which polymerize in air and in nonpolar solvents, and are inhibitors of mitochondrial respiration in fungi, yeasts, and insects (Kaken: Japan Kokai 75-132183, 1974/1975). The four members of each group of piericidins differ in their alkylation pattern in the same way. The "A" series consists of the 10-alcohols, with the "C" compounds being the corresponding 11,12-epoxides. Similarly the "D" series are the 11,12-epoxides of the 10-methoxy "B" compounds.

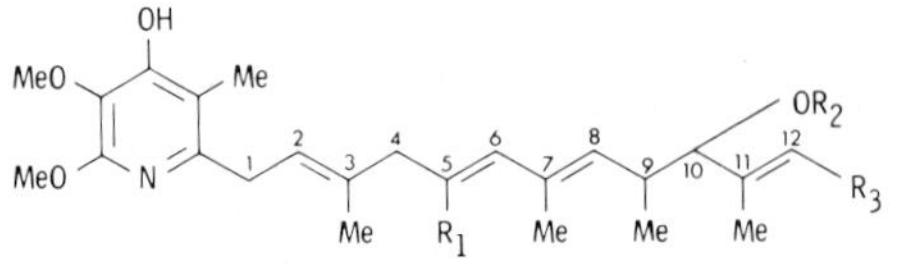

	R_1	R_2	R_3
a	H	H	Me
b	Me	H	Me
c	H	H	$CHMe_2$
d	Me	H	$CHMe_2$
e	H	Me	Me
f	Me	Me	Me
g	H	Me	$CHMe_2$
h	Me	Me	$CHMe_2$

(CLVIII) piericidin

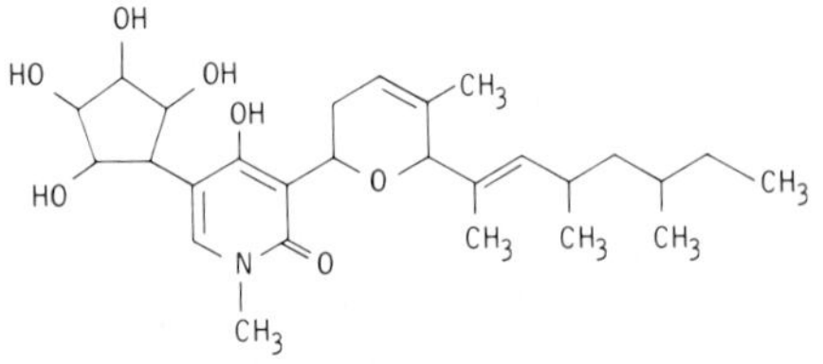

(CLIX) funiculosin

Funiculosin is an *N*-methyl-4-hydroxy-2-pyridone antibiotic, the structure (CLIX) and absolute configuration of which have been determined by X-ray crystallographic analysis of the tetrahydro derivative; it is antiviral and antifungal and has been isolated from *Penicillium funiculosum* (Ando *et al.*, 1978). It has several unique features. In particular, it is the only natural example with a cyclopentanetetraol group. This may enable it to function as a possible nucleoside mimic, though a distant analogy can also be drawn with the structure of blasticidin S (see later). Funiculosin is especially active against dermatophytes, with modest activity against yeasts over a 3-day period; most fungi however can develop in the presence of relatively high concentrations of antibiotic over a 7-day growth period. A 0.5% hydrophilic ointment gave excellent control of *T. mentagrophytes* in guinea pigs, comparable with or superior to 3% topical preparations of griseofulvin, pyrrolnitrin, naphthiomate, undecylenic acid, or its iodo-derivative. The acute toxicity of funiculosin is very species specific; it is well absorbed orally and very toxic (LD_{50} 5–7 mg/kg) to mice and rats by all routes, causing lung congestion. By contrast, guinea pigs and rabbits tolerated an oral dose of 2000 mg/kg, and the former withstood 500 mg/kg ip.

The isolation of ilicicolin H (CLX) from *Cylindrocladium ilicicola* MFC-870 has been described by Matsumoto (1979). Like funiculosin it is a 4-hydroxy-2-pyridone derivative, this time with a *p*-hydroxyphenol and a bicyclic sesquiterpene group attached. Like other ilicicolins, it is very active *in vitro* against *C. albicans* and moderately active against gram-positive bacteria.

Another group of antifungal 2-pyridones bear an *N*-hydroxyl, and are thus cyclic hydroxamates. The simplest of these, antibiotic G-1549 (identical to BN-227; XXXII), has been mentioned earlier; it is topically active in guinea pigs infected with *M. canis* but is toxic to mice when given

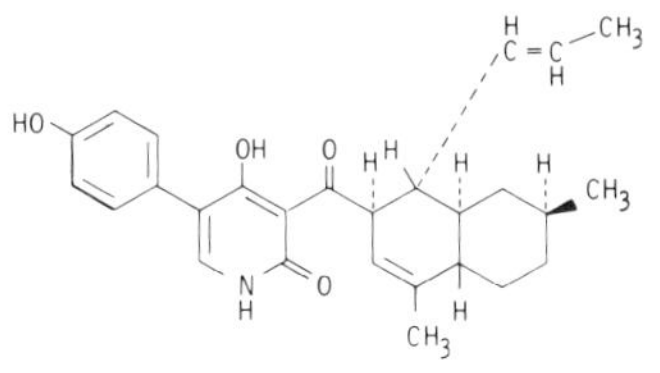

(CLX) ilicicolin H

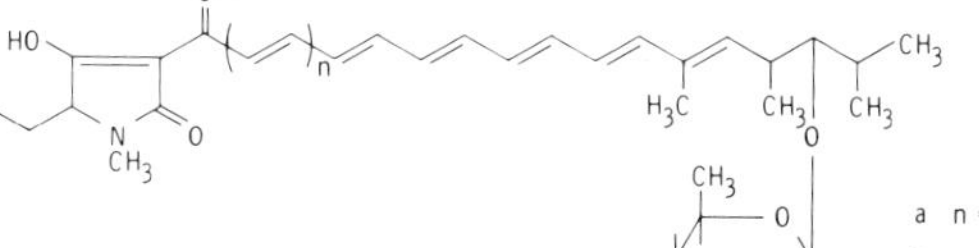

(CLXI) tenellin (a) ; bassianin (b)

(CLXII) oleficin (a) ; α-lipomycin (b)

systemically (Itoh *et al.*, 1979). Two other cyclic hydroxamates, closely related to ilicicolin H and funiculosin, are tenellin and bassianin (CLXIa,b; Wat *et al.*, 1977). They are produced by the fungi *Beauvaria tenella* and *B. bassiana*, and are derived from phenylalanine and tyrosine with tetraketide and pentaketide side-chains, respectively.

Several tetramic acids deserve mention as 5-ring homologs of the pyridones, and together with them, the cyclized form of cerulenin (CXXXIV) in protic solvents. Oleficin (CLXIIa) is a metabolite of *Streptomyces parvulus* (Gyimesi *et al.*, 1978), and the lower vinylogue α-lipomycin (CLXIIb) was isolated from *Streptomyces aureofaciens* by Kunze *et al.* (1972). Biological activity is confined to gram-positive bacteria and Yoshida sarcoma and appears to be due to alterations in cell membrane permeability, since it is antagonized by lecithin and by some sterols.

F. Acetylenic Compounds

Straight-chain acetylenes are fairly common products of both higher plants and fungi; dicotyledons, especially the *Compositae*, most frequently produce C_{13} compounds, while *Basidiomycetes* give C_9 and C_{10} chain lengths (Anchel, 1967). The detection of polyacetylenes has been facilitated by their antibacterial and antifungal properties. The simplest member is probably acetylene dicarboxamide (CLXIII), which as cellocidin was found in broths of *Streptomyces chibaensis* by Suzuki *et al.* (1958). Its antibacterial activity has been exploited to a limited extent in Japan in the control of rice bacterial leaf blight caused by *Xanthomonas oryzae*, a solution of 100–200 μg/ml providing protection. At greater concentrations, problems of phytotoxicity are encountered, and the LD_{50} in mice of 11 mg/kg iv precludes any possible application in mammals (Dekker, 1971). It has been shown to inhibit strongly the conversion of β-ketoglutarate to succinate in *Xanthomonas oryzae* and the uptake of thymidine into DNA in *Bacillus subtilis* (Yoneyama *et al.*, 1978). It is antagonized by sulfhydryl

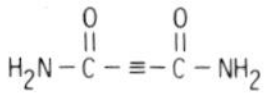

$H_2N-C(=O)-C\equiv C-C(=O)-NH_2$

(CLXIII) cellocidin

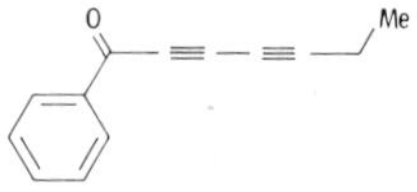

(CLXIV) capillin

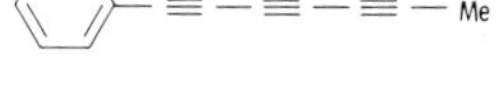

(CLXV)

compounds, and adds two molecules of, for example, cysteine in a Markownikoff manner.

The antifungal diacetylene capillin (CLXIV; MIC 0.25 μg/ml against *T. purpureum*) from the essential oils of *Artemisia capillaris* has been known for some time (Imai *et al.*, 1956). More recently the leaves of a tropical weed *Bidens pilosa* (*Asteraceae*) have been the source of a related compound, 1-phenyl-heptatriyne (CLXV), the activity of which against gram-positive bacteria, yeasts, fungi, and human fibroblasts is dependent on the presence of light (Wat *et al.*, 1979). The phytoalexin wyerone (CXXXVIIb) has been discussed earlier (Section IV,D,1), but the enynone side chain of the furan ring bears an obvious similarity to the aryl diynone of capillin (CLXIV).

Several related C_{17} polyacetylenes are fairly widely occurring and seem to play a protective role against phytopathogens, though they are not phytoalexins in the strict sense. Falcarindiol (CLXVIa) has been reported together with the much less potent falcarinol (CLXVIb) in extracts of young shoots of ground elder, *Aegopodium podagraria* (Kemp, 1978). Growth of *Alternaria brassicicola* and *Septoria nodorum* was totally inhib-

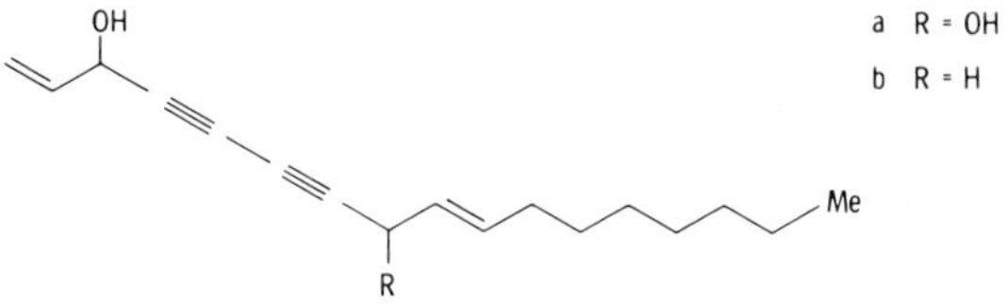

OH R Me

a R = OH
b R = H

(CLXVI) falcarindiol (a); falcarinol (b)

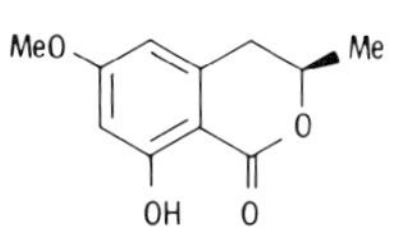

MeO Me O OH O

(CLXVII)

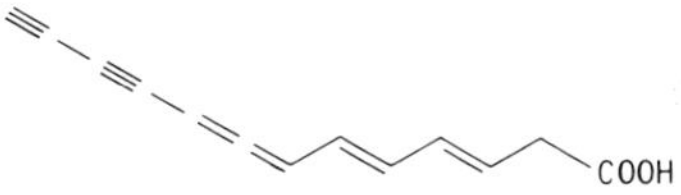

COOH

(CLXVIII) mycomycin

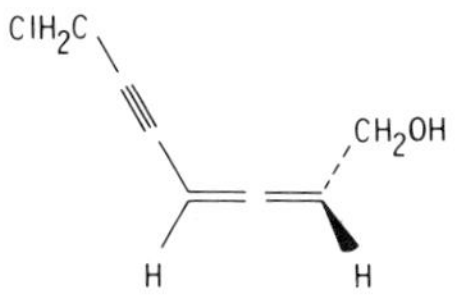

ClH_2C CH_2OH H H

(CLXIX) scorodin

ited at 20 μg/ml, and this activity has been shown to be comparable to that of wyerone and safynol. Falcarindiol and 6-methoxymellein (CLXVII) also occur in carrot roots. The periderm, in which concentrations are particularly high, is very resistant to liquorice rot caused by *Mycocentrospora acerina*. Although toxic to this organism, falcarindiol also disrupts membranes of the host cells, and it is postulated that localization in extracellular hydrophobic oil droplets (75 μg/gm) insulates the host from the toxic effects of the compound (Garrod and Lewis, 1979). A further plant source is "seven finger" *Schefflera digitata* (*Araliaceae*), which was used by the Maori people to treat ringworm and other skin infections; falcarindiol has been shown to possess potent antidermatophyte properties and this specificity may be related to the unusual cell wall composition of dermatophytes (Muir and Walker, 1979; Muir *et al.*, 1979). An improved yield (0.11%) of a heptadeca-1,9-diene-4,6-diyne-3,8-diol from cowbane (*Cicuta virosa*) has been the subject of a patent (Ermakova, V. A. *et al.*: U.S.S.R. 642286, 1977/1979); it is claimed as only weakly toxic, presumably to the host. The 9,10-epoxide of falcarinol has been isolated by Poplawski *et al.* (1980) together with the parent compound from roots of *Panax ginseng*, and subsequently the 9,10-epoxide of heptadec-16-ene-4,6-diyn-8-ol has been recognized as a constituent of *Cirsium japonicum* (Yano, 1980). Other similar compounds are known, but no antifungal properties have been ascribed to them.

In connection with the polyacetylenes, isomeric allenes are also known. Mycomycin (CLXVIII) exhibits both antibacterial and antifungal activity *in vitro*, but is inactive and nontoxic *in vivo* (Celmer and Solomons, 1952). A more recent example is the halogenated allenic antibiotic scorodin (CLXIX), a metabolite of *Marasmius scorodonius* (Anke *et al.*, 1980). It shows antibacterial and antifungal properties (MICs against *C. albicans* and *S. cerevisiae* 10–25 and 8–50 μg/ml) and inhibits DNA and RNA synthesis. Chlorinated acetylenes are also found in the *Compositae* and in some algae. The above mentioned allenes isomerize fairly readily to the corresponding acetylenes. Although many polyacetylenes are extremely toxic to higher animals (oenanthotoxin and cicutoxin from members of the *Umbelliferae* are well-known as sheep poisons), it is not beyond the bounds of possibility that a relatively nontoxic one may be found. In general however they are also deactivated by serum, which mitigates against systemic usefulness.

G. Phytoalexins

Higher plants of more than 20 genera respond to fungal infection by the release of antifungal principles of which more than 85 are now known. Of these, the "post inhibitins" are normally stored in healthy tissue in a suitably protected and bound form ready to be called upon when required, while the "phytoalexins" arise when the synthesis of specific enzymes which make them is elicited. It is this second response with which this section will be mainly concerned. An excellent review by Harborne and Ingham (1978) deals with the mechanism of disease resistance in plants, and comprehensively surveys the various genera and structural types involved. Several other articles may also be recommended (Stoessl, 1972; Gross, 1977; Grisebach and Ebel, 1978). It is our intention to discuss the potential of phytoalexins as antifungal agents, and to update these reviews with reports of new phytoalexins that have appeared in the literature in the 1976–1980 period.

In addition to living microorganisms, phytoalexin formation can be provoked by exposure to compounds of microbial origin (elicitors), by stress (cold, UV light), and by heavy metal salts. Yoshikawa (1978) has studied the accumulation of glyceollin (CLXXa) in soybean, and has shown that

	R	R^1	R^2	R^3	R^4	R^5	R^6
a glyceollin I	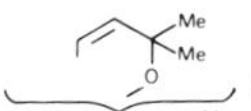 O, Me, Me (R + R^1)		H	H	OH	H	OH
b glyceollin II	H	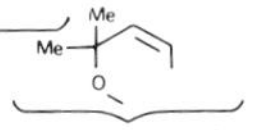 Me, Me, O (R^1 + R^2)		H	OH	H	OH
c (-)-phaseollin	H	OH	H	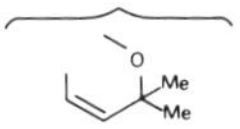 O, Me, Me (R^3 + R^4)		H	H
d medicarpin	H	OH	H	H	OMe	H	H
e maackiain	H	OH	H	H	—O—CH_2—O— (R^4 + R^5)		H
f cristacarpin	H	OH	H	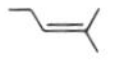 (prenyl)	OMe	H	OH
g hydroxyphaseollin	H	OH	H	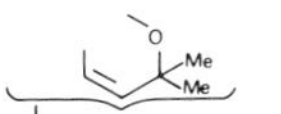 O, Me, Me (R^3 + R^4)		H	OH
h phaseollidin	H	OH	H	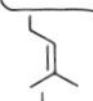 (prenyl)	OH	H	H
i phaseollidin hydrate	H	OH	H	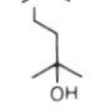 OH	OH	H	H
j nissolin	H	OH	H	OMe	OH	H	H
k methylnissolin	H	OH	H	OMe	OMe	H	H
l sparticarpin	H	OMe	OMe	H	OH	H	H
m neodunol	H	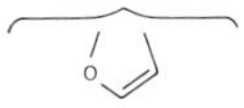 O (R^1 + R^2)		H	OH	H	H

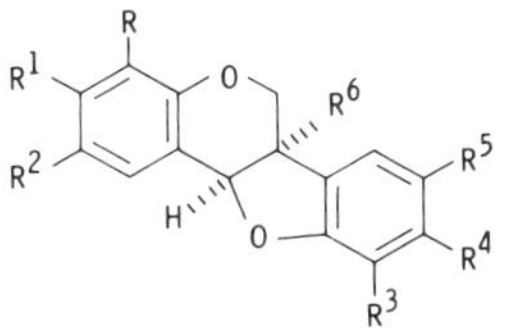

(CLXX)

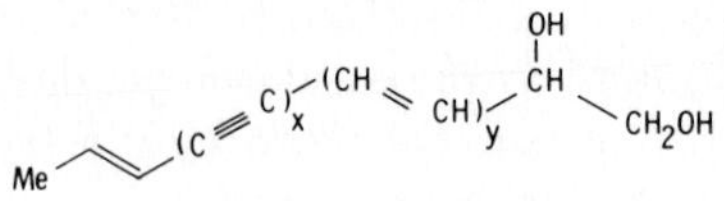

$$\mathrm{Me-CH{=}CH-(C{\equiv}C)_x-(CH{=}CH)_y-CH(OH)-CH_2OH}$$

a x = 3 ; y = 1 safynol
b x = 4 ; y = 0 dehydrosafynol

(CLXXI)

biotic elicitors—e.g., the highly pathogenic *Phytophthora megasperma* var. *sojae*—stimulated glyceollin biosynthesis without greatly affecting its rate of degradation. Abiotic elicitors on the other hand appeared to have little effect on synthesis, but strongly inhibited the degradation. As a result, the overall effect of these quite different actions was comparable.

Phytoalexins are of interest in the search for new antifungal agents since they represent a *natural* response to fungal infection aimed at limiting or eliminating that infection, and although this type of response to infection is concerned with plants and plant pathogens, nevertheless the hope is that a study of phytoalexins will lead to agents of medical or veterinary significance. It should be noted that the types of phytoalexin produced depend more on the plant producing them than on the eliciting pathogen, and that although they have antifungal activity, they also produce effects on the host plant. Thus diseased tissue is destroyed and eliminated—along with the infecting fungus—and the net result is somewhat akin to that produced by Whitfield's ointment in the treatment of human dermatophyte infections.

In very approximate terms there are four main plant families from which phytoalexins have been isolated, and each produces in general one principal structural type: *Compositae,* polyacetylenes; *Leguminosae,* isoflavonoids; *Solanaceae,* sesquiterpenes; *Orchidaceae,* dihydrophenanthrenes.

1. *Polyacetylenes*

As indicated above, polyacetylenic phytoalexins usually originate from species of the *Compositae,* e.g., safynol (CLXXIa) and dehydrosafynol (CLXXIb) from safflower, *Carthamus tinctorius* infected with *Phytophthora drechsleri* (Allen and Thomas, 1971a,b). Other polyacetylenes have been discussed in Section IV,F. The furanoacetylenes related to wyerone (CXXXVIIb), produced by *Vicia faba* infected with *Botrytis,* have been mentioned earlier. Wyerol (the corresponding 8-alcohol) and the 11,12-dihydro derivatives of wyerol, wyerone and wyeronic acid, are also known, though concentrations are always less than the unsaturated compounds (Mansfield *et al.*, 1980). Acetate, malonate, and oleate are all incorporated into the *Vicia faba* phytoalexins following infection with *B. cinerea* (Cain and Porter, 1979).

2. *Isoflavonoids*

Although the antifungal activity of phytoalexins against certain parasitizing fungi, and in particular the eliciting organism, has usually received attention, very little is known concerning their effect on human pathogenic fungi. This has been partially rectified in the case of seven isoflavonoids: three isoflavans, (−)-phaseollinisoflavan (CLXXIIa), (±)-sativan (CLXXIIb), (±)-vestitol (CLXXIIc); and four pterocarpans, (+)-pisatin (CLXXIIIa), (−)-phaseollin (CLXXc), (±)-medicarpin (CLXXd), and (±)-maackiain (CLXXe; Gordon *et al.*, 1980). The results from broth dilution assays with a number of pathogens are shown in Table IV, the vast

	R	R^1	R^2	R^3	R^4	R^5
a (−) phaseollinisoflavan	H	OH	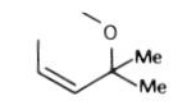 O–C(Me)(Me)–CH=CH– (ring)		H	H
b sativan	H	OMe	H	OMe	H	H
c vestitol	H	OH	H	OMe	H	H
d demethylvestitol	H	OH	H	OH	H	H
e 5-methoxyvestitol	OMe	OH	H	OMe	H	H
f astraciceran	H	OMe	H	$O\text{-}CH_2\text{-}O$		H
g mucronulatol	H	OMe	OH	OMe	H	H
h "3-hydroxymaackiainisoflavan"	H	OH	H	$O\text{-}CH_2\text{-}O$		OH

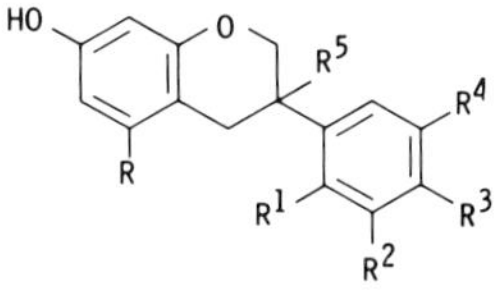

(CLXXII)

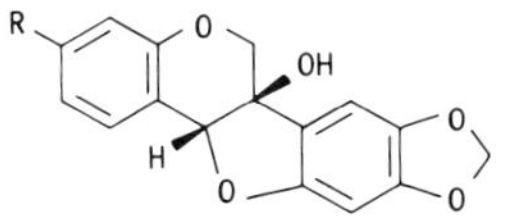

	R
a (+)-pisatin	OMe
b demethylpisatin	OH

(CLXXIII)

majority being sensitive to one or more phytoalexin between 12.5 and 50 μg/ml; phaseollinisoflavan was the most effective. Oxygen substituents and lipophilic groups seem to be particularly desirable for activity. Attempts to rationalize structure–activity relationships on the basis of three-dimensional shape (Perrin and Cruickshank, 1969) have since been

TABLE IV

ANTIFUNGAL ACTIVITY OF PHYTOALEXINS[a]

Test organism	Isoflavans			Pterocarpans			
	Phaseollinisoflavan (CLXXIIa)	Sativan (CLXXIIb)	Vestitol (CLXXIIc)	Pisatin (CLXXIIIa)	Phaseollin (CLXXc)	Maackiain (CLXXe)	Medicarpin (CLXXd)
Aspergillus fumigatus	100	>100	100	50	100	>100	>100
Candida albicans	50	>100	>100	>100	100	>100	>100
Coccidioides immitis	25	—	—	50	100	—	—
Cryptococcus neoformans	12.5	>100	100	50	12.5	>100	>100
Histoplasma capsulatum	50	>100	50	>100	100	25	>100
Petriellidium boydii	50	—	—	100	50	—	—
Rhizopus oryzae	50	—	—	>100	50	—	—
Sporothrix schenckii	25	>100	25	100	50	>100	>100
Trichophyton rubrum	12.5	25	25	50	25	100	>100

[a] MICs in μg/ml. Adapted from Gordon *et al.* (1980).

refuted (Van Etten, 1976). There are indications that these phytoalexins act upon the plasma membrane or upon some process necessary for its function, but in a way different from that of the polyenes. Although they may induce lysis of human erythrocytes—as do the polyenes—toxicity studies in mammals reveal a relative tolerance to phytoalexins. It is thus not beyond the bounds of possibility that a suitably modified phytoalexin be synthesized with a more promising profile.

Isoflavans, at least 14 of which have been isolated from the *Papilionoideae* (*Leguminosae*), are usually associated with the corresponding oxygenated pterocarpans. An exception is the tribe *Lotae*. Ingham and Dewick (1979) have examined leaflets of *Lotus hispidus* infected with *Helminthosporium carbonum* and found demethylvestitol, vestitol, sativan, and the new member 5-methoxyvestitol (CLXXIIe), the second 5-oxygenated isoflavan to be found in nature. Vestitol is the only one to accumulate in concentrations greater than its ED_{50} against *H. carbonum* (17 μg/ml). *Astragalus cicer* (*Galegeae*) has furnished the methylenedioxyisoflavan, astraciceran (CLXXIIf), together with mucronulatol (CLXXIIg), previously isolated from *A. gummifer* (Ingham and Dewick, 1980a). The biosynthesis of isoflavan, pterocarpan, and coumestan metabolites has been studied in *Medicago sativa* (Dewick and Martin, 1979). The pterocarpan, medicarpin (CLXXd), and the isoflavan vestitol (CLXXIIc) are interconvertible, and sativan is probably derived by methylation of the latter. A 3-hydroxyisoflavan (CLXXIIh) is a pisatin metabolite produced by *Fusarium oxysporum* after prior demethylation to CLXXIIIb. A strain of *F. oxysporum* not pathogenic to peas was not capable of this transformation.

An isoflavanone, kievitone (CLXXIVa), is one of the major phytoalexins of the kidney bean *Phaseolus vulgaris* (Smith *et al.*, 1973). Other related compounds, including 5-deoxykievitone (CLXXIVb) and the isoflavone 2,3-dehydrokievitone (CLXXVa), arise after infection with *Monilia fructicola* (Woodward, 1979b). The latter is indicative of a second biosynthetic pathway leading to kievitone via isoflavone prenylation. That the isomeric antifungal phaseoluteone (CLXXVb) is also found in the plant supports this postulate (Woodward, 1979a). A related antimicrobial,

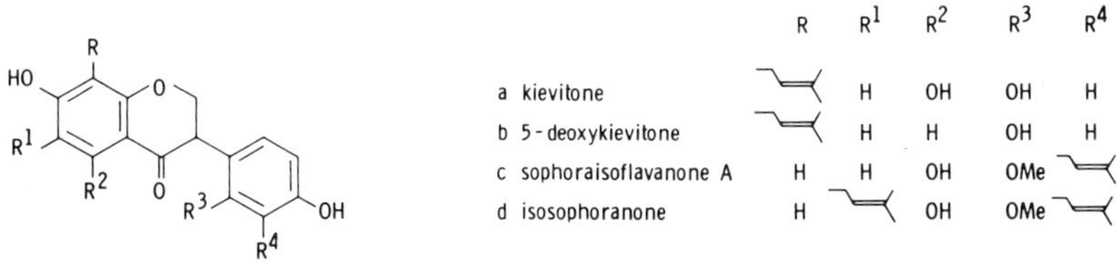

	R	R^1	R^2	R^3	R^4
a kievitone		H	OH	OH	H
b 5-deoxykievitone		H	H	OH	H
c sophoraisoflavanone A	H	H	OH	OMe	
d isosophoranone	H		OH	OMe	

(CLXXIV)

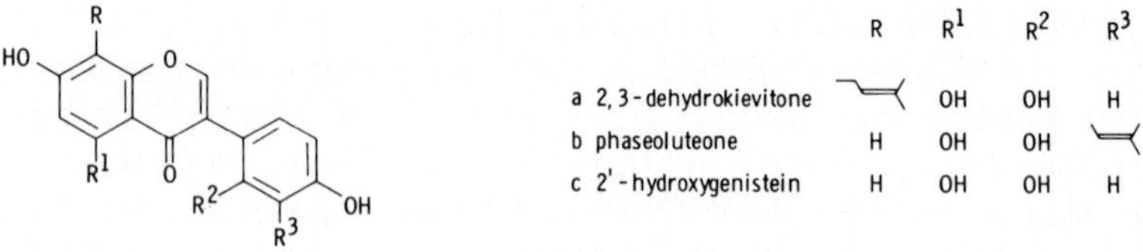

	R	R^1	R^2	R^3
a 2,3-dehydrokievitone		OH	OH	H
b phaseoluteone	H	OH	OH	
c 2'-hydroxygenistein	H	OH	OH	H

(CLXXV)

sophoraisoflavanone A (CLXXIVc) has been isolated by Komatsu *et al.* (1978) from the aerial parts of *Sophora tomentosa* together with isosophoranone, the 6-prenyl compound, and several flavanones. Sophoraisoflavanone A would appear to be a natural plant product as distinct from a phytoalexin. At 2 mg/ml it inhibits the growth of *C. albicans, Penicillium citrinum,* gram-positive and to a lesser extent gram-negative bacteria, but is without effect on *Aspergillus niger, A. fumigatus,* and *Saccharomyces sake*. Other isoflavone natural products which have alternative oxygenation and prenylation patterns are known, such as osajin and pomiferin from the osage orange *Maclura pomifera,* but although we have found that these show slight antiprotozoal activity *in vitro,* yeasts and dermatophytes were not affected by them.

Isoflavones are biosynthetic precursors of the principal legume phytoalexins, the pterocarpans, e.g., medicarpin (CLXXd) and maackiain (CLXXe) (Dewick and Ward, 1978; Woodward, 1980). There are two enantiomeric *cis*-fused series of pterocarpans, many of which bear a hydroxyl group at the ring junction (6a position) and are typified by (+)-pisatin (CLXXIIIa) and (−)-cristacarpin (CLXXf), isolated by Ingham and Markham (1980) from infected *Erythrina* species. 6a-Hydroxyphaseollin (CLXXg) is less fungitoxic than the parent system and may be another example of a detoxification product of fungal metabolism. A further instance is the conversion of phaseollidin (CLXXh) to the tertiary alcohol (CLXXi) by *Fusarium solani* with a 5- to 10-fold reduction in potency (Smith *et al.,* 1980).

New pterocarpan phytoalexins to be discovered include nissolin (CLXXj) and methylnissolin (CLXXk) from *Lathyrus nissolia* (Robeson and Ingham, 1979), and sparticarpin (CLXXl) from Spanish broom, *Spartium junceum,* following exposure to UV light or *H. carbonum* (Ingham and Dewick, 1980b); all three are active against *Cladosporium herbarum.* The yam bean *Pachyrrhizus erosus* produces the furanopterocarpan neodunol (CLXXm) having an ED_{50} of 27 μg/ml against *H. carbonum,* and in general lower activity against other phytopathogens, especially *Botrytis cinerea* (100 μg/ml) which is known to be capable of detoxification. Activity among pterocarpans seems to be highest for the phenolic ones (Ingham, 1979).

Although much rarer, a few examples of antifungal flavanoids being produced postinfection are known. The three hydroxyflavans (CLXXVIa,b,c) are found in daffodil bulb scales after attack by *B. cinerea* (Coxon *et al.*, 1980). Much more potent however is the first chlorinated flavone to be

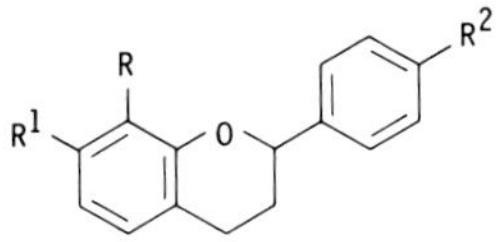

	R	R¹	R²
a	H	OH	H
b	H	OH	OH
c	Me	OH	OH

(CLXXVI)

isolated, chlorflavonin (CLXXVII), a metabolite of *Aspergillus candidus*, which is very active against several *Aspergilli* (0.08 μg/ml) and against *B. cinerea* and *Paecilomyces variotii* (5 μg/ml; Richards *et al.*, 1969). Again, however, chlorflavonin is not a phytoalexin but a natural product.

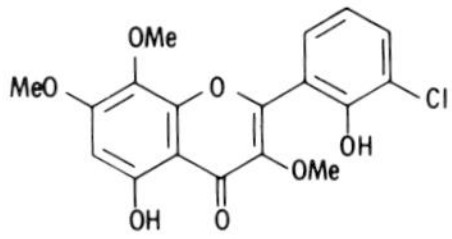

(CLXXVII) chlorflavonin

The furanopterocarpan neodunol (CLXXm) could equally be considered with another structural type, the benzofurans, the biosynthetic origins of which can be diverse. The phytoalexin vignafuran (CLXXVIIIa) from leaves of the cowpea *Vigna unguiculata* infected with *Colletotrichum lindemuthianum* and from diseased *Lablab niger* is derived from phenylalanine via an isoflavanoid precursor (Martin and Dewick, 1979);

	R	R¹	R²	R³	R⁴	R⁵	R⁶
a vignafuran	H	H	OMe	OMe	H	OH	H
b demethylvignafuran	H	H	OH	OMe	H	OH	H
c isopterofuran	H	H	OH	OMe	OMe	OH	H
d moracin A	OMe	H	OMe	H	OH	H	OH
e moracin B	H	OH	OMe	H	OMe	H	OH
f moracin M	H	H	OH	H	OH	H	OH

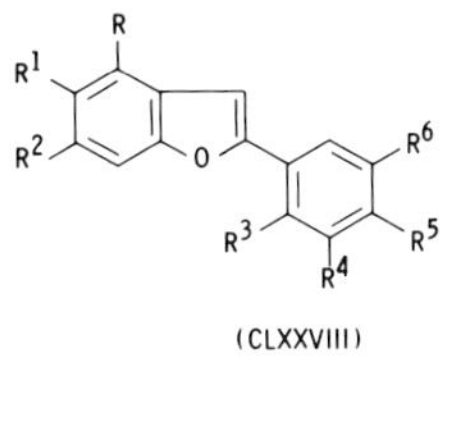

(CLXXVIII)

C-3 of the amino acid is lost and the aromatic residue becomes the 2-aryl group. The antifungal activity of 6-demethylvignafuran (CLXXVIIIb), a phytoalexin of *Tetragonolobus maritimus* and other *Leguminosae,* is considerably greater than the pterocarpan medicarpin (CLXXd) against *Cladosporium herbarum in vitro* (Ingham and Dewick, 1978). Infected *Coronilla emerus* also produces 6-demethylvignafuran together with the 3′-methoxy derivative isopterofuran (CLXXVIIIc) which is highly fungitoxic (Dewick and Ingham, 1980). A rather different oxygenation pattern is seen in the isomeric mulberry phytoalexins, moracins A and B (CLXXVIIId,e), from *Morus alba* infected with *Fusarium solani.* Interestingly moracin A is marginally but consistently more active against tested organisms than moracin B (Takasugi *et al.,* 1978). Further examination has enlarged this group to include moracins C–L, moracin M (CLXXVIIIf), the known stilbene oxyresveratrol (CLXXIXa), and the new derivative CLXXIXb. The healthy epidermis contains three new antifungal compounds, together with kuwanon C and morusin (Takasugi *et al.,* 1979).

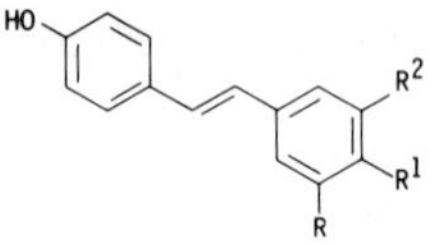

HO R² R¹ R

	R	R^1	R^2
a oxyresveratrol	OH	OH	OH
b	OH	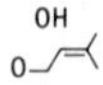 O	OH
c pterostilbene	OMe	H	OMe
d resveratrol	OH	H	OH

(CLXXIX)

Stilbenes are possible biosynthetic precursors of benzofurans via an oxidative cyclization of hydroxy derivatives. They are certainly precursors of the oligomeric viniferins which occur in the vine *Vitis vinifera* after inoculation with *B. cinerea* and which have a 2,3-dihydrobenzofuran structure (Langcake and Pryce, 1977; Pryce and Langcake, 1977). Pterostilbene (CLXXIXc), a minor vine phytoalexin, is a more potent antifungal than resveratrol (CLXXIXd) or the viniferins (Langcake *et al.,* 1979).

3. *Sesquiterpenes*

These compounds fall into two main types, each produced by a different genus; furanoterpenes from the *Convolvulaceae* and bicyclic sesquiterpenes from the *Solanaceae.* The sweet potato *Ipomoea batatas* on treatment with mercuric chloride gives rise to a series of stress metabolites which occur as normal products of secondary metabolism in other plants. Myoporone (CXXXVIII) has already been mentioned. 4-Hydroxy and 7-hydroxymyoporone are also known (Burka and Iles, 1979), the latter having been synthesized by a short sequence using a propargyl phenylselenide dianion (Reich *et al.,* 1979). Two keto-alcohols, corresponding to reduction of each ketone group of myoporone, have been isolated and resolved by HPLC. The 6-alcohol is 2–3 times as hepatotoxic as ipomeamarone (CLXXX), and is of obvious importance with respect to contaminated foodstuffs. Ten antifungal sesquiterpenes and norsesquiterpenes have been identified in potato tubers infected with microorganisms, and these include rishitin (CLXXXI), a bicyclo[4.4.0]decane, and lubimin (CLXXXII), a spirobicyclo[4.5]decane. The conversion of (−)-rishitin to (+)-glutinosine (CLXXXIIIa) has allowed the absolute configuration of this compound and of (+)-oxyglutinosine (CLXXXIIIb) to be established (Murai *et al.,* 1980a). The former is produced by *Nicotiana glutinosa* infected with tobacco mosaic virus, whereas the latter arises after the attack of potato by *Phytophthora infestans.* Racemic glutinosone has also been synthesized by two routes (Murai *et al.,* 1980b). Solavetivone (CLXXXIV) was the first vetispirane to be found in a *Nicotiana* species

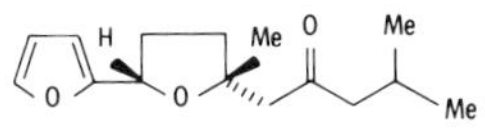

(CLXXX) ipomeamarone

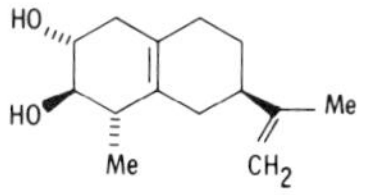

(CLXXXI) (−)-rishitin

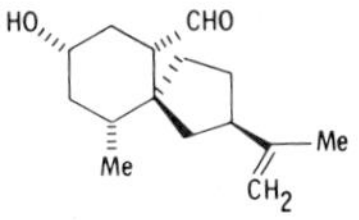

(CLXXXII) lubimin

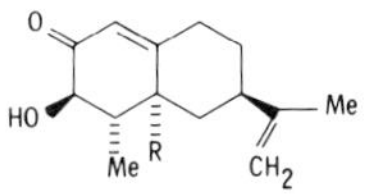

a (+)-glutinosone R = H
b (+)-oxyglutinosone R = OH

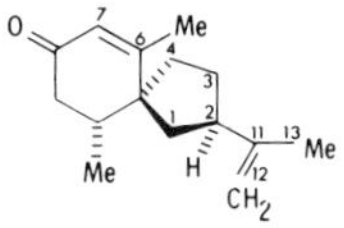

(CLXXXIII)

(CLXXXIV) solavetivone

(suffering viral necrosis; Fujimori *et al.,* 1979). Subsequently a report describing the isolation of four coumarins and seven isoprenoid phytoalexins induced by *Phoma exigua* in *Solanum tuberosum* has appeared (Malmberg and Theander, 1980). One of these was a mixture of two diastereoisomers of a 12-*O*-β-glucopyranoside of an 11,12-diol based on the solavetivone skeleton. The tricyclic sesquiterpenes phytuberol (CLXXXVa; Uegaki *et al.,* 1980a) and its acetate phytuberin (CLXXXVb; Hammerschmidt and Kuć, 1979; Uegaki *et al.,* 1980b) have also been detected in diseased *Nicotiana* species.

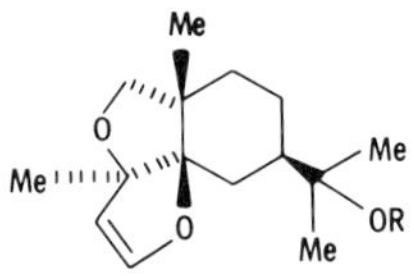

a phytuberol R = H
b phytuberin R = Ac

(CLXXXV)

Holland and Taylor (1979) have described the transformation of various steroids and of solanine by *Phytophthora infestans* as part of investigations into stress metabolites provoked by the potato blight organism. No hydroxylations were observed, but 3β-, 6α-, 11α-, and 17β-hydroxysteroids were oxidized to the corresponding ketones, whereas solanine was deacetylated to solanidine.

Diterpenoid phytoalexins such as casbene produced by the *Euphorbiaceae,* and the momilactones found in the *Graminae,* are known (Harborne and Ingham, 1978). This review also mentions terpenes, e.g., myrcene from infected *Abies grandis,* and the isoprenoid glycosides tuliposides A and B which are bound toxins of the *Liliiflorae* and act as sources of post-inhibitins. The enzymes responsible for phytoalexin synthesis have received some attention as illustrated by the purification and characterization of casbene synthetase (Dueber, 1979).

4. *Dihydrophenanthrenes*

The phenolic 9,10-dihydrophenanthrenes orchinol (CLXXXVIa), hircinol (CLXXXVIb), and loroglossol (CLXXXVIc) are phytoalexins produced by members of the *Orchidaceae* (Fisch *et al.,* 1973) which help to limit the extent of fungal development of the mycorrhizal relationship. *In vitro* activity against *Candida lipolytica* BY17 has been demonstrated at 50–100 μg/ml. Other examples of dihydrophenanthrenes and phenanthrenes bearing additional alkyl and thioalkyl substituents (e.g., De Alvarenga *et al.,*

	R	R^1	R^2	R^3	R^4	R^5
a orchinol	H	OMe	OMe	H	H	OH
b hircinol	H	OH	OMe	OH	H	H
c loroglossol	H	OMe	OMe	OH	H	H
d juncusol	Me	OH	H	$CH=CH_2$	Me	OH
e juncunol	Me	OH	H	H	Me	$CH=CH_2$
f juncunol (revised)	Me	OH	H	$CH=CH_2$	H	Me
g effusol	Me	OH	H	$CH=CH_2$	H	OH

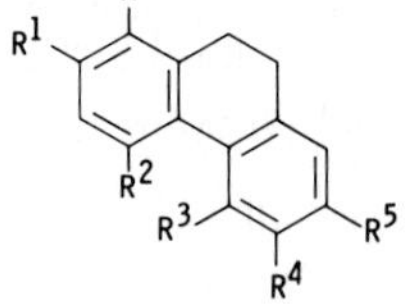

(CLXXXVI)

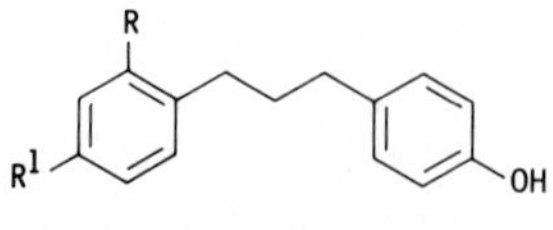

	R	R^1
a broussonin A	OH	OMe
b broussonin B	OMe	OH

(CLXXXVII)

1976) have been isolated from *Euphorbiaceae*. More recently species of *Juncaceae* have furnished variants with vinyl substituents. Juncusol (CLXXXVId) was detected in *Juncus roemerianus* by its cytotoxicity, and its structure confirmed by X-ray diffraction on the diacetate (Miles *et al.*, 1977). Being from an estuarine marsh plant which thrives in areas of high fungal growth, the possibility exists that juncusol is a phytoalexin. Structure–activity relationships have been investigated (Miles *et al.*, 1978) and total syntheses have appeared (Kende and Curran, 1978, 1979; McDonald and Martin, 1978). A mono-hydroxy cometabolite juncunol has also been described (Bhattacharyya and Miles, 1977). The tentatively assigned structure CLXXXVIe has been revised to CLXXXVIf as a result of synthetic studies (Cossey *et al.*, 1980). ^{13}C-NMR spectra have also been reported (Pelletier *et al.*, 1978). A lower homolog of juncusol, 6-norjuncusol or effusol (CLXXXVIg), has been found in the common rush *J. effusus* (Bhattacharyya, 1980). By using an antifungal bioassay we have independently isolated juncusol and effusol from common rush and from hard rush. *J. inflexus* and found activity against *C. albicans* and dermatophytes. The abundance of juncusol in these sources (around 0.5 g/kg dried plant) probably mitigates against it being a phytoalexin.

5. *The Role of Phytoalexins*

The role of phytoalexins and the induction of their formation are still subjects of considerable speculation despite almost 20 years of research in this area. Novel types of phytoalexins are continually being reported—as for example the diphenylpropanes, broussonins A and B (CLXXXVIIa,b) from infected paper mulberry *Broussonetia papyrifera* (Takasugi *et al.*, 1980). It has been hypothesized that since a wide variety of microbial metabolites, many of which are protein synthesis inhibitors, results in the stimulation of phytoalexin production requiring *de novo* RNA and protein synthesis, they must do so by interfering with the negative gene control mechanisms of the host. Genes are thus activated with subsequent dramatic changes in host metabolism (Schwochau and Hadwiger, 1972). That glucans and glycoproteins associated with the microbial cell wall can act as elicitors has also started a search for the molecular basis of the specificity in the "gene-for-gene" relationship between plant cultivars and physiological races of a pathogen. Evidence concerning these concepts is usefully summarized by Dixon and Lamb (1980) and by Grisebach and Ebel (1978).

H. Grisans

The term "grisan" is applied to the spiro-cyclohexanodihydrobenzofuran skeleton present in the well-known antifungal antibiotic griseofulvin

(II). Initially of interest in the control of plant pathogens, griseofulvin has occupied a valuable place in the oral treatment of human and animal dermatophyte diseases for some 20 years; its incorporation into keratin makes it particularly useful in hair and nail infections. Despite the rather large doses for long periods that are sometimes required owing to the fungistatic nature of its action and the need for infected tissue to grow out and regenerate, serious side-effects are of low frequency. The narrow spectrum of activity of griseofulvin is its main limitation, and much effort was expended in the 1960s in searching for improved compounds either in nature or by synthesis or by a combination of both. Incorporation of (+)-griseofulvin, dehydrogriseofulvin or the 1-thia-1-deoxa analog in cultures of *Streptomyces cinereocrocatus* NRRL 3443 for example gave rise to the (+)-5′-hydroxy compounds (II: R = OH, X = O or S) which in addition showed slight activity against *Candida* (Cyanamid: U.S. 3557151, 1968/1971). A marine grisan thelepin (CLXXXVIII)—from the annelid

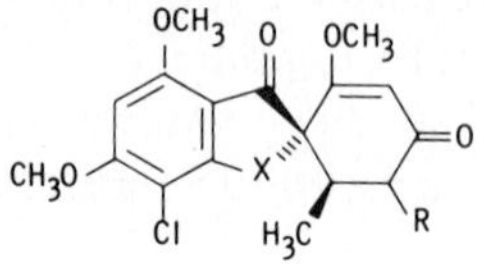

(II) griseofulvin X = O, R = H

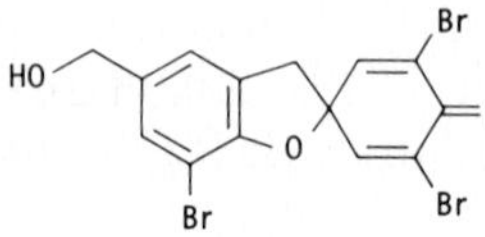

(CLXXXVIII) thelepin

Thelepus setosus—has been reported with biological activity comparable to that of griseofulvin itself (Higa and Scheuer, 1975).

Davies (1980) gives a useful review on the history, toxicology, and pharmacology of griseofulvin and summarizes some of the numerous modes of action which have been attributed to the drug. Of interest in connection with the antimitotic effects of griseofulvin is the demonstration by Roobol *et al.* (1976, 1977) that it is able to inhibit microtubule assembly *in vitro* and that it does this by binding to a microtubule associated protein. Mir *et al.* (1978) have produced somewhat tenuous evidence—correlating inhibition of microtubule polymerization with antifungal and *in vivo* effects of griseofulvin and four of its derivatives—in support of the hypothesis that microtubule proteins are the primary pharmacological target of griseofulvin.

I. Nucleosides

1. *Polyoxins, Neopolyoxins, and Nikkomycins*

The polyoxins are a group of closely related pyrimidine nucleoside peptide antibiotics isolated from *Streptomyces cacaoi* var. *asoensis*

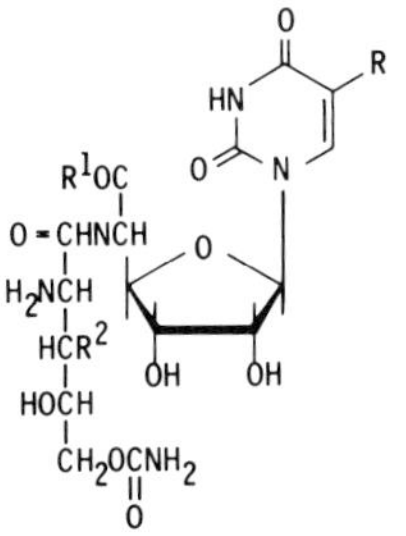

	R	R^1	R^2
a polyoxin A	CH_2OH	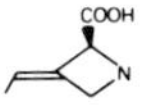 COOH N	OH
b polyoxin B	CH_2OH	HO	OH
d polyoxin D	COOH	HO	OH
e polyoxin E	COOH	HO	H
f polyoxin F	COOH	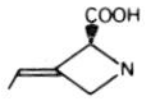 COOH N	OH
g polyoxin G	CH_2OH	HO	H
h polyoxin H	CH_3	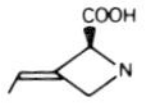 COOH N	OH
j polyoxin J	CH_3	HO	OH
k polyoxin K	H	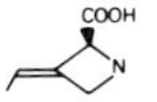 COOH N	OH
l polyoxin L	H	HO	OH
m polyoxin M	H	HO	H

(CLXXXIX)

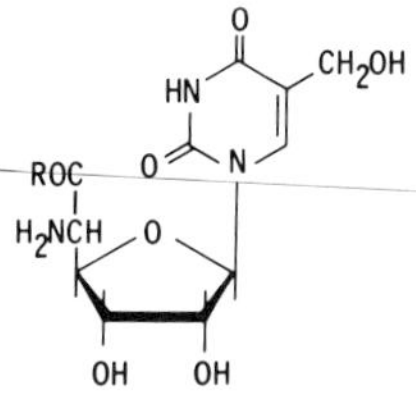

	R
a polyoxin C	HO
b polyoxin I	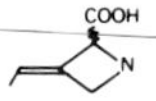 COOH N

(CXC)

(CLXXXIX; CXC; Isono *et al.,* 1969). The compounds act as competitive inhibitors of the fungal enzyme chitin synthetase which is located in or close to the cell wall. This action is probably due to their similarity to the enzyme's natural substrate UDP-*N*-acetylglucosamine (CXCI), and synthesis of the vital cell wall constituent chitin (poly-*N*-acetylglucosamine) is thus blocked. The polyoxins are fungicides effective against certain plant pathogens, particularly *Piricularia oryzae* and *Alternaria kikuchiana,* and this has resulted in their wide-spread commercialization in Japan. The polyoxins are the subject of a comprehensive review by Isono and Suzuki (1979). Although the compounds are active against chitin synthetase isolated from a great variety of species including *Candida,* the activity is not necessarily expressed against the intact organism—as is the case with some yeasts and other resistant species. This may be due to a failure of the polyoxins to penetrate the cell wall, and chemical modification aimed at overcoming this obstacle might well furnish an agent useful in human chemotherapy. Considerable structure–activity work was undertaken by the Japanese after their discovery of the polyoxins, and among the key features identified for binding to chitin synthetase are the terminal peptide residue, the pendant free amino and carboxyl groups, and the uracil base. A synthesis of the basic nucleoside skeleton 1-(5-amino-5-deoxy-β-D-allofuranosyluronic acid)-uracil (polyoxin C) has been reported (Damodaran *et al.*, 1971).

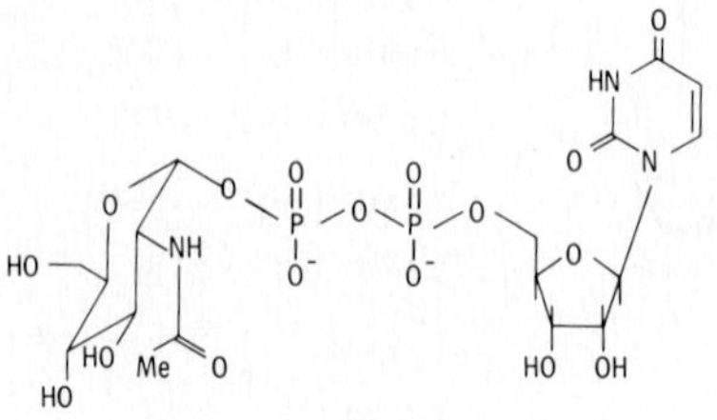

(CXCI) UDP-N-acetylglucosamine

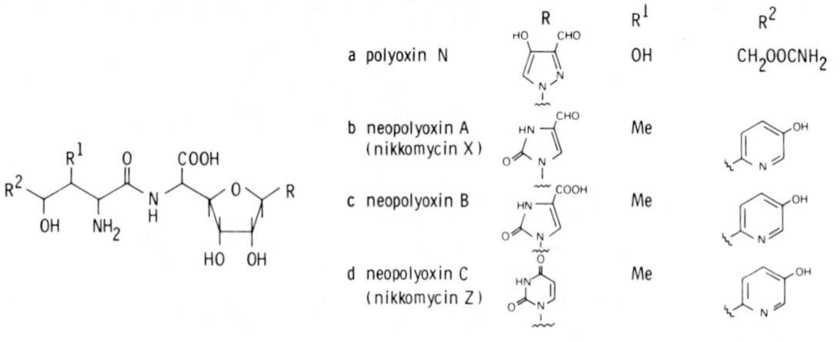

(CXCII)

More recently the production of isomeric neopolyoxins or nikkomycins by other strains of *Streptomyces* has been demonstrated. Polyoxin N (CXCIIa) differs from the other polyoxins in having 3-formyl-4-hydroxypyrazole as the base rather than a pyrimidine (Uramoto *et al.*, 1978). Neopolyoxin A (CXCIIb) has an isomeric nucleobase, and in addition a new peptide amino acid having a 3-hydroxypyridine ring (Kobinata *et al.*, 1980); surprisingly it is active against *C. albicans*. Neopolyoxin B (CXCIIc) has the same peptide side chain but 2-oxo-4-imidazoline-4-carboxylic acid as base, and is inactive against *C. albicans*. Structure CXCIIb has also been isolated as nikkomycin X (Hagenmaier *et al.*, 1979). Nikkomycins Z (CXCIId) and X are also active against fungal chitin synthetases, and open up new vistas in the established structure–activity relationships. Among other structural variations which have been carried out, a transglycosylation reaction was used to prepare the adenine nucleoside corresponding to polyoxin C. Like the latter, it was inactive, but even aminoacyl derivatives only exhibited weak antifungal properties (Azuma and Isono, 1977; Azuma *et al.*, 1977).

Blasticidin S (CXCIIIa) is a cytosine nucleoside peptide in which the sugar is a Δ^2-4-amino-2,3,4-trideoxyglucuronic acid bearing the blastidoyl chain (CXCIIIa: R^2). Although it is active against experimental candidosis in mice, no activity was detected *in vitro*. It does however inhibit protein synthesis in intact cells of *Candida* in contrast to puromycin and cycloheximide, which are effective only in cell-free systems. Blasticidin S is therefore able—like 5-FC—to penetrate the cell wall. Despite fairly high

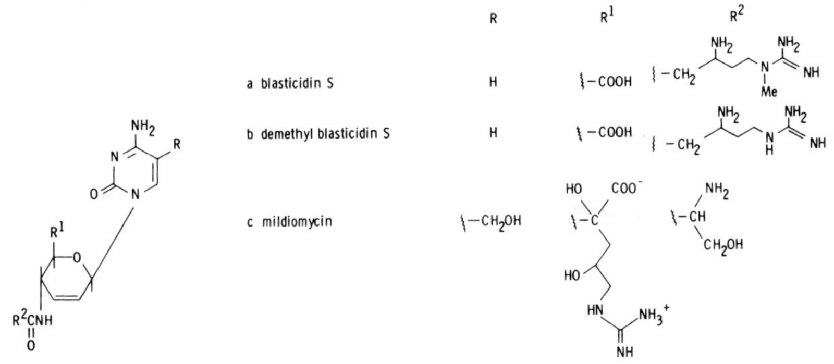

	R	R^1	R^2
a blasticidin S	H	$-COOH$	$-CH_2$–CH(NH_2)–CH$_2$–CH$_2$–N(Me)–C(NH_2)=NH
b demethyl blasticidin S	H	$-COOH$	$-CH_2$–CH(NH_2)–CH$_2$–CH$_2$–NH–C(NH_2)=NH
c mildiomycin	$-CH_2OH$	–C(HO)(COO$^-$)–CH$_2$–CH(HO)–CH$_2$–HN–C(=NH)–NH_3^+	–CH(NH_2)–CH_2OH

(CXCIII)

	R	R^1	R^2
a blasticidin H	OH	$-CH_2$–CH(NH_2)–CH$_2$–CH$_2$–N(Me)–C(NH_2)=NH	H
b gougerotin	NH_2	MeHN–CH$_2$–C(=O)–NH–CH(CH$_2$OH)–	OH

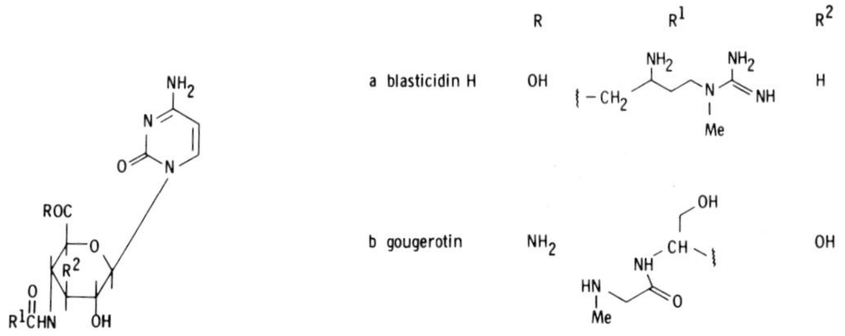

(CXCIV)

mammalian and plant toxicity, it has found wide use in Japan in the control of rice blast caused by *Piricularia oryzae* (Dekker, 1971; Arai, 1974). The homolog in which the guanidine group is not methylated (CXCIIIb) is equiactive and with similar toxicity in mice (Seto and Yonehara, 1977b). *Streptomyces griseochromogenes* also produces blasticidin H (CXCIVa), differing from blasticidin S only by hydration of the sugar Δ^2-double bond (Seto and Yonehara, 1977a). This change however results in a loss of most of the biological activity. Gougerotin (CXCIVb), a cytosine glucuronic acid derivative, shows only very weak antibacterial properties (Dolak, 1979). Another related compound, mildiomycin (CXCIIIc) from *Streptoverticillium rimofaciens* B-98891, has 5-hydroxymethylcytosine as base. It is remarkably nontoxic to mammals and fish, but is only of significant antifungal interest in the control of powdery mildews such as *Erysiphe graminis* (Iwasa *et al.*, 1978).

Ezomycin A_1 and A_2 (CXCVa,d) are cytosine-based, but ezomycins B_1 and B_2, C_1 and C_2 (CXCVb,e,c,f), and D_1 and D_2 (CXCVIa,b) are the first examples of C–C linked pseudouridine nucleoside antibiotics. The ezomycins A–C have a bicyclic anhydrooctose uronic acid instead of ribose attached to 3-amino-3,4-dideoxyglucuronic acid, usually bearing L-cystathionine (Sakata *et al.*, 1977a,b). Interestingly, the first examples of naturally occurring bicyclic anhydrooctose uronic acid nucleosides were

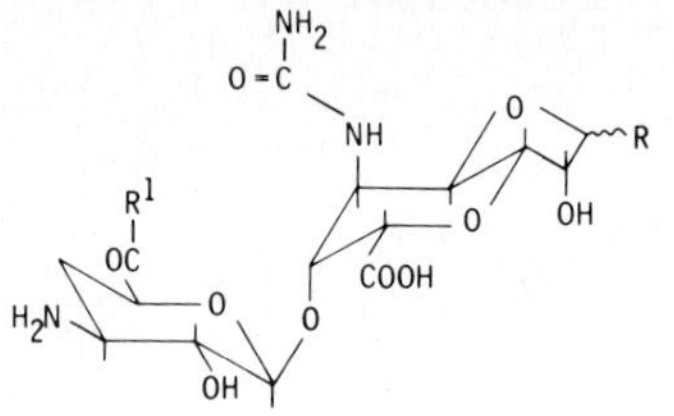

		R	R^1
a	ezomycin A_1	β-1-cytosine	$HOOC-CH(NH_2)-CH_2-S-CH_2-CH_2-CH(COOH)-NH-$
b	ezomycin B_1	β-5-uracil	"
c	ezomycin C_1	α-5-uracil	"
d	ezomycin A_2	β-1-cytosine	OH
e	ezomycin B_2	β-5-uracil	OH
f	ezomycin C_2	α-5-uracil	OH

(CXCV)

		R	R^1
a	ezomycin D_1	5-uracil	$HOOC-CH(NH_2)-CH_2-S-CH_2-CH_2-CH(COOH)-NH-$
b	ezomycin D_2	5-uracil	OH

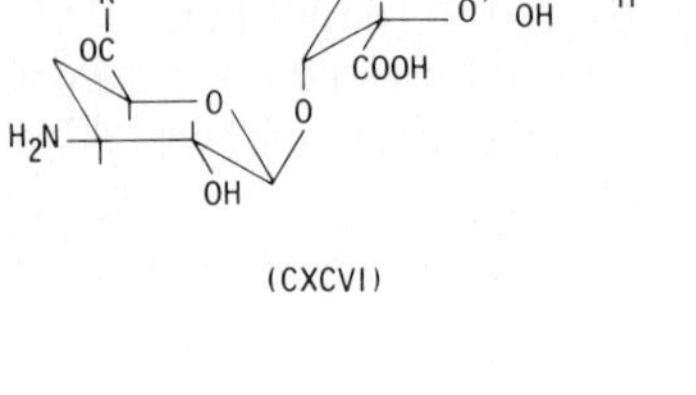

(CXCVI)

the analogous octosyl acids A, B, and C, which are cometabolites of the polyoxins (Isono *et al.,* 1975); ezomycins and polyoxins share a common sugar skeleton. Ablastmycin, bulgerin, antibiotic SF-1508, and ileumycin are nucleoside antibiotics which share the limited antifungal spectrum of the ezomycins, and whose complete structures remain to be determined (Kawakami *et al.,* 1978).

2. *Tunicamycins*

Another family of uridine nucleoside antibiotics of *Streptomyces* origin which interferes with a different aspect of fungal metabolism—peptidoglycan synthesis—is the tunicamycin (tsunikamycin) complex, initially isolated from *S. lysosuperificus.* Four components A–D (CXCVIIe,g,b,j) were eventually characterized, differing from each other by the length of the α,β-unsaturated fatty acid of the *iso* series they contain (Takatsuki *et al.,* 1977). HPLC has now enabled 10 tunicamycins to be separated and identified (CXCVIIa–j; Ito *et al.,* 1980). All have a common tunicaminyl uracil residue (CXCVIII) bearing *N*-acetylglucosamine via a 1″, 1‴-saccharide bond and the fatty acid as an amide function. Tunicaminyl uracil itself is an acid hydrolysis product of tunicamycins (Ito *et al.,* 1979). The tunicamycins have been found in several distinct species of *Streptomyces,* including the clavulanic acid producer *S. clavuligerus* (Currie *et al.,* 1979; Kenig and Reading, 1979). It now appears that the mycospodins are identical to tunicamycins and that antibiotics 24010 and

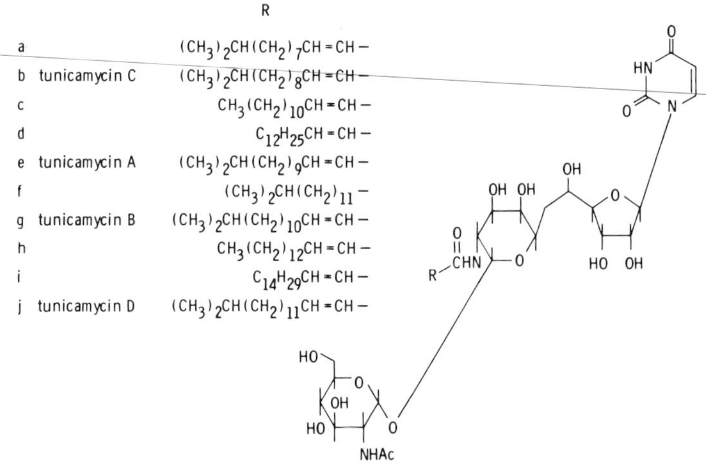

		R
a		$(CH_3)_2CH(CH_2)_7CH=CH-$
b	tunicamycin C	$(CH_3)_2CH(CH_2)_8CH=CH-$
c		$CH_3(CH_2)_{10}CH=CH-$
d		$C_{12}H_{25}CH=CH-$
e	tunicamycin A	$(CH_3)_2CH(CH_2)_9CH=CH-$
f		$(CH_3)_2CH(CH_2)_{11}-$
g	tunicamycin B	$(CH_3)_2CH(CH_2)_{10}CH=CH-$
h		$CH_3(CH_2)_{12}CH=CH-$
i		$C_{14}H_{29}CH=CH-$
j	tunicamycin D	$(CH_3)_2CH(CH_2)_{11}CH=CH-$

(CXCVII)

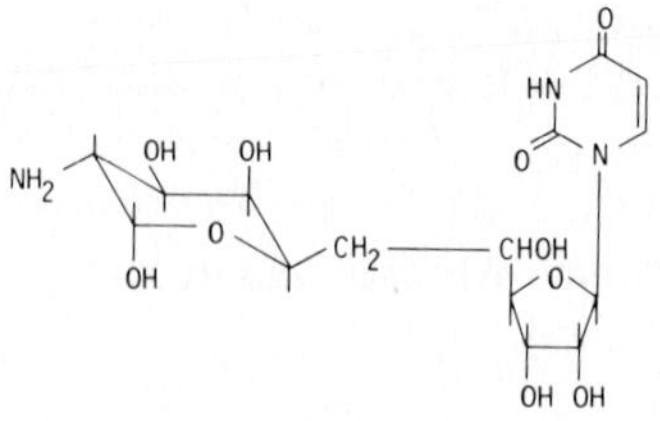

(CXCVIII) tunicaminyl uracil

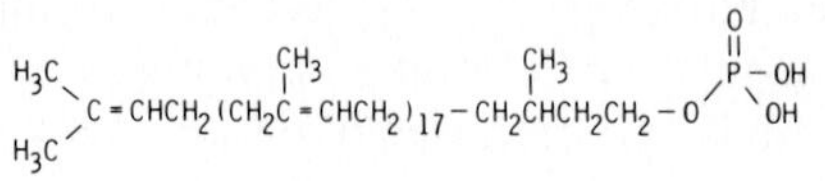

(CIC) dolichol phosphate

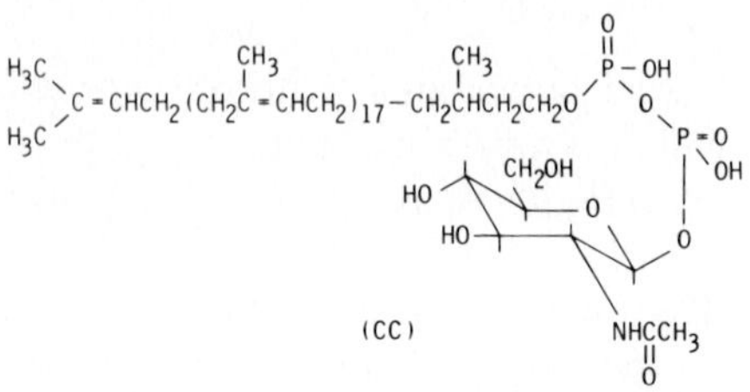

(CC)

MM 19290 are members of this family, as are the streptovirudins (Eckardt *et al.,* 1975) which contain smaller hydrophobic groups (Tkacz, 1980).

In addition to inhibiting the growth of yeasts and fungi—especially the rice pathogen *Piricularia oryzae*—the tunicamycins are active against gram-positive bacteria, viruses, and murine leukemia L1210, and their activity against coccidia has been patented (Meiji: JAP. 79055737, 1977/1979). Their main interest however is as a biochemical tool since they specifically inhibit the first step in the lipid-linked oligosaccharide pathway via dolichol phosphate (CIC) to *N*-acetylglucosaminylpyrophosphoryldolichol (CC) (Heifetz *et al.,* 1979). Evidence points to irreversible inhibition of the *N*-acetylglucosaminyl-1-pyrophosphate transferase by way of a substrate–product transition state analogy. The tunicamycins have activity in avian and mammalian systems, and transformed cells are markedly more sensitive than normal cells (Kohno *et al.,* 1979). The development of tunicamycins toward clinical use as antifungal agents appears to have been halted.

3. *Purine Derivatives*

The two major antibiotics produced by *Streptomyces griseolus* contain an L-ornithine residue linked by the δ-carbon atom to C-5′ of adenosine. Sinefungin (CCIa) is highly active *in vitro* against *C. albicans* and is equipotent with amphotericin B in mice, whereas the 4′,5′-didehydroanalog of CICa, factor C, is somewhat less so (Berry and Abbott, 1978). *Streptomyces incarnatus* can be fermented to give antibiotic RP 32232, seemingly identical to sinefungin (Rhône-Poulenc: DT. 2736238, 1977/1979), together with its cyclic lactam derivative antibiotic

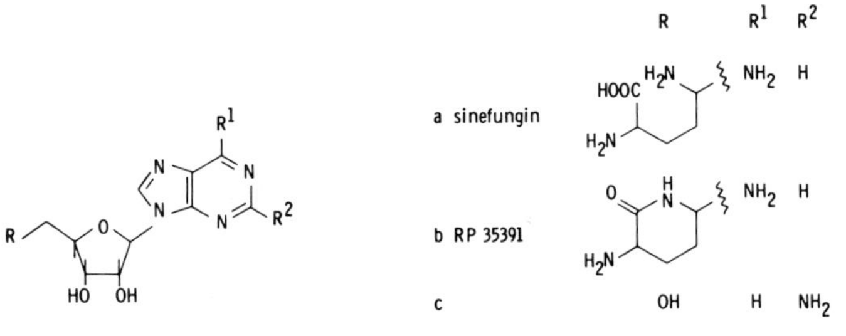

	R	R^1	R^2
a sinefungin		NH_2	H
b RP 35391		NH_2	H
c	OH	H	NH_2

(CCI)

RP 35391 (CCIb). *In vitro* and *in vivo* activity against *Candida* and systemic mycoses is claimed, with low acute oral toxicity in mice. Unfortunately sinefungin produces bone marrow toxicity, precluding its use clinically. Sinefungin is a "carba" structural analog of *S*-adenosylmethionine and *S*-adenylhomocysteine. In chick embryo fibroblasts it is a competitive inhibitor of tRNA methylases and of protein methylases (Vedel *et al.*, 1978). Calf thymus and bovine adrenal protein *O*-methyl transferases are also inhibited (Borchardt *et al.*, 1979). Other systems, e.g., viral mRNA (guanine-7) methyl transferase, viral mRNA (nucleoside 2′) methyl transferase, norepinephrine and histamine *N*-methyl transferases, and catechol-*O*-methyl transferases, have also been studied (Pugh *et al.*, 1978).

Amipurimycin is an antibiotic from *Streptomyces novoguineensis* with *in vitro* activity against *T. mentagrophytes* (10 μg/ml), and against phytopathogens *in vitro* and *in vivo* (Iwasa *et al.*, 1977). It is the first natural product example of a 2-aminopurine nucleoside and has been compared with 2-aminopurine-9-β-D-riboside (CCIc), a product obtained biosynthetically using cell-free systems from *E. coli*. Amipurimycin has high toxicity to rats and mice both iv and orally.

J. Peptides

Few peptides have found a place in human chemotherapy. In the treatment of deep-seated fungal infections, saramycetin—a polyacidic peptide of molecular weight around 14000 isolated from *Streptomyces saraceticus*—has had limited trials in man. Administered subcutaneously at a dose of 4–8 mg/kg daily, it was studied in cases involving *Histoplasma capsulatum, Blastomyces dermatitidis, Coccidioides immitis,* and *Sporothrix schenckii* (D'Arcy and Scott, 1978). Saramycetin hydrolyses to give the amino acids aspartic acid, glycine, proline, threonine, cystine, and a thiazolidine derivative.

1. *Diketopiperazines*

Of the lower molecular weight compounds, cyclic dipeptides provide numerous examples with biological activity; these fall into two main types, diketopiperazines and the 3,6-epi-dithia-bridged compounds. Epicorazine A (CCII) from the fungus *Epicoccum nigrum* is an elaborate example based on a modified phenylalanylphenylalanine (Deffieux *et al.*, 1978). More interesting antifungal properties have been described for hyalodendrin (CCIII) and for antibiotic A-30641 (CCIV). Hyalodendrin is a simple relative of phenylalanylserine—obtained from a *Hyalodendron* species —which has been found to prevent the germination of sporangia of *Phytophthora infestans* and to be active *in vitro* against *T. mentagrophytes*

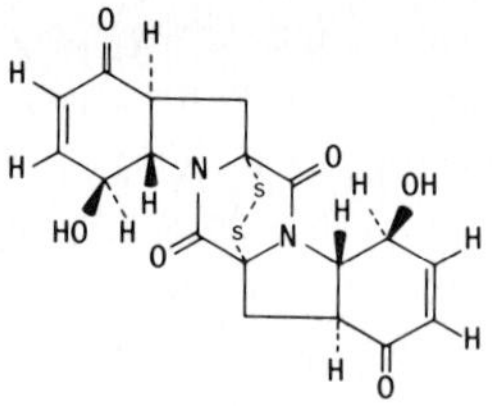

(CCII) epicorazine A

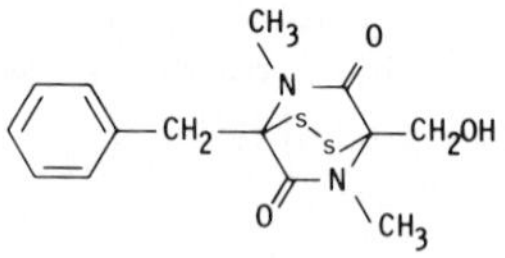

(CCIII) hyalodendrin

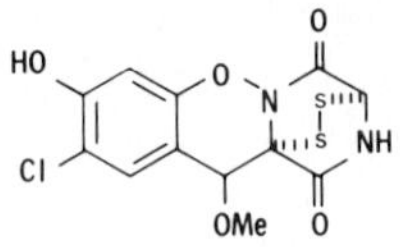

(CCIV) antibiotic A-30641

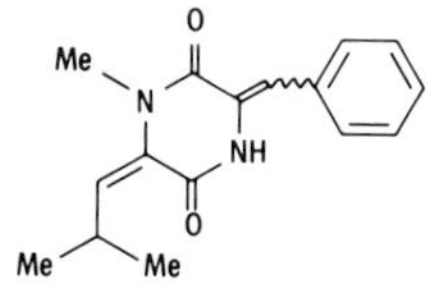

(CCV) N-methylalbonoursin

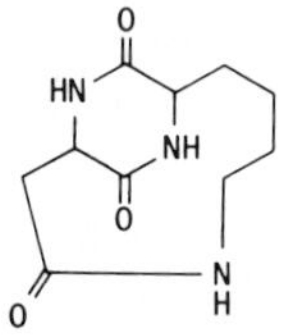

(CCVI) cairomycin

(12.5 μg/ml) and *C. albicans* (25 μg/ml; Stillwell *et al.*, 1974). Conversion to the acetate does not affect its antifungal properties, whereas a cometabolite in which the disulfide bridge has been replaced by two methylthio groups is devoid of activity. *Aspergillus tamarii* is the source of antibiotic A-30641, a curious tetracyclic compound with only marginal antiviral properties but with good activity against yeasts and fungi (Berg *et al.*, 1976). In general the absence of the disulfide bridge results in greatly reduced antimicrobial potency. *N*-Methylalbonoursin (CCV), isolated in these laboratories from an unidentified *Streptomyces*, is a cyclic dehydroleucinyldehydrophenylalanine with a very modest effect on dermatophytes. Similarly cairomycin B (CCVI), a lactam related to lysylaspartic acid, has limited antimicrobial activity (Shimi *et al.*, 1977).

2. *Other Cyclic Peptides*

This group includes some of the most interesting antifungal antibiotics. Benz *et al.* (1974) described the isolation from *Aspergillus nidulans* var.

echinulatus of a novel polypeptide complex with potent activity specifically against growing yeasts. The major component echinocandin B (MIC 0.2–0.35 μg/ml against *C. albicans*) was later shown to be identical to antibiotic SL 7810 from *A. rugulosus,* and the structure CCVIIb deduced for it from X-ray crystallographic studies of an ether derivative of tetrahydroechinocandin B (Keller-Juslén *et al.,* 1976). In addition to

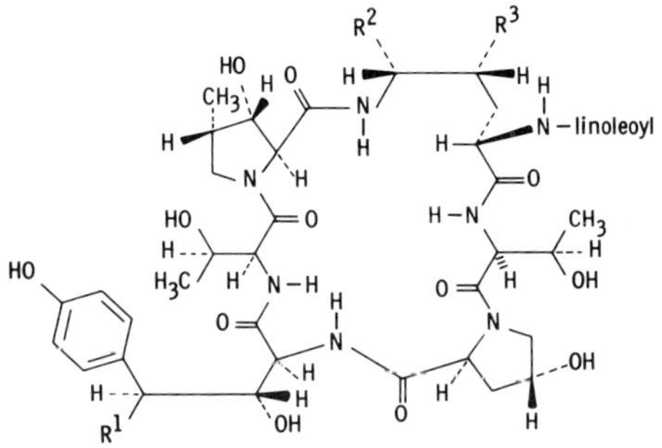

		R^1	R^2	R^3
b	echinocandin B	OH	OH	OH
c	echinocandin C	H	OH	OH
d	echinocandin D	H	H	H

(CCVII)

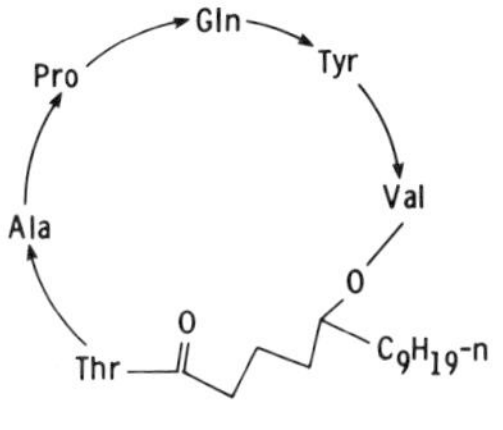

(CCVIII) MSD-A43F

linoleic acid, echinocandin B contains six amino acids, of which 4,5-dihydroxyornithine, 3,4-dihydroxyhomotyrosine, and 3-hydroxy-4-methylproline are unusual. Echinocandins C and D (CCVIIc,d) contain less hydroxyl groups (Traber *et al.,* 1979). A series of patents covering aminoalkyl ethers of tetrahydroechinocandin B and related compounds (including aculeacin A) has appeared (Sandoz: DT. 2704030, 1976/1977; DT. 2742435, 1976/1978; DT. 2803581, 1978/1979; DT. 2803584, 1978/1979). The effect of these antibiotics on yeast cell wall synthesis has been investigated (Baguley *et al.,* 1979). Using *Saccharomyces cerevisiae* it was found that echinocandin B caused a selective inhibition of glucose incorporation into alkali-insoluble glucan. A mutant of *C. albicans* resistant to papulacandin B (CILb) was also insensitive to echinocandin B, and no effect on glucan synthesis by this mutant was observed.

Aculeacins A–G are produced by *Aspergillus aculeatus* (Satoi *et al.,*

1977). They are closely related to the echinocandins but liberate palmitic rather than linoleic acid on alkaline hydrolysis; their biological spectrum follows a close parallel: they are virtually inactive against bacteria, extremely potent fungicides against yeasts (except *C. tropicalis*), and are fungistatic at very low concentrations to filamentous fungi such as dermatophytes. No fungicidal effect was observed even at 25 μg/ml. The LD_{50} of aculeacin A in mice is 350 mg/kg iv, and experimental infections in mice have confirmed interest (Mizuno *et al.*, 1977). Aculeacin D is two to four times more active than aculeacin A against yeasts *in vitro*. Like echinocandins, aculeacin A has been shown to inhibit glucan synthesis—which occurs particularly at the tips of the buds of growing yeasts—resulting in lysis (Mizoguchi *et al.*, 1977). By contrast, 2-deoxyglucose inhibits both UDP-glucose mediated glucan synthesis and GDP-mannose/dolichol phosphate mediated mannan synthesis. An antifungal peptide of unknown structure, antibiotic K-73, which hydrolyses to give alanine, aspartic acid, glutamic acid, glycine, isoleucine, threonine, and valine, has also been reported from *A. rugulosus* (Dasgupta *et al.*, 1970).

Cultures of *Verticillium lamellicola* produce another cyclic hexapeptide MSD-A43F (CCVIII; Albers-Schönberg *et al.*, 1979). A 5-hydroxymyristic acid group forms a bridge across the peptide by acylating a threonine hydroxyl and esterifying a valine carboxylic acid group; its biological activity is however of a low order. *Aeromonas* sp. W-10 produces a mixture of up to six antifungal antibiotics—referred to as the W-10 complex—from which two substances have been isolated and identified (Schering Corp.: U.S. 4137224, 1977/1979). Antibiotics 20561 and 20562

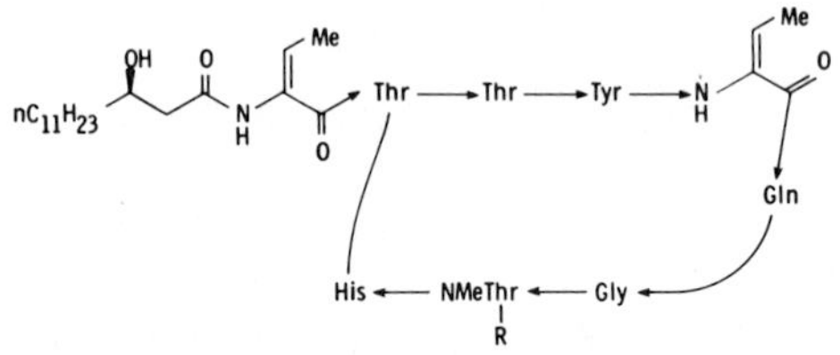

		R
	antibiotic 20561	H
(CCIX)	antibiotic 20562	glucosyl

(CCIX) are both cyclic octapeptides, the *N*-methylthreonine component of 20562 being glucosylated. Antibiotic 20562 is active *in vitro* against *C. albicans* at 0.075 μg/ml, and a single dose of 4 mg/kg sc or 25 mg/kg by mouth protects mice against a lethal systemic infection with *C. albicans;* toxicity is low, the LD_{50} in mice being 600 mg/kg sc or 800 mg/kg by mouth. *Candida* vaginitis in hamsters and *T. mentagrophytes* infections in guinea pigs were controlled by topical treatment with antibiotic 20562, but no indication is given as to whether these infections would respond to systemic medication. In fact the inventors see these antibiotics as potential topical rather than systemic remedies. Lipopeptin A from *Streptomyces violaceochromogenes* is a cyclic octapeptide with a C_{15} fatty side-chain and a similar structure (Isono *et al.,* 1980). Again toxicity is low, but so is activity. It inhibits peptidoglycan synthesis in *E. coli* at 150 μg/ml and incorporation of mannose from GDP-mannose into proteoglycan (mannan) in *Piricularia oryzae* (Tsuda *et al.,* 1980). Fermentation of *Erwinia herbicola* in carbohydrate-rich media produces herbicolins A and B; they are inactive against bacteria, but highly active against *Candida* and dermatophytes. Other eukaryotic cells are also affected by herbicolins, and since their activity is reversed by sterols and cardiolipins, they would appear to be membrane-active. Herbicolin A consists of seven amino acid residues—2 glycines, L-threonine, D-*allo*-threonine, D-glutamine, D-leucine, and L-arginine—and 3-hydroxymyristic acid (Winkelmann *et al.,* 1980).

Bacillus subtilis has furnished several series of antifungal cyclic peptidolipids (Shoji, 1978), e.g., the iturin group characterized by a highly lipophilic β-amino acid linked to a peptide, again consisting of both D- and L-α-amino acids (Besson *et al.,* 1978, 1979). It includes iturin A (CCX), bacillomycin L (CCXI), and with a slightly larger nine component ring and longer β-amino acid, mycosubtilin (CCXII). Investigation of the antifun-

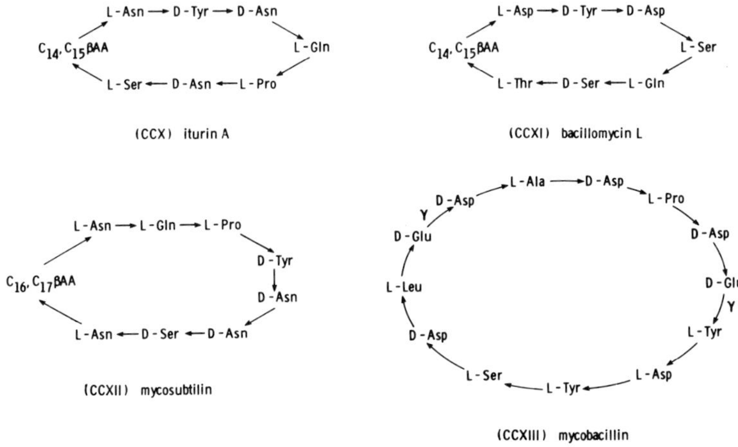

gal activity of these antibiotics and some derivatives has underlined the importance of the hydroxyl and phenolic groups (Peypoux *et al.,* 1979). They may act via an interaction with lipid components of the cytoplasmic membrane, being particularly strongly antagonized by cholesterol, and to a varying degree by some phospholipids. Thirteen residues comprised of seven different α-amino acids make up the ring of mycobacillin (CCXIII)—also from *B. subtilis* (Banerjee and Bose, 1963). It has been mainly evaluated as an agricultural fungicide (Nandi *et al.,* 1975). Although mycobacillin contains no long-chain fatty acid units, its antifungal activity is antagonized by cholesterol—as with the iturin group—and by oleic acid—in which the *cis*-configuration of the 9,10-double bond is essential. Derivatives in which the tyrosine phenol groups are acylated retain some antifungal properties, but are no longer antagonized in the same way (Mukherjee and Bose, 1978); the serine hydroxyl and the seven carboxylic acid groups do not appear to be involved in the antagonism. Elucidation of the structures of several *B. subtilis* antifungal peptides is still awaited. Subsporin A contains 14 amino acids (Ebata *et al.,* 1969), and like manilosporins C_1 and C_2 (Hoechst: DT. 2732467, 1977/1979), is active against phytopathogenic fungi and dermatophytes. Alboleutin is the most recent of these peptides, acid hydrolysis furnishing leucine, aspartic acid, glutamic acid, and valine in a ratio of 4 : 1 : 1 : 1 (Omura *et al.,* 1980b).

In addition to lipopeptin A, a number of other cyclic peptide antibiotics is elaborated by *Streptomyces,* ranging in complexity from griseoviridin (from *S. griseus*) to stendomycin (from *S. endus*). Griseoviridin is a tricyclic compound derived from a δ-hydroxyhexanoic acid and the amino acids D-cysteine, serine, and an ω-aminodecanoic acid (Birnbaum and Hall, 1976), whereas stendomycin has 14 amino acids. Seven of these are in a ring and include L-stendomycidine (L-(1-methyl-2-methylamino-1,4,5,6-tetrahydropyrimidin-6-yl)glycine); the side chain terminates in a proline residue *N*-acylated with one of several iso-series fatty acids (Bodanszky *et al.,* 1969). Pantomycin, recently isolated from *S. hygroscopicus,* gives a very similar hydrolysate to stendomycin with the additional presence of carbohydrate (Gurusiddaiah *et al.,* 1979).

3. *Other Peptides*

Fungal fruiting bodies often contain physiologically active metabolites and toxins. Thus hypelcins A and B have been obtained from the fruiting bodies of *Hypocrea peltata* (Fujita *et al.,* 1979). Hypelcin A (CCXIV) is a linear peptide of 20 residues with a high content of α-aminoisobutyric acid (Aib), and having *N*-acetyl-Aib as N-terminal and leucinol as C-terminal

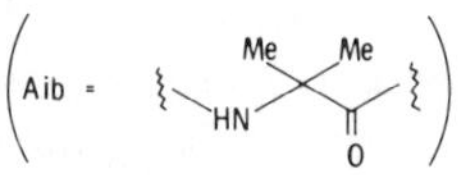

(Aib = –HN–C(Me)(Me)–C(=O)–)

$CH_3C(=O)$–Aib-Pro-Aib-Ala-Aib-Aib-Gln-Leu-Aib-Gly-Aib-Aib-Aib-Pro-Val-Aib-Aib-Gln-Gln-Leuol

(CCXIV) hypelcin A

residues. Trichopolyns A and B (Fuji *et al.,* 1978), trichotoxin A-40 (Irmscher *et al.,* 1978), and alamethicins (Pandey *et al.,* 1977) also contain Aib, the latter having phenylalaninol as the C-terminus. The hypelcins and trichopolyns inhibit the growth of the Japanese edible fungus *Lentinus eddodes,* and the trichopolyns have good *in vitro* activity against *C. albicans* (MIC 6.25 μg/ml) and *T. mentagrophytes* (MIC 0.78 μg/ml). These peptides appear to be membrane-exciting or pore-forming antibiotics.

K. Aminoglycosides and Other Sugars

1. *Aminoglycosides*

The use of antibiotics composed of unusual sugars, particularly aminodeoxy derivatives, is well-known in the treatment of gram-negative bacterial infections, and a great deal of effort has been devoted to semisynthetic modification in order to minimize side effects such as nephro- and oto-toxicity in mammals. Many of the antifungal antibiotics discussed in preceding sections contain a sugar or aminodeoxy sugar; e.g., mycosamine (3-amino-3,6-dideoxy-D-mannose) and perosamine (4-amino-4,6-dideoxy-D-mannose) occur in the polyenes where they may be very important for activity. Candihexins E and F do not have a mycosamine unit and are inactive, while candihexins A and B which do contain mycosamine are highly active as antifungals (Martín and Gil, 1979). Oleficin (CLXIIa), ambruticin (CXLVII), and papulacandins (CIL) all bear modified sugar units which contribute in different degrees to their antifungal activity. In one case the sugar may be important simply to confer the right distribution properties on the molecule, while in another it may be absolutely critical for recognition by the target enzyme(s), e.g., glucan synthetase. The nucleoside antibiotics also contain a sugar—frequently ribose, but sometimes modified—attached to the nucleobase. The sugar often carries an elaborate chain which can be variously regarded as an oxidized aminodeoxysugar or as a polyfunctional amino acid [e.g., the polyoxins (CLXXXIX)]; alternatively it may bear other sugars [e.g., tunicamycin (CXCVII), ezomycins (CXCV)]. It is well known that certain sugars, e.g., 2-deoxyglucose, are competitive inhibitors of cell wall synthesis enzymes. The aminoglycoside antibacterials have a totally different point of intervention—that of protein synthesis at the 70 S ribosome level. They inhibit the nonenzymatic binding of aminoacyl RNA to messenger RNA-containing ribosomes. The basic aminocyclitol kasugamycin (CCXV) seems to have this mode of action in *Piricularia oryzae*. Kasugamycin is obtained from *Streptomyces kasugensis,* and has become an important agricultural fungicide for the treatment of rice blast.

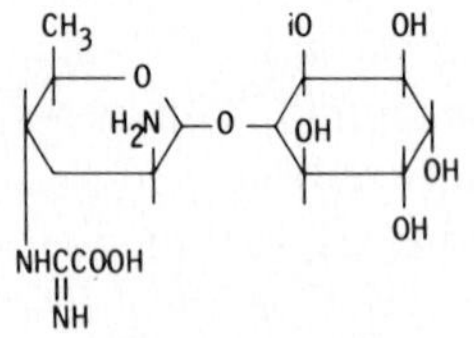

(CCXV) kasugamycin

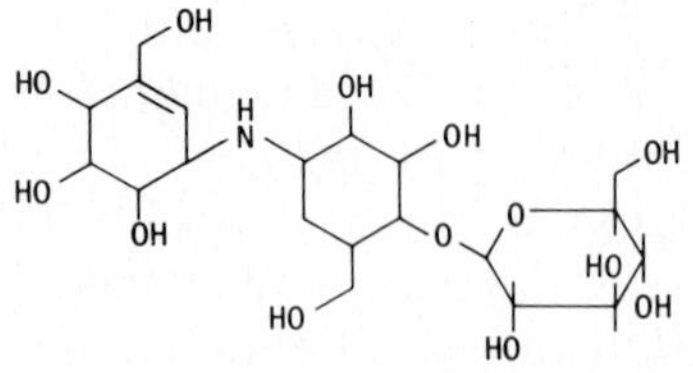

(CCXVI) validamycin

It is relatively nontoxic to mammals and to fish and thus has some clear advantages over blasticidin S (CXCIIIa) which it is replacing.

Streptomyces hygroscopicus produces the validamycin aminoglycosides, the structures of which have recently been revised (Suami *et al.,* 1980). Validamycin A (CCXVI) has β-D-glucopyranose attached to the 4-position of the validoxylamine A nucleus. In order to improve antifungal potency against rice sheath blight, *Pellicularia oryzae,* and to elucidate the biological significance of differences in the glycosidic component, microbial glucosidation and galactosidation of validoxylamine A have been investigated (Kameda *et al.,* 1980). Inhibition of *Rhizoctonia solani* is antagonized by a hyphal extract of *R. solani,* i.e., possibly by a factor involved in hyphal extension (Shibata *et al.,* 1980).

N-Carbamoyl-D-glucosamine (CCXVII) is a metabolite of *Streptomyces halstedii* and is active against gram-negative bacteria and some fungi (Omoto *et al.,* 1979). Unlike the antibiotic nojirimycin, it does not inhibit glucosidase. On standing at room temperature for several days, it cyclizes to the inactive imidazolinone CCXVIII. Another inhibitor of protein synthesis of *Streptomyces* origin is prumycin (CCXIX), a 4-D-alanyl

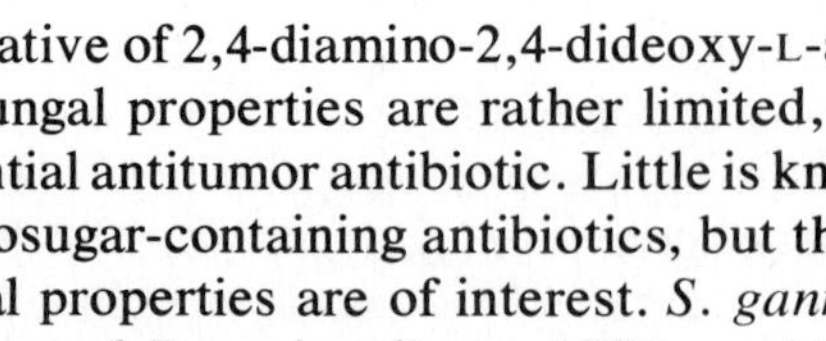

(CCXVII) (CCXVIII) 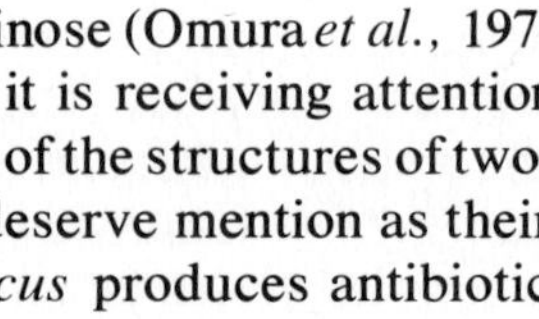 (CCXIX) prumycin

derivative of 2,4-diamino-2,4-dideoxy-L-arabinose (Omura *et al.,* 1974). Its antifungal properties are rather limited, but it is receiving attention as a potential antitumor antibiotic. Little is known of the structures of two other aminosugar-containing antibiotics, but they deserve mention as their antifungal properties are of interest. *S. ganmycicus* produces antibiotic S-15 (Sinha and Basuchaudhary, 1977), and *S. yokosukaensis* produces antibiotic H-537-SY2, which contains three amino sugars and is active against *Candida* (Kondo *et al.,* 1976).

2. *Other Sugar Derivatives*

A novel fungus of the genus *Pyrenochaeta* has been reported to give the unusual D-mannitol-1,6-diester, antibiotic A 32390A (CCXX; Turner *et al.*, 1978). It is the acyl groups which make this compound particularly striking, since they are derived from 2-isocyano-3-methylcrotonic acid; isonitrile is usually considered a fairly reactive and unpleasant group. This compound is active against gram-positive bacteria and against *C. albicans* *in vitro* (MIC 20 μg/ml) and *in vivo* (at doses down to 12.5 mg/kg × 3 in mice, sc or ip, but not oral), and although it inhibits dopamine β-hydroxylase and lowers blood pressure in hypertensive rats, it is well tolerated by mice. The 6-mono- and 2,6-diacetyl derivatives of 4-*O*-β-D-3′-palmitoylmannopyranosyl-D-erythritol have been isolated from a smut fungus parasitic on a *Carex* species, *Schizonella melanogramma*, and named schizonellins A and B (CCXXIa,b; Deml *et al.*, 1980). They have a detergent-like action and are strongly hemolytic to bovine erythrocytes.

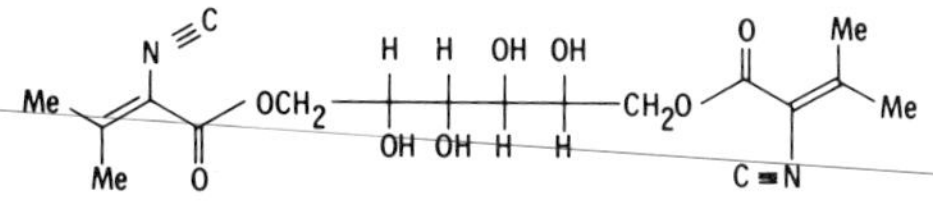

(CCXX) antibiotic A 32390A

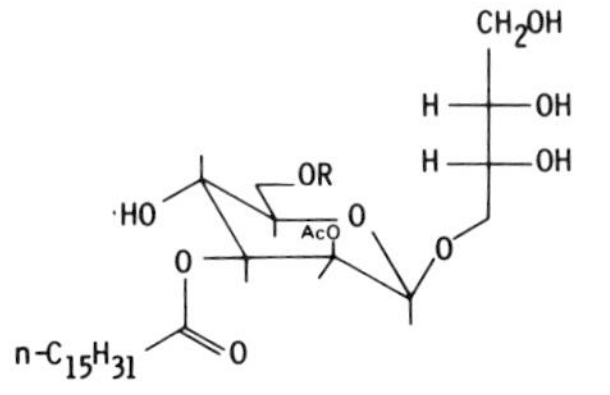

	R
a schizonellin A	H
b schizonellin B	Ac

(CCXXI)

L. Miscellaneous Compounds

1. *β-Lactams*

Fifty years have elapsed since Fleming's original observation, which has led to the antibacterial penicillins, cephalosporins, carbapenems, and beyond. It is only in the last few years however that a few semisynthetic β-lactams have been found to have antifungal activity. The only example in the penicillin series is a patent covering a phenylglycylamino side chain *N*-acylated with pteridine-6-carboxylic acid derivatives (Mitsubishi: JAP. 78124296, 1977/1978). Several patents addressed to cephems (Asahi: JAP. 78124283, 1977/1978), some with isothiourea branching on an otherwise normal arylacylamido side chain (Yeda: U.S. 4125715, 1977/1978), have appeared. 3-Trifluoromethylcephem-4-carboxylic acids are specifically covered for use against fungi (Sankyo: JAP. 78124287, 1977/1978). Several cephems related to cephalexin, but with a 2-methylmercaptopyridine-*N*-oxide substituent at the 3-position inhibit the growth of *T. mentagrophytes* and *C. albicans in vitro* (Uri *et al.,* 1978). No protection is afforded against *C. albicans in vivo,* however, although these compounds exhibit broad-spectrum antibacterial activity both *in vitro* and *in vivo.* Another patent describes 2-keto-oxacepham and 2-ketocepham and ceph-3-em-4-carboxylic acids as antifungal agents (Fujisawa: G.B. 2022092A, 1978/1979). Workers at Glaxo have now found three antifungal β-lactams from *S. clavuligerus*—better known for producing the β-lactamase inhibitor clavulanic acid. The active compounds are the clavams CCXXIIa,b,c, which are particularly effective against plant fun-

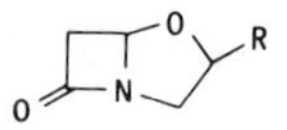

	R
a	CH_2OH
b	CH_2OCOH
c	CO_2H

(CCXXII)

gal pathogens, but also have activity against *C. albicans* and dermatophytes (Brown *et al.,* 1979).

2. *Inhibitors of Steroid Biosynthesis*

Ergosterol and its congeners are important constituents of the fungal membrane. Interference with these sterols, either by association—as occurs with the polyenes—or by inhibition of their synthesis—as is the case with the imidazoles—results in membrane disruption and eventual lysis. Clearly these effects could be antagonistic if both types of agent were used together. There are several biosynthetic steps leading to sterols which may be blocked. The rate-limiting enzyme in mammalian hepatocytes is 3-hydroxy-3-methylglutaryl-CoA reductase (3HMGCoA-reductase), an early step in the sequence to cholesterol. The *Pythiaceae* is a family of fungi which do not make detectable amounts of sterols, but rather contain squalene, though not squalene oxide. It may be presumed therefore that the natural biosynthetic block in this case is at the squalene oxidase level (Gottlieb *et al.,* 1978). *N*-Dodecylimidazole interferes specifically with 2,3-oxidosqualene cyclase in the rat, and in *Ustilago maydis* it inhibits C-14 demethylation, 2,3-oxidosqualene cyclization, and subsequent transmethylation, probably by binding to a sterol carrier protein. Miconazole (VII) and a number of other imidazoles have been assayed for their ability to inhibit ergosterol biosynthesis in *C. albicans* at the C-14 demethylation step (Marriott, 1980).

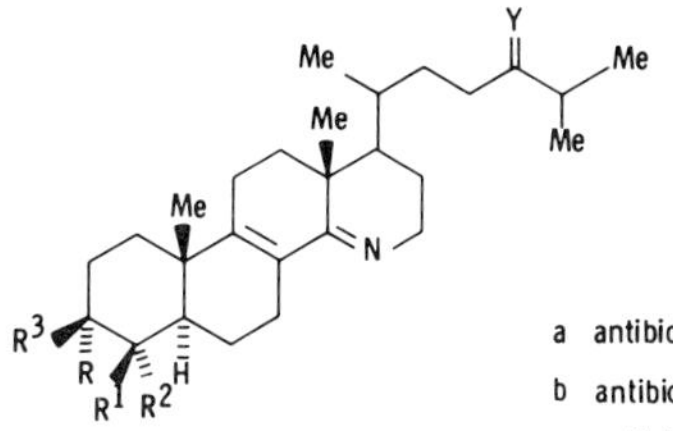

	R^1	R^2	R^3	R	Y
a antibiotic A25822 A	Me	Me	OH	H	CH_2
b antibiotic A25822 B	H	H	OH	H	CH_2
c antibiotic A25822 M	H	H	OAc	H	CH_2
d antibiotic A25822 N	H	H	=O		CH_2

(XXII)

The fungus *Geotrichum flavo-brunneum* produces a complex of 15-aza-24-methylene-D-homocholestadienes, antibiotics A 25822 A, B, D, H, L, M, and N, referred to in Section III,C. Antibiotic A 25822 B (XXIIb) is the major factor and is active against *Candida, Trichophyton,* and other pathogenic fungi both *in vitro* and *in vivo* (Michel *et al.,* 1975; Gordee and Butler, 1975); high toxicity and percutaneous absorption however preclude its development as a therapeutic agent. At subinhibitory concentrations, ignosterol (ergosta-8,14-dien-3β-ol) accumulates in *S. cerevisiae* (Hays *et al.,* 1977), while at higher concentrations its analogy to fecosterol probably enables it to act as a competitive inhibitor of 24(28)-methylene reductase. However 14,15,24,28-tetrahydro derivatives are also very active (MIC against *C. albicans* 1.25 μg/ml; *T. mentagrophytes* 0.078 μg/ml; Lilly: U.S. 4039547, 1976/1977).

Inhibitors of 3-HMGCoA-reductase have been considered of potential interest as hypocholesterolemic agents, antifungals, and for their antitumour activity. 3-Hydroxy-3-methylglutaric acid is itself an inhibitor. So too are certain hydroxylated steroids: 25-hydroxycholesterol (CCXXIIIa; Kandutsch and Chen, 1974); 7-ketocholesterol (CCXXIIIb);

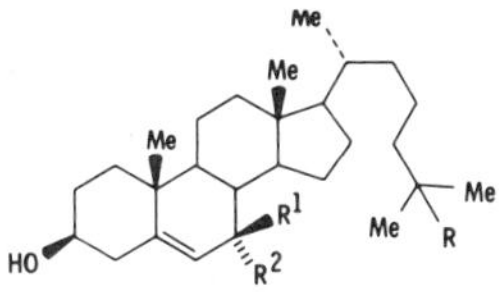

	R	R^1	R^2
a 25-hydroxycholesterol	OH	H	H
b 7-ketocholesterol	H	=O	
c 7β-hydroxycholesterol	H	OH	H

(CCXXIII)

7β-hydroxycholesterol (CCXXIIIc) and the 7α-epimer (Kandutsch and Chen, 1973). 7β-, 7α-, and 7-keto-derivatives of campesterol, stigmasterol, and sitosterol have been found in roots of *Euphorbia fischeriana,* a traditional Chinese medicine used for its antitumor properties (Schroeder *et al.,* 1980). 7β-Hydroxycampesterol and CCXXIIIc were obtained by

Cheng *et al.* (1977) as the active constituents of another Chinese antitumor remedy, *Bombyx-cum-Botryte,* and this has led to considerable synthetic work around hydroxylated steroids (Nagano *et al.,* 1977; Cheng *et al.,* 1979). The 24,25-dihydro derivative of inotodiol [(22R)-22-hydroxylanosterol], a sterol from the wood-rotting fungus *Inonotus obliquus* used as a Russian antitumor drug "chaga," is also a potent inhibitor of sterol biosynthesis (Poyser *et al.,* 1974). There is a marked selective toxicity for hepatoma cells compared to healthy fibroblasts. Some 25-alkyl-7-keto- and 25-alkyl-22-hydroxycholesterols have been patented as inhibitors of 3-HMGCoA reductase (Searle: DT. 2837414, 1977/1979). Interestingly they are also active against *Trichomonas vaginalis.* Synthetic ether analogs such as 21-nor-7-keto-20-oxacholesterol inhibit the enzyme *in vitro* but not *in vivo* orally in rats (Dygos and Desai, 1979). This contrasts with the potent hypocholesterolemic fungal metabolites monacolin

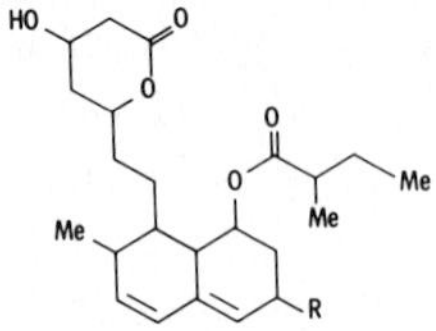

		R
a	monacolin K	Me
b	ML-236B (compactin)	H

(CCXXIV)

K (CCXXIVa) and ML-236B (compactin; CCXXIVb) which are active *in vitro* and *in vivo.* Monacolin K from *Monascus ruber* differs from compactin—a *Penicillium citrinum* metabolite—only by an additional methyl group. This is sufficient however to raise the level of activity by a factor of four to five (Kuroda *et al.,* 1979; Endo, 1979, 1980). Although relatively nontoxic, these antibiotics do not seem to have excited interest as antifungal agents.

3. *Alkaloids*

Apart from phenolic compounds, saponins and phytoalexins, antifungal agents from plants are relatively rare. Pipermethystine (CXLIII) has already been discussed in Section IV,D. The indigo plants *Strobilanthes cusia, Polygonium tinctorium,* and *Isatis tinctoria* have all been found to contain tryptanthrin (CCXXV), an indolo(2,1-*b*)quinazoline first isolated from *C. lipolytica* fed large amounts of L-tryptophan (Schindler and Zähner, 1971). It is active against dermatophytes at 3.1–6.3 μg/ml *in vitro,* which supports the traditional use of the plants in Taiwan folklore to treat athlete's foot (Honda and Tabata, 1979; Honda *et al.,* 1980). Canthin-6-one from *Hibiscus syriacus* (Yokota *et al.,* 1978) has a structure not unlike CCXXV, and is active against *T. interdigitale.* The alkaloid sanguinarine (CCXXVIa) from *Sanguinaria canadensis, Conydalis ophiocarpa,* and oth-

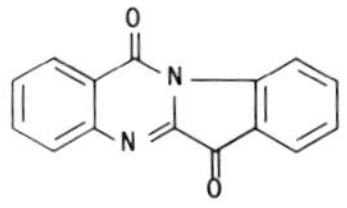

(CCXXV) tryptanthrin

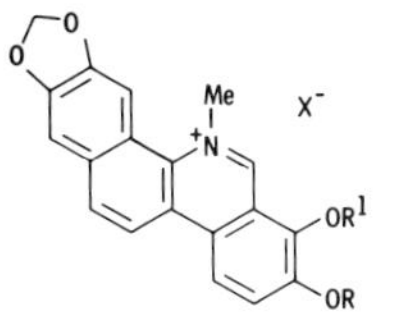

	R	R^1
a sanguinarine	—CH_2—	
b chelerythrine	Me	Me

(CCXXVI)

ers and the closely related chelerythrine (CCXXVIb) are used in the USSR as topical antifungal agents (Tin-Wa *et al.*, 1970; Vichkanova and Adgina, 1973). They induce glaucoma however when dosed to animals (Hakim *et al.*, 1961). Recently some pseudoalcoholates of sanguinarine have been isolated from *Hunnemannia fumariaefolia* and are claimed to be dramatically more active than the parent compound (Mitscher *et al.*, 1978). Some synthetic copper-chelating 8-hydroxyquinolines (XCIV) were discussed in Section III,O. Compounds of this type—such as 4-formyl-8-hydroxyquinoline from *Broussonetia zeylanica* (*Moraceae*)—are natural products and possess antibacterial and antifungal properties (Gunatilaka *et al.*, 1979). The steroidal saponins based on tomatidine may be considered as antifungal alkaloids, and one example is tomatine from *Lycopersicon pimpinellifolium* (Fontaine *et al.*, 1948). Such compounds are cytotoxic however since they interact with membranes containing sterols.

Phenazines on the other hand are fairly common metabolites of microorganisms. Myxin (1-hydroxy-6-methoxy-9,10-dihydrophenazine-9,10-dioxide) is obtained from a species of *Sorangium* (a myxobacterium). It is very active *in vitro* against a number of species of *Candida, B. dermatitidis, C. immitis,* and *Sporothrix schenckii;* it is also effective topically against *T. mentagrophytes* in guinea pigs (Sekhon and Hargesheimer, 1975), and as a copper derivative is used in a cream for treating dermal infections in horses. Simple phenazines such as tubermycin B (phenazine-1-carboxylic acid) and oxychlororaphin (phenazine-1-carboxamide) have been detected in these laboratories by following antidermatophyte activity extractable from the culture of an unidentified bacterium. Lomofungin (5-formyl-4,6,8-trihydroxyphenazine-1-carboxamide) produced by *Streptomyces lomendensis* has broad antibacterial and antifungal properties. It rapidly inhibits RNA synthesis in yeast protoplasts prior to any effect on protein synthesis (Kuo *et al.*, 1973) and it does this by inhibition of DNA-dependent RNA polymerase (Cano *et al.*, 1973).

4. *Isonitriles*

Since the determination of the structure of xanthocillin—a metabolite of *Penicillium notatum* (Hagedorn and Tönjes, 1957)—several other natural products containing the isonitrile group have been discovered. Antibiotic

A 32390A (CCXX) has already been discussed, and great interest was shown in its antifungal properties for some considerable time. Marine sources, especially sponges, have furnished several other examples—of which the amphilectene derivative CCXXVII is fairly typical. It is a diter-

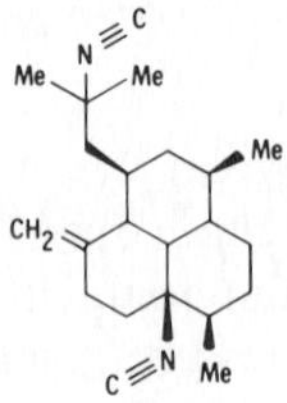

(CCXXVII)

penoid di-isonitrile with antimicrobial activity against *Staphylococcus aureus, B. subtilis,* and *C. albicans* (Wratten *et al.*, 1978). Other antimicrobial isocyanides have been isolated from *Adocia* species (Kazlauskas *et al.*, 1980). The biosynthetic origin of the isonitrile group does not appear to be via *N*-formylation and dehydration, at least in the case of xanthocillin.

5. *Glutarimides*

Cycloheximide or actidione (CCXXVIII) is the most important member of the glutarimide antifungal antibiotics. The group is characterized by a glutarimide ring, and this is usually joined from C-4′ by a two carbon bridge to C-6 of a 2,4-dimethylcyclohexanone ring. Upward of 17 variants are naturally occurring, including 3 of the 16 possible stereoisomers of cycloheximide. Compounds of this type act by inhibition of protein syn-

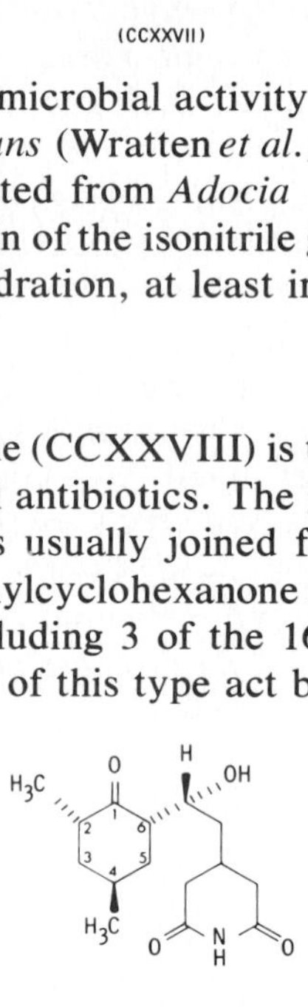

(CCXXVIII) cycloheximide (actidione)

thesis at the 80 S ribosome level, preventing the transfer of aminoacyl tRNA to the ribosomes, and thus formation of the peptide bond. They are inactive against bacteria, but toxic to many yeasts, filamentous fungi, protozoa, plants, and animals (Dekker, 1971). Lack of penetration of the intact organism is responsible for the ineffectiveness of cycloheximide against *C. albicans*. Phytotoxicity has prevented exploitation of its powerful inhibitory activity against powderey mildews, though it has found some application on noncrop plants. 4-Acetoxycycloheximide, antibiotic

E-73, has the most potent antitumor activity, but is less active against yeasts (Rao and Cullen, 1960). Protomycin, in which the cyclohexanone ring has been replaced by an open form, retains activity against yeasts and is well-tolerated iv by rodents (Sugawara, 1963). The glutarimides are exclusively metabolites of *Streptomyces* origin (Johnson, 1971).

6. *Pyrrolnitrins*

3-Arylpyrroles are unusual in nature. Pyrrolnitrin (CCXXIX) is an antibiotic from the fermentation of a *Pseudomonas* species which is mainly active against the common species of *Trichophyton,* but also against systemic candidosis and cryptococcosis in mice; it is not effective against

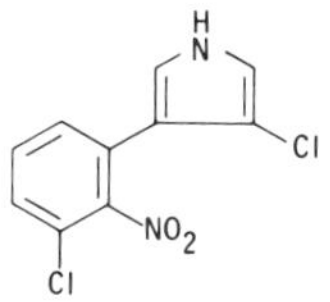

(CCXXIX) pyrrolnitrin

blastomycosis and histoplasmosis. The LD_{50} ip in mice is 680 mg/kg. In *S. cerevisiae* it has been shown to inhibit terminal electron transport between succinate or NADH and coenzyme Q (Tripathi and Gottlieb, 1969). It is used in Japan and some European countries as ''Pyro-ace'' for the topical treatment of dermatophyte infections. Umio *et al.* (1970) have claimed that the compound lacking the nitro function is even more active and has a broader spectrum of activity *in vitro* at least. As pyrrolnitrin is a metabolic derivative of tryptophan, synthetic derivatives of tryptophan have been used as nutrients to give rise to unnatural pyrrolnitrins; an alternative approach has been to supplement the medium with potassium or ammonium bromide.

Some 2-aryl- and aroyl-pyrroles are also *Pseudomonas* metabolites. Pyoluteorin (CCXXXa) is one of the latter type which has some plant fungicidal and herbicidal activity, and has recently been obtained using *n*-paraffins as the carbon source in cultures of *Ps. aeruginosa* (Ohmori *et al.,* 1978). The pentachloro-2-phenylpyrrole, antibiotic A 15104Y (CCXXXb) has general antimicrobial properties. Antibiotic A 15104Z

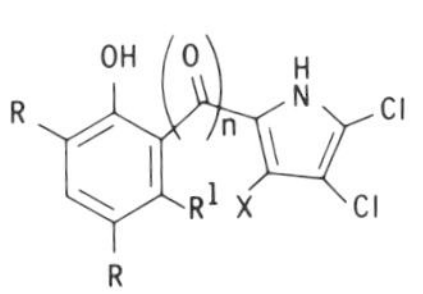

	X	n	R	R^1
a pyoluteorin	H	1	H	OH
b antibiotic A15104Y	Cl	0	Cl	H

(CCXXX)

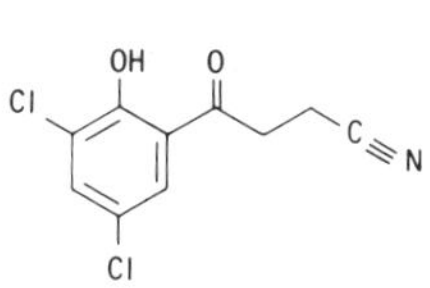

(CCXXXI) antibiotic A15104Z

(CCXXXI) is a cometabolite and possible precursor with a more limited spectrum; ip toxicity is high (LD_{50} around 5 mg/kg; Cavalleri *et al.*, 1978). The pentabromo isostere of CCXXXb has also been found from marine bacterial sources, and is a very potent inhibitor of gram-positive organisms (MIC 0.0063 μg/ml; Burkholder *et al.*, 1966; Wratten *et al.*, 1977).

7. *Plants and Marine Life as Sources of Antifungals*

Although terrestrial microorganisms, particularly the *Streptomycetes*, have provided the majority of antifungal antibiotics, other forms of life are also potential sources of useful activity. Traditional medicine based on plants and herbs must in many instances have a chemotherapeutic basis, and it is to be hoped that closer chemical investigation of many of these products will soon be carried out. We have already mentioned tryptanthrin extracted from Taiwanese plants used in the treatment of athlete's foot and falcarindol isolated from "seven finger," used by the Maoris to treat ringworm. Among the many other instances which could be cited, we may mention that ether extracts of "Choti dudhi" plants *Euphorbia prostrata* and *E. thymifolia* have recently been shown to have curative effects when applied topically to various experimental ringworm infections in rabbits and goats (Pal and Gupta, 1979), and that allicin, the volatile principle of *Allium sativum* responsible for potent *in vitro* activity against *Candida, Cryptococcus,* and dermatophytes, is the monoxide of diallyl disulfide (Yamada and Azuma, 1977).

Marine organisms too, although they do not seem to have the same place in traditional remedies, are a potential source of antifungals worth further investigation. We have already mentioned aplidiasphingosine and thelepin. A remarkable product containing 75% by weight of bromine (2(1′,1′-dibromopropyl)-3,5,6-tribromo-γ-pyrone) has been isolated from *Ptilonia australasica;* not surprisingly perhaps it is active against bacteria, yeasts, and filamentous fungi (Kazlauskas *et al.*, 1978). Cycloeudesmol is a sesquiterpene alcohol containing a fused cyclopropyl ring which has been isolated from *Chondria oppositiclada* and is inhibitory to *C. albicans* (Fenical and Sims, 1974). The sesquiterpene quinone methide puupehenone—obtained from an unidentified sponge—has a broader spectrum, being active against *Trichophyton* and *Trichomonas* as well as *Candida* (Ravi *et al.*, 1979). A metabolite of unknown structure ($C_{43}H_{58}O_{11}$)—very active against *Cryptococcus* and *Trichophyton in vitro,* and less so against *C. albicans*—has been obtained from a Puerto Rican species of the marine dinoflagellate *Goniodoma* and named goniodomin (Sharma *et al.*, 1968), while an antifungal polysaccharide of molecular weight around 30,000 has been obtained from *Chaetoceros lauderi*

(Pesando *et al.*, 1980). Doubtless the wide oceans contain very many more organisms producing antifungal activity—some of which might have really practical applications. "Seek and ye shall find. . . . !"

V. What of the Future?

Although in this article we have covered a vast array of diverse chemical structures which display some sort of antifungal activity—in many cases limited to activity *in vitro*—the number of types which are in current clinical use is limited. It is fortunate that at this stage drug resistance in the antifungal field is not a problem of major significance. The only compound where the occurrence or development of drug resistance may need to be considered during clinical management of the patient is 5-FC; the most recent and authoritative discussion of this problem with 5-FC is given by Scholer (1980). Parasitic fungi—like their hosts—are eukaryotes, and theoretically it should be more difficult to discover antifungals showing differential toxicity than in a prokaryote–eukaryote situation (e.g., antibacterial chemotherapy). The most obvious difference between the fungal and mammalian cell is the fungal cell wall. Many of the components of the wall and the reactions by which they are produced are unique to the fungus, and several compounds have been mentioned which interfere with this cell wall synthesis, and consequently display antifungal activity—at an experimental level at least. Biochemical studies on the wall and its synthesis are continuing in a number of centers, with antagonism of these processes being constantly in mind. That the fungal cell wall is a structure vital to the parasite may be inferred from the consequences of its destruction *in vivo* by polysaccharidase enzymes such as mycolase (Davies and Pope, 1978); mice infected systemically with a fatal inoculum of *Aspergillus fumigatus* could be protected by treatment with mycolase given iv or the fungus could be rendered more susceptible to amphotericin B following less vigorous enzyme treatment. The fungal cell wall is not however the only potential target for chemotherapeutic attack; we have mentioned in passing a number of other modes of drug action, and some of these are summarized in Fig. 2—the basis for which we are indebted to Professor D. Pappagianis. Even the fungal nucleus—which is the organelle responsible by definition for the basic distinction between eukaryote and prokaryote—is susceptible to differential chemotherapeutic attack. Griseofulvin for example produces a greater effect on the dermatophyte than on the host cell nucleus by interfering with its microtubule-associated protein. In designing a drug however, it is not only necessary to identify a system in the fungal parasite which is more sensitive to a particular agent

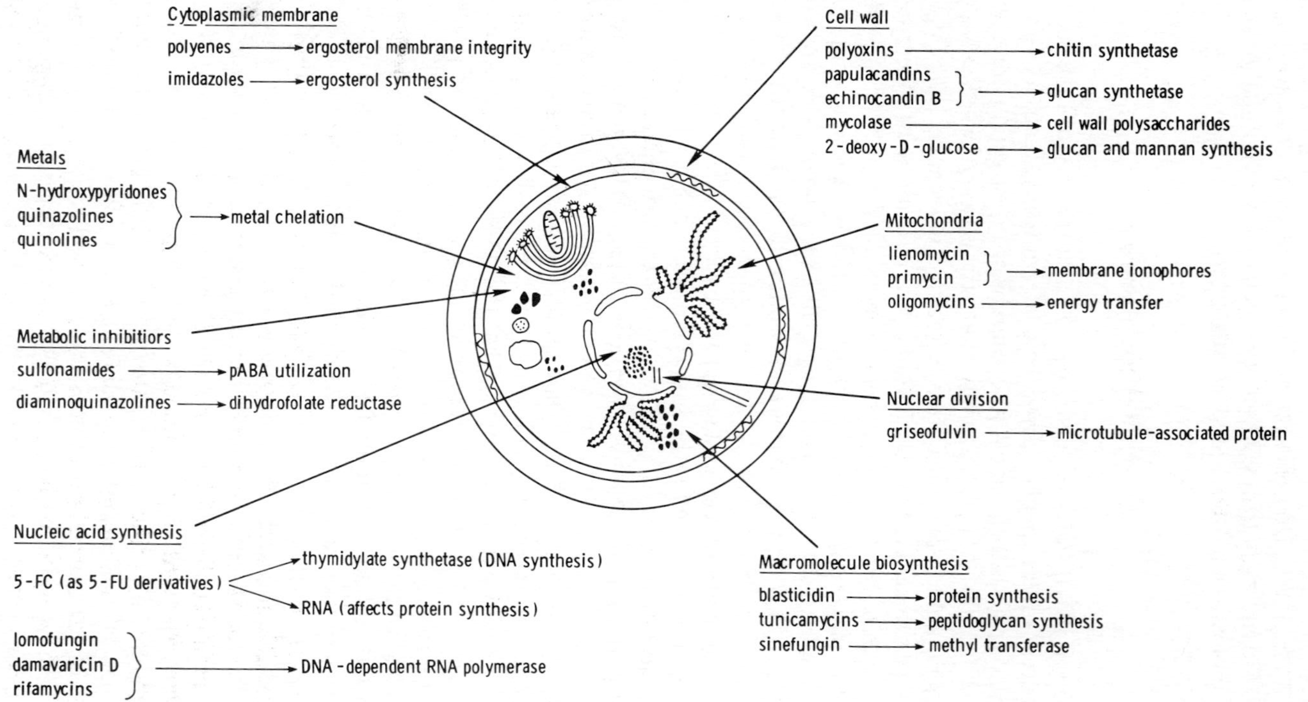

FIG. 2. Mode of action of some antifungal natural products.

than the analogous system in the host; the potential drug also has to have the right pharmacological properties to enable it to reach its target site in the host–parasite complex. That this is an even more difficult undertaking than the initial discovery of activity is evident from the multitude of compounds reviewed which display *in vitro* but not *in vivo* activity.

Directed research—whether it be against an identified biochemical target or inspired by already known activity—will always need to be supplemented by the empirical approach of drug screening; this is especially true in the case of natural product research. We hope nevertheless that this article, by drawing attention to antifungal activity in molecules which themselves have not become drugs, will nevertheless inspire rational chemical synthesis which seeks to improve and extend this activity. There is a continuing and urgent need for new antifungal drugs with both a wider spectrum of activity and suitable pharmacology and lack of toxicity to enable them to be used by the oral route.

References

Abbott, B. J., Horton, D. R., and Whitney, J. G. (1980). *J. Antibiot.* **33,** 506.

Aberhart, J., Fehr, T., Jain, R. C., de Mayo, P., Motl, O., Baczynskyj, L., Gracey, D. E. F., MacLean, D. B., and Szilágyi, I. (1970). *J. Am. Chem. Soc.* **92,** 5816.

Actor, P., Berkoff, C. E., Craig, P. N., Julius, M., Redl, G., Grout, R. J., Hynam, B. M., and Partridge, M. W. (1974). *Arzneim. Forsch.* **24,** 8.

Aerts, F., De Brabander, M., Van den Bossche, H., Van Cutsem, J., and Borgers, M. (1980). *Mykosen* **23,** 53.

Ajello, E. (1971). *J. Heterocycl. Chem.* **8,** 1035.

Albers-Schönberg, G., Arison, B. H., Bennett, C. D., Douglas, A. W., Miller, J. E., Onishi, J. C., Rowin, G. L., and Smith, J. L. (1979). *Int. Congr. Chemother., 11th, Intersci. Conf. Antimicrob. Ag. Chemother., 19th, Boston* Abstr. 151.

Allen, E. H., and Thomas, C. A. (1971a). *Phytochemistry* **10,** 1579.

Allen, E. H., and Thomas, C. A. (1971b). *Phytopathology* **61,** 1107.

Allison, M. J., Gerszten, E., Shadomy, H. J., Munizaga, J., and Gonzalez, M. (1979). *Bull. N.Y. Acad. Med.* **55,** 670.

Anchel, M. (1967). *In* "Antibiotics. Vol. II, Biosynthesis" (D. Gottlieb and P. D. Shaw, eds.), pp. 189–215. Springer-Verlag, Berlin and New York.

Ando, K., Matsuura, I., Nawata, Y., Endo, H., Sasaki, H., Okytomi, T., Saehi, T., and Tamura, G. (1978). *J. Antibiot.* **31,** 533.

Anghel, C., and Silberg, A. (1971). *Stud. Univ. Babes Bolyai, Ser. Chem.* **16,** 9.

Anke, T., Oberwinkler, F., Steglich, W., and Schramm, G. (1977). *J. Antibiot.* **30,** 806.

Anke, T., Hecht, H. J., Schramm, G., and Steglich, W. (1979). *J. Antibiot.* **32,** 1112.

Anke, T., Kupka, J., Schramm, G., and Steglich, W. (1980). *J. Antibiot.* **33,** 463.

Arai, T. (1974). *Postepy Hig. Med. Dosw.* **28,** 649.

Arcamone, F., Franceschi, G., Gioia, B., Penco, S., and Vigevani, A. (1972). *J. Am. Chem. Soc.* **95,** 2009.

Arison, B. H., and Omura, S. (1974). *J. Antibiot.* **27,** 28.

Azuma, T., and Isono, K. (1977). *Chem. Pharm. Bull.* **25,** 3347.

Azuma, T., Isono, K., Crain, P. F., and McCloskey, J. A. (1977). *J. Chem. Soc. Chem. Commun.* 159.

Baguley, B. C., Rommele, G., Gruner, J., and Wehrli, W. (1979). *Eur. J. Biochem.* **97,** 345.

Baker, H., Sidorowicz, A., Sehgal, S. N., and Vézina, C. (1978). *J. Antibiot.* **31,** 539.

Baloniak, S., Mroczkicwicz, A., and Cagara, M. (1975). *Acta Pol. Pharm.* **32,** 445.

Banerjee, A. B., and Bose, S. K. (1963). *Nature (London)* **200,** 471.

Barker, W. R., Callaghan, C., Hill, L., Noble, D., Acred, P., Harper, P. B., Sowa, M. A., and Fletton, R. A. (1979). *J. Antibiot.* **32,** 1096.

Bartlett, P. A., and Green, F. R., III (1978). *J. Am. Chem. Soc.* **100,** 4858.

Baum, G. L. (1979). *Postgrad. Med. J.* **55,** 587.

Bennett, J. E., Dismukes, W., Duma, R., Medoff, G., Saude, M., Gallis, H., Cate, T., Cobbs, G., Haywood, H., Leonard, J., McGee, Z., Fields, B., Bradshaw, M., Williams, T., Warner, J., and Alling, D. (1976). *Intersci. Conf. Antimicrob. Ag. Chemother., 16th, Chicago* Abstr. 308.

Benz, F., Knüsel, F., Nüesch, J., Treichler, H., Voser, W., Nyfeler, R., and Keller-Schierlein, W. (1974). *Helv. Chim. Acta* **57,** 2459.

Berg, D. H., Massing, R. P., Hoehn, M. M., Boeck, L. D., and Hamill, R. L. (1976). *J. Antibiot.* **29,** 394.

Bergman, S. (1955). *Acta Pathol. Microbiol. Scand.* **37,** Suppl. 104, 8.

Berry, D. R., and Abbott, B. J. (1978). *J. Antibiot.* **31,** 185.

Besson, F., Peypoux, F., Michel, G., and Delcambe, L. (1978). *J. Antibiot.* **31,** 284.

Besson, F., Peypoux, F., Michel, G., and Delcambe, L. (1979). *J. Antibiot.* **32,** 828.

Betina, V., Baráthova, H., Nemec, P., and Barath, Z. (1969). *J. Antibiot.* **22,** 129.

Bhattacharyya, J. (1980). *Experientia* **36,** 27.

Bhattacharyya, J., and Miles, D. H. (1977). *Tetrahedron Lett.* 2749.

Bianchi, M., Cotta, E., Ferny, G., Grein, A., Julita, P., Mazzoleni, R., and Spalla, C. (1974). *Arch. Microbiol.* **98,** 289.

Biere, H., and Redmann, N. (1976). *Eur. J. Med. Chem.* **11,** 351.

Birnbaum, G. I., and Hall, S. R. (1976). *J. Am. Chem. Soc.* **98,** 1926.

Blinov, N. O., Onoprienko, V. V., Rodina, T. M., Againa, S. I., and Khlebarova, E. I. (1974). *Antibiotiki* **19,** 579 (*Chem. Abst.* **82,** 15178f, 1975).

Block, E. R., Jennings, A. E., and Bennett, J. E. (1973). *Antimicrob. Ag. Chemother.* **4,** 392.

Bodanszky, M., Izdebski, J., and Muramatsu, I. (1969). *J. Am. Chem. Soc.* **91,** 2351.

Boeckman, R. K., Jr., and Thomas, E. W. (1977). *J. Am. Chem. Soc.* **99,** 2805.

Böhme, H., and Ahrens, K. H. (1974). *Arch. Pharm. (Weinheim, Ger.)* **307,** 828.

Borchardt, R. T., Eiden, L. E., Wu, B., and Rutledge, C. O. (1979). *Biochem. Biophys. Res. Commun.* **89,** 919.

Borgers, M., De Brabander, M., and Van den Bossche, H. (1979). *Congr. Int. Soc. Human Animal Mycol., 7th, Jerusalem* Abstr. p. 73.

Borowski, E., Golik, J., Zielínski, J., Falkowski, L., Kolodziejczyk, P., Pawlak, J., and Shenin, Y. (1978). *J. Antibiot.* **31,** 117.

Botter, A. A., Dethier, F., Mertens, R. L. J., Morias, J., and Peremans, W. (1979). *Mykosen* **22,** 274.

Boyer, J. M. (1976). *Antimicrob. Ag. Chemother.* **9,** 1070.

Brantsevich, L. G., Miroshnichenko, N. S., Stetsenko, A. V., Slabospitskaya, A. T., and Chekmachava, V. V. (1975). *Mikrobiol. Zh. (Kiev)* **37,** 635 (*Chem. Abst.* **84,** 25886r, 1976).

Brass, C., Shainhouse, J. Z., and Stevens, D. A. (1979). *Antimicrob. Ag. Chemother.* **15,** 763.

Brown, D., Evans, J. R., and Fletton, R. A. (1979). *J. Chem. Soc. Chem. Commun.* 282.

Brufani, M., Cellai, L., Musu, C., and Keller-Schierlein, W., von (1972). *Helv. Chim. Acta* **55,** 2329.

Buchel, K. H., Draber, W., Regel, E., and Plempel, M. (1972). *Drugs Made Ger.* **15,** 77.

Burka, L. T., and Iles, J. (1979). *Phytochemistry* **18,** 873.

Burkholder, P. R., Pfister, R. M., and Leitz, R. M. (1966). *Appl. Microbiol.* **14,** 649.

Cain, R. O., and Porter, A. E. A. (1979). *Phytochemistry* **18,** 322.

Cano, F. R., Kuo, S.-C., and Lampen, J. O. (1973). *Antimicrob. Ag. Chemother.* **3,** 723.

Capek, A., Simek, A., Leiner, J., and Weichet, J. (1973). *Folia Microbiol.* **18,** 142.

Carter, G. T., and Rinehart, K. L., Jr. (1978). *J. Am. Chem. Soc.* **100,** 7441.

Carter, S. B., Franklin, T. J., Jones, D. F., Leonard, B. L., Mills, S. D., Turner, R. W., and Turner, W. B. (1969). *Nature (London)* **223,** 848.

Cartwright, R. Y. (1975). *J. Antimicrob. Chemother.* **1,** 141.

Cartwright, R. Y. (1978a). *In* "Medicinal Chemistry VI. Proceedings of the 6th. International Symposium on Medicinal Chemistry. Brighton" (A. Simkin, ed.), pp. 433–436. Cotswold Press, Oxford.

Cartwright, R. Y. (1978b). *Br. Med. J.* **2,** 108.

Cassone, A., Kerridge, D., and Gale, E. F. (1979). *J. Gen. Microbiol.* **110,** 339.

Castaldo, R. A., Gump, D. W., and McCormack, J. J. (1978). *Intersci. Conf. Antimicrob. Ag. Chemother., 18th, Atlanta* Abstr. 52.

Castaldo, R. A., Gump, D. W., and McCormack, J. J. (1979). *Antimicrob. Ag. Chemother.* **15,** 81.

Cavalleri, B., Volpe, G., Tuan, G., Berti, M., and Parenti, F. (1978). *Curr. Microbiol.* **1,** 319.

Celmer, W. D., and Solomons, I. A. (1952). *J. Am. Chem. Soc.* **74,** 1870.

Chakrabarti, S., and Chandra, A. L. (1979). *Indian J. Exp. Biol.* **17,** 313.

Cheng, K. P., Nagano, H., Bang, L., Ourisson, G., and Beck, J. P. (1977). *J. Chem. Res.* **(S)** 217, **(M)** 2501.

Cheng, K. P., Bang, L., Ourisson, G., and Beck, J. P. (1979). *J. Chem. Res.* **(S)** 84. **(M)** 1101.

Cheung, S. C., Medoff, G., Schlessinger, D., and Kobayashi, G. S. (1975). *Antimicrob. Ag. Chemother.* **8,** 426.

Clayton, Y. M., and Connor, B. L. (1973). *Br. J. Dermatol.* **89,** 297.

Connor, D. T., and Strandtmann, M., von (1978). *J. Org. Chem.* **43,** 4606.

Connor, D. T., and Strandtmann, M., von (1979). *J. Med. Chem.* **22,** 1055, 1144.

Connor, D. T., Klutchko, S., and Strandtmann, M., von (1979). *J. Antibiot.* **32,** 368.

Cope, J. E. (1980). *J. Gen. Microbiol.* **119,** 245.

Corey, E. J., and Williams, D. R. (1977). *Tetrahedron Lett.* 3847.

Cossey, A. L., Gunter, M. J., and Mander, L. N. (1980). *Tetrahedron Lett.* **21,** 3309.

Coxon, D. T., O'Neill, T. M., Mansfield, J. W., and Porter, A. E. A. (1980). *Phytochemistry* **19,** 889.

Crank, G., Neville, M., and Ryden, R. (1973). *J. Med. Chem.* **16,** 1402.

Craveri, R., Manachini, P. L., and Aragozzini, F. (1972). *Experientia* **28,** 867.

Currie, S. A., Flor, J. E., Monaghan, R. L., and Tejera, E. (1979). *Int. Congr. Chemother., 11th, Intersci. Conf. Antimicrob. Ag. Chemother., 19th, Boston,* Abstr. 508.

Damodaran, N. P., Jones, G. H., and Moffatt, J. G. (1971). *J. Am. Chem. Soc.* **93,** 3812.

D'Arcy, P. F., and Scott, E. M. (1978). *In* "Drug Research" (E. Jucker, ed.), pp. 93–147. Birkhauser-Verlag, Basel and Stuttgart.

Dasgupta, J., Khannan, L. V., Mehdi, I., Vora, V. C., and Dhar, M. M. (1970). *Indian J. Biochem.* **7,** 81.

Davies, D. A. L., and Pope, A. M. S. (1978). *Nature (London)* **273,** 235.

Davies, R. R. (1980). *In* "Antifungal Chemotherapy" (D. C. E. Speller, ed.), pp. 149–182. Wiley, New York.

Davis, A. L., Hulme, K. L., Wilson, G. T., and McCord, T. J. (1977). *Annu. Meet. Am. Soc. Microbiol., 77th, New Orleans* Abstr. A40.
De Alvarenga, M. A., Gottlieb, O. R., and Magalhàes, M. T. (1976). *Phytochemistry* **15,** 844.
Deffieux, G., Baute, M. A., Baute, R., and Filleau, M. J. (1978). *J. Antibiot.* **31,** 1102.
Dekker, J. (1971). *World Rev. Pest Contr.* **10,** 9.
Deml, G., Anke, T., Oberwinkler, F., Giannetti, B. M., and Steglich, W. (1980). *Phytochemistry* **19,** 83.
De Nollin, S., and Borgers, M. (1974). *Sabouraudia* **12,** 341.
De Nollin, S., and Borgers, M. (1976). *Mykosen* **19,** 317.
De Nollin, S., Van Belle, H., Gossens, F., Thone, F., and Borgers, M. (1977). *Antimicrob. Ag. Chemother.* **11,** 500.
Deshmukh, P. V., Kakinuma, K., Ameel, J. J., Rinehart, K. L., Jr., Wiley, P. F., and Li, L. H. (1976). *J. Am. Chem. Soc.* **98,** 870.
Destro, R., and Colombo, A. (1979). *J. Chem. Soc. Perkin Trans.* **II,** 896.
Dewick, P. M., and Ingham, J. L. (1980). *Phytochemistry* **19,** 289.
Dewick, P. M., and Martin, M. (1979). *Phytochemistry* **18,** 591, 597.
Dewick, P. M., and Ward, D. (1978). *Phytochemistry* **17,** 1751.
Dimmock, J. R., Turner, W. A., and Baker, H. A. (1975). *J. Pharm. Sci.* **64,** 995.
Dimmock, J. R., Qureshi, A. M., Noble, L. M., Smith, P. J., and Baker, H. A. (1976). *J. Pharm. Sci.* **65,** 38.
Dittmar, W., and Lohaus, G. (1973). *Arzneim. Forsch.* **23,** 670.
Dittmar, W., Druckrey, E., and Urbach, H. (1974). *J. Med. Chem.* **17,** 753.
Dixon, R. A., and Lamb, C. J. (1980). *Nature (London)* **283,** 135.
Dixon, D. M., Wagner, G. E., Shadomy, S., and Shadomy, H. J. (1978a). *Chemotherapy* **24,** 364.
Dixon, D. M., Shadomy, S., Shadomy, H. J., Espinel-Ingroff, A., and Kerkering, T. M. (1978b). *J. Infect. Dis.* **138,** 245.
Doerfler, D. L., Ernst, L. A., and Campbell, I. M. (1980). *J. Chem. Soc. Chem. Commun.* 329.
Dolak, L. (1979). *J. Antibiot.* **32,** 1346.
Doorenbos, N. J., and Aboul-Enein, H. Y. (1974a). *J. Heterocycl. Chem.* **11,** 557.
Doorenbos, N. J., and Aboul-Enein, H. Y. (1974b). *Pharm. Acta Helv.* **49,** 320.
Doorenbos, N. J., and Bossle, P. C. (1970). *Chem. Ind.* 1660.
Doorenbos, N. J., and Solomons, W. E. (1973). *J. Pharm. Sci.* **62,** 638.
Doorenbos, N. J., and Solomons, W. E. (1974). *J. Pharm. Sci.* **63,** 19.
Dornberger, K., Thrum, H., and Radics, L. (1979). *Tetrahedron* **35,** 1851.
Dueber, M. T. (1979). Ph.D. Thesis, University of California, Los Angeles. *Diss. Abstr. Int.* **B** (1980). **40,** 3706.
Dufour, J. P., Boutry, M., and Goffeau, A. (1980). *J. Biol. Chem.* **255,** 5735.
Dygos, J. H., and Desai, B. P. (1979). *J. Org. Chem.* **44,** 1590.
Ebata, M., Miyazaki, K., and Takahashi, Y. (1969). *J. Antibiot.* **22,** 467.
Eckardt, K., Thrum, H., Brandler, G., Tonew, E., and Tonew, M. (1975). *J. Antibiot.* **28,** 274.
Eisele, K. (1975a). *Z. Naturforsch.* **30c,** 541.
Eisele, K. (1975b). *Experientia* **31,** 764.
Emmons, C. W., Chapman, H. B., Utz, J. P., and Kwon-Chung, K. J. (1977). "Medical Mycology," 3rd Ed. Lea & Febiger, Philadelphia, Pennsylvania.
Endo, A. (1979). *J. Antibiot.* **32,** 852.
Endo, A. (1980). *J. Antibiot.* **33,** 334.

Ericsson, H. M., and Sherris, J. C. (1971). *Acta Pathol. Microbiol. Scand.* **79,** Suppl. 217, 67.

Falkowski, L., Zieliński, J., Golik, J., Bylec, E., and Borowski, E. (1978). *J. Antibiot.* **31,** 742.

Falkowski, L., Stefanska, B., Zieliński, J., Bylec, E., Golik, J., Kolodziejczyk, P., and Borowski, E. (1979). *J. Antibiot.* **32,** 1080.

Falkowski, L., Jarzebski, A., Stefanska, B., Bylec, E., and Borowski, E. (1980). *J. Antibiot.* **33,** 103.

Fang, J. N., Hua, J. C., and Hu, Y. L. (1979). *Wei Sheng Wu Hsueh Pao* **19,** 76 (*Chem. Abstr.* **90,** 200157b, 1979).

Fenical, W., and Sims, J. J. (1974). *Tetrahedron Lett.* 1137.

Fisch, M. H., Flick, B. H., and Arditti, J. (1973). *Phytochemistry* **12,** 437.

Fisher, B. D., and Armstrong, D. (1977). *Antimicrob. Ag. Chemother.* **12,** 614.

Fisher, M. H., and Lusi, A. (1972). *J. Med. Chem.* **15,** 982.

Fontaine, T. D., Irving, G. W., Jr., Ma, R., Poole, J. B., and Doolittle, S. P. (1948). *Arch. Biochem.* **18,** 467.

Fuji, K., Fujita, E., Takaishi, Y., Fujita, T., Arita, I., Komatsu, M., and Hiratsuka, H. (1978). *Experientia* **34,** 237.

Fujimori, T., Uegaki, R., Takagi, Y., Kubo, S., and Kato, K. (1979). *Phytochemistry* **18,** 2032.

Fujita, T., Takaishi, Y., and Shiromoto, T. (1979). *J. Chem. Soc. Chem. Commun.* 413.

Furusaki, A., Matsumoto, T., Nakagawa, A., and Omura, S. (1980). *J. Antibiot.* **33,** 781.

Galgiani, J. N., and Stevens, D. A. (1976). *Antimicrob. Ag. Chemother.* **10,** 721.

Garrod, B., and Lewis, B. G. (1979). *Trans. Br. Mycol. Soc.* **72,** 515.

Gauri, K. K. (1970). *Chemotherapy* **15,** 201.

Gauri, K. K., and Meyer-Rohn, J. (1974). *Biochem. Pharmacol.* **23,** 1231.

Gentles, J. C. (1958). *Nature* (*London*) **182,** 476.

Georgopoulos, A. (1978). *Mykosen* **21,** 19.

Gershon, H. (1974). *J. Med. Chem.* **17,** 824.

Gershon, H., McNeil, M. W., Parmegiani, R., and Godfrey, P. K. (1972a). *J. Med. Chem.* **15,** 105.

Gershon, H., McNeil, M. W., Parmegiani, R., and Godfrey, P. K. (1972b). *J. Med. Chem.* **15,** 987.

Gershon, H., Parmegiani, R., and Godfrey, P. K. (1972c). *Antimicrob. Ag. Chemother.* **1,** 373.

Gershon, H., McNeil, M. W., and Bergmann, E. D. (1973). *J. Med. Chem.* **16,** 1407.

Giori, P., Guarneri, M., Mazzotta, D., Vertuani, G., and Branca, C. (1979). *Farmaco Ed. Sci.* **34,** 277.

Godefroi, E. F., Heeres, J., Van Cutsem, J., and Janssen, P. A. J. (1969). *J. Med. Chem.* **12,** 784.

Gordee, R. S., and Butler, T. F. (1975). *J. Antibiot.* **28,** 112.

Gordon, M. A., Lapa, E. W., Fitter, M. S., and Lindsay, M. (1980). *Antimicrob. Ag. Chemother.* **17,** 120.

Gottlieb, D., and Shaw, P. D. (1970). *Annu. Rev. Phytopathol.* **8,** 371.

Gottlieb, D., Knaus, R. J., and Wood, S. G. (1978). *Phytopathology* **68,** 1168.

Granade, T. C., and Artis, W. M. (1980). *Antimicrob. Ag. Chemother.* **17,** 725.

Grier, N. (1979). *J. Pharm. Sci.* **68,** 407.

Grinev, A. N., Druzhinina, A. A., Sorokina, I. K., Guskova, T. A., Berlyand, E. A., Pershin, G. N., and Sizova, T. N. (1977). *Khim.-Farm. Zh.* **11,** 67 (*Chem. Abst.* **88,** 22525u, 1978).

Grisebach, H., and Ebel, J. (1978). *Angew. Chem. Int. Ed.* **17,** 635.

Gross, D., von (1977). *Fortschr. Chem. Org. Naturst.* **34,** 187.

Grye, W., Dabrowska, M., and Tomicka, B. (1979). *Pol. J. Chem.* **53,** 1085.

Gunatilaka, A. A. L., Perera, J. S. H. Q., Sultanbawa, M. U. S., Brown, P. M., and Thomson, R. H. (1979). *J. Chem. Res.* (S) 61.

Gupta, S. P., and Sarita, R. (1978). *J. Indian Chem. Soc.* **55,** 483.

Gupta, R. C., Nath, R., Shanker, K., Bhagarva, K. P., and Kishor, K. (1978). *J. Indian Chem. Soc.* **55,** 832.

Gurusiddaiah, S., Winward, L. D., Burger, D., and Graham, S. O. (1979). *Mycologia* **71,** 103.

Gyimesi, J., Méhesfalvi-Vajna, Z., and Horváth, G. (1978). *J. Antibiot.* **31,** 626.

Hagedorn, I., and Tönjes, H. (1957). *Pharmazie* **12,** 567.

Hagenmaier, H., Keckeiser, A., Zähner, H., and König, W. A. (1979). *Justus Liebigs Ann. Chem.* 1494.

Hairi, A. R., and Larsh, H. W. (1976). *Proc. Soc. Exp. Biol.* **151,** 173.

Hakim, S. A. E., Mijović, V., and Walker, J. (1961). *Nature* (*London*) **189,** 198.

Haller, I. (1979a). *Postgrad. Med. J.* **55,** 681.

Haller, I. (1979b). *Mykosen* **22,** 423.

Hammerschmidt, R., and Kuć, J. (1979). *Phytochemistry* **18,** 874.

Hammond, S. M. (1977). *Prog. Med. Chem.* **14,** 105.

Harborne, J. B., and Ingham, J. L. (1978). *In* "Biochemical Aspects of Plant and Animal Co-evolution" (J. B. Harborne, ed.), pp. 343–405. Academic Press, New York.

Harefeld, W., and Hinz, W. (1980). *Arch. Pharm.* (*Weinheim, Ger.*) **313,** 20.

Hargreaves, J. A., Mansfield, J. W., Coxon, D. T., and Price, K. R. (1976). *Phytochemistry* **15,** 1119.

Haupt, I., Spata, L., Thrum, H., and Weber, H. (1979). *Z. Allg. Mikrobiol.* **19,** 89.

Hays, P. R., Neal, W. D., and Parks, L. W. (1977). *Antimicrob. Ag. Chemother.* **12,** 185.

Heeres, J., Backx, L. J. J., and Van Cutsem, J. M. (1976). *J. Med. Chem.* **19,** 1148.

Heeres, J., Mostmans, J. H., and Van Cutsem, J. (1977). *J. Med. Chem.* **20,** 1511, 1516.

Heeres, J., Backx, L. J. J., Mostmans, J. H., and Van Cutsem, J. (1979). *J. Med. Chem.* **22,** 1003.

Heifetz, A., Keenan, R. W., and Elbein, A. D. (1979). *Biochemistry* **18,** 2186.

Heindl, J., Schroder, E., and Kelm, H. W. (1975a). *Eur. J. Med. Chem.* **10,** 121.

Heindl, J., Schroder, E., and Kelm, H. W. (1975b). *Eur. J. Med. Chem.* **10,** 551.

Higa, T., and Scheuer, P. J. (1975). *Tetrahedron* **31,** 2379.

Higashide, E., Asai, M., Ootsu, K., Tanida, S., Kozai, Y., Hasegawa, T., Kishi, T., Sugino, Y., and Yoneda, M. (1977). *Nature* (*London*) **270,** 721.

Hiremath, S. P., Mruthyunjayaswamy, B. M. M., and Purohoit, M. G. (1978). *Indian J. Chem.* **16B,** 789.

Hoeprich, P. D., and Finn, P. D. (1972). *J. Infect. Dis.* **126,** 353.

Holland, H. L., and Taylor, G. J. (1979). *Phytochemistry* **18,** 437.

Holt, R. J. (1975). *J. Clin. Pathol.* **28,** 767.

Honda, G., and Tabata, M. (1979). *Planta Med.* **36,** 85.

Honda, G., Tosirisuk, V., and Tabata, M. (1980). *Planta Med.* **38,** 275.

Hynes, J. B., Hough, L. V., Smith, A. B., and Gali, G. R. (1976). *Proc. Soc. Exp. Biol. Med.* **153,** 230.

Ikawa, M., McGrattan, C. J., Burge, W. R., Iannitelli, R. C., Uebel, J. J., and Noguchi, T. (1978). *J. Antibiot.* **31,** 158.

Imai, K., Ikeda, N., Tanaka, K., and Sugawara, S. (1956). *Yakugaku Zasshi* (*J. Pharm. Soc. Jpn.*) **76,** 397.

Ingham, J. L. (1979). *Z. Naturforsch.* **34c,** 683.
Ingham, J. L., and Dewick, P. M. (1978). *Phytochemistry* **17,** 535.
Ingham, J. L., and Dewick, P. M. (1979). *Phytochemistry* **18,** 1711.
Ingham, J. L., and Dewick, P. M. (1980a). *Phytochemistry* **19,** 1767.
Ingham, J. L., and Dewick, P. M. (1980b). *Z. Naturforsch.* **35c,** 197.
Ingham, J. L., and Markham, K. R. (1980). *Phytochemistry* **19,** 1203.
Irmscher, G., Bovermann, G., Boheim, G., and Jung, G. (1978). *Biochim. Biophys. Acta* **507,** 470.
Isono, K., and Suzuki, S. (1979). *Heterocycles* **13,** 333.
Isono, K., Asahi, K., and Suzuki, S. (1969). *J. Am. Chem. Soc.* **91,** 7490.
Isono, K., Crain, P. F., and McCloskey, J. A. (1975). *J. Am. Chem. Soc.* **97,** 943.
Isono, K., Nishii, M., and Kihara, T. (1980). *Intersci. Conf. Antimicrob. Ag. Chemother., 20th, New Orleans* Abstr. 468.
Ito, T., Kodama, Y., Kawamura, K., Suzuki, K., Takatsuki, A., and Tamura, G. (1979). *Agric. Biol. Chem.* **43,** 1187.
Ito, T., Takatsuki, A., Kawamura, K., Sato, K., and Tamura, G. (1980). *Agric. Biol. Chem.* **44,** 695.
Itoh, J., Miyadoh, S., Takahashi, S., Amano, S., Ezaki, N., and Yamada, Y. (1979). *J. Antibiot.* **32,** 1089.
Iwasa, T., Kishi, T., Matsuura, K., and Wakae, O. (1977). *J. Antibiot.* **30,** 1.
Iwasa, T., Suetomi, K., and Kusaka, T. (1978). *J. Antibiot.* **31,** 511.
Jadhav, K. D., Shingare, M. S., and Ingle, D. B. (1978). *Acta Cienc. Indica* **4,** 141.
Jakubowski, A. A., Guziec, F. S., Jr., and Tishler, M. (1977). *Tetrahedron Lett.* 2399.
Jevons, S., Gymer, G. E., Brammer, K. W., Cox, D. A., and Leeming, M. R. G. (1979). *Antimicrob. Ag. Chemother.* **15,** 597.
Johnson, F. (1971). *Fortschr. Chem. Org. Naturst.* **29,** 140.
Just, G., and Payette, D. (1980). *Tetrahedron Lett.* **21,** 3219.
Just, G., and Potvin, P. (1981). *Can. J. Chem.* **58,** 2173.
Kameda, Y., Asano, N., Wakae, O., and Isawa, T. (1980). *J. Antibiot.* **33,** 764.
Kandutsch, A. A., and Chen, H. W. (1973). *J. Biol. Chem.* **248,** 8408.
Kandutsch, A. A., and Chen, H. W. (1974). *J. Biol. Chem.* **249,** 6057.
Kawakami, Y., Matsuwaka, S., Otani, T., Kondo, H., and Nakamura, S. (1978). *J. Antibiot.* **31,** 112.
Kazlauskas, R., Lidgard, R. O., and Wells, R. J. (1978). *Tetrahedron Lett.* 3165.
Kazlauskas, R., Murphy, P. T., Wells, R. J., and Blount, J. F. (1980). *Tetrahedron Lett.* **21,** 315.
Keller-Juslén, C., Kuhn, M., Loosli, H. R., Petcher, T. J., Weber, H. P., and Wartburg, A. von (1976). *Tetrahedron Lett.* 4147.
Keller-Schierlein, W., von, and Gerlach, H. (1968). *Fortschr. Chem. Org. Naturst.* **26,** 161.
Kemp, M. S. (1978). *Phytochemistry* **17,** 1002.
Kende, A. S., and Curran, D. P. (1978). *Tetrahedron Lett.* 3003.
Kende, A. S., and Curran, D. P. (1979). *J. Am. Chem. Soc.* **101,** 1857.
Kenig, M., and Reading, C. (1979). *J. Antibiot.* **32,** 549.
Kitahara, M., Seth, V. K., Medoff, G., and Kobayashi, G. S. (1976). *Antimicrob. Ag. Chemother.* **9,** 909.
Kitao, C., Ikeda, H., Hamada, H., and Omura, S. (1979). *J. Antibiot.* **32,** 593.
Kluepfel, D., Bagli, J., Baker, H., Charest, M.-P., Kudelski, A., Sehgal, S. N., and Vézina, C. (1972). *J. Antibiot.* **25,** 109.
Kobayashi, G. S., and Medoff, G. (1977). *Annu. Rev. Microbiol.* **31,** 291.

Kobinata, K., Uramoto, M., Nishii, M., Kusakabe, H., Nakamura, G., and Isono, K. (1980). *Agric. Biol. Chem.* **44,** 1709.

Kohno, K., Hiragun, A., Mitsui, H., Takatsuki, A., and Tamura, G. (1979). *Agric. Biol. Chem.* **43,** 1553.

Komatsu, M., Yokoe, I., and Shirataki, Y. (1978). *Chem. Pharm. Bull.* **26,** 3863.

Kondo, H., Vehara, M., Nakama, S., Otani, T., and Nakamura, S. (1976). *J. Antibiot.* **29,** 847.

Kondo, H., Sumomogi, H., Otani, T., and Nakamura, S. (1979). *J. Antibiot.* **32,** 13.

Konev, Y. E., Shenin, Y. D., Severinets, L. Y., and Kamyshko, O. P. (1977). *Antibiotiki* **22,** 7 (*Chem. Abstr.* **86,** 68176t, 1977).

Konev, Y. E., Efimova, V. M., Etingov, E. D., and Zavalnaya, N. M. (1978). *Antibiotiki* **23,** 143 (*Chem. Abstr.* **88,** 168434k, 1978).

Korytnyk, W., and Ahrens, H. (1971). *J. Med. Chem.* **14,** 947.

Korytnyk, W., and Paul, B. (1970). *J. Med. Chem.* **13,** 187.

Korytnyk, W., Angelino, N., Lachmann, B., and Potti, P. G. G. (1972). *J. Med. Chem.* **15,** 1262.

Kotler-Brajtburg, J., Medoff, G., Kobayashi, G. S., Boggs, S., Schlessinger, D., Pandey, R. C., and Rinehart, K. L. Jr. (1979). *Antimicrob. Ag. Chemother.* **15,** 716.

Kreutzberger, A., and Schimmelpfennig, H. (1980). *Arch. Pharm.* (*Weinheim, Ger.*) **313,** 260.

Kulalaeva, Z. I., Gibalov, V. I., Poltorak, V. A., and Silaev, A. B. (1978). *Bioorg. Khim.* **4,** 1244 (*Chem. Abstr.* **90,** 54795q, 1979).

Kunze, B., Schabacher, K., Zähner, H., and Zeeck, A. (1972). *Arch. Mikrobiol.* **86,** 147.

Kuo, S.-C., Cano, F. R., and Lampen, J. O. (1973). *Antimicrob. Ag. Chemother.* **3,** 716.

Kuroda, M., Tsujita, Y., Tanzawa, K., and Endo, A. (1979). *Lipids* **14,** 585.

Lambert, P. A. (1978). *Prog. Med. Chem.* **15,** 87.

Langcake, P., and Pryce, R. J. (1977). *Experientia* **33,** 151.

Langcake, P., Cornford, C. A., and Pryce, R. J. (1979). *Phytochemistry* **18,** 1025.

Leiner, J., Simek, A., and Capek, A. (1970). *Pharm. Ind.* **32,** 940.

Levine, H. B. (1977). *Chest* **70,** 755.

Levine, H. B., and Cobb, J. M. (1978). *Amnu. Rev. Resp. Dis.* **118,** 715.

Levine, H. B., Ringel, S. M., and Cobb, J. M. (1978). *Chest* **73,** 202.

Lew, M. A., Beckett, K. M., and Levin, M. J. (1978). *Antimicrob. Ag. Chemother.* **14,** 465.

Lipkin, A. E., and Bespalova, Zh. P. (1970). *Khim.-Farm. Zh.* **4,** 24 (*Chem. Abstr.* **72,** 111193w, 1970).

Liu, C. M., Evans, R., Jr., Fern, L., Hermann, T., Jenkins, E., Liu, M., Palleroni, N. J., Prosser, R. L., Sello, L. H., Stempel, A., Tabenkin, B., Westley, J. W., and Miller, P. A. (1976). *J. Antibiot.* **29,** 21.

Loebenberg, D., Parmegiani, R., Miller, G. H., and Wright, J. J. (1980). *Intersci. Conf. Antimicrob. Ag. Chemother., 20th, New Orleans* Abstr. 471.

McDonald, E., and Martin, R. T. (1978). *Tetrahedron Lett.* 4723.

Malmberg, A. G., and Theander, O. (1980). *Phytochemistry* **19,** 1739.

Manachini, P. L., and Aragozzini, F. (1972). *Ann. Microbiol. Enzimol.* **22,** 55.

Mandrichenko, B. E., Tkachenko, G. E., Mazur, I. A., and Steblyuck, P. N. (1978). *Khim.Farm. Zh.* **12,** 64 (*Chem. Abstr.* **90,** 38864f, 1979).

Mansfield, J. W., Porter, A. E. A., and Smallman, R. V. (1980). *Phytochemistry* **19,** 1057.

Marriott, M. S. (1980). *J. Gen. Microbiol.* **117,** 253.

Marks, M. I., and Eickhoff, T. C. (1970). *Antimicrob. Ag. Chemother.* 491.

Martel, R. R., Klicius, J., and Galet, S. (1977). *Can. J. Physiol. Pharmacol.* **55,** 48.

Martín, J. F. (1979). *In* "Secondary Products of Metabolism: Economic Microbiology" (A. H. Rose, ed.), Vol. III, pp. 355–387. Academic Press, New York.

Martín, J. F., and Gil, J. A. (1979). *Jpn. J. Antibiot.* **32,** Suppl., S-122.
Martin, M., and Dewick, P. M. (1979). *Phytochemistry* **18,** 1309.
Massarani, E., Nardi, D., Tajana, A., Leonardi, A., and Degen, L. (1974). *Arzneim. Forsch.* **24,** 1545.
Matsumae, A., Nomura, S., and Hata, T. (1972). *J. Antibiot.* **25,** 365.
Matsumoto, M. (1979). *J. Sci. Hiroshima Univ. Ser. A* **43,** 47.
Mazens, M. F., Andrews, G. P., and Bartlett, R. C. (1979). *Antimicrob. Ag. Chemother.* **15,** 475.
Mazzone, G., and Bonina, F. (1979). *Farmaco Ed. Sci.* **34,** 390.
Mechlinski, W., and Schaffner, C. P. (1980). *J. Antibiot.* **33,** 591.
Medoff, G., and Kobayashi, G. S. (1980a). *N. Engl. J. Med.* **302,** 145.
Medoff, G., and Kobayashi, G. S. (1980b). *In* "Antifungal Chemotherapy" (D. C. E. Speller, ed.), pp. 3–33. Wiley, New York.
Mehta, K. J., and Parikh, A. R. (1978). *Indian J. Chem.* **16B,** 836.
Mehta, K. J., Parikh, K. S., and Parikh, A. R. (1978). *J. Inst. Chem. (Calcutta)* **50,** 210.
Mészáros, L., König, T., Paróczai, M., Náhm, K., and Horváth, I. (1979). *J. Antibiot.* **32,** 161.
Mészáros, L., Hoffmann, L., Paróczai, M., König, T., and Horváth, I. (1980). *J. Antibiot.* **33,** 523.
Michel, K. H., Hamill, R. L., Larsen, S. H., and Williams, R. H. (1975). *J. Antibiot.* **28,** 102.
Miles, D. H., Bhattacharyya, J., Mody, N. V., Atwood, J. L., Black, S., and Hedin, P. A. (1977). *J. Am. Chem. Soc.* **99,** 618.
Miles, D. H., Pelletier, S. W., Bhattacharyya, J., Mody, N. V., and Hedin, P. A. (1978). *J. Org. Chem.* **43,** 4371.
Minato, H., Katayama, T., Hayakawa, S., and Katagiri, K. (1972). *J. Antibiot.* **25,** 315.
Mir, L., Oustrin, M.-L., Lecointe, P., and Wright, M. (1978). *FEBS Lett.* **88,** 259.
Mitscher, L. A., Park, Y. H., Clark, D., Clark, G. W., Hammesfahr, P. D., Wu, W.-N., and Beal, J. L. (1978). *J. Nat. Prod.* **41,** 145.
Mizoguchi, J., Saito, T., Mizuno, K., and Hayano, K. (1977). *J. Antibiot.* **30,** 308.
Mizuno, K., Yagi, A., Satoi, S., Takada, M., Hayashi, M., Asano, K., and Matsuda, T. (1977). *J. Antibiot.* **30,** 297.
Montesano, R. (1979). *Nature (London)* **280,** 328.
Morozumi, S. (1978). *Shinkin Shinkinsho* **19,** 172 (*Chem. Abstr.* **90,** 76463g, 1979).
Muir, A. D., and Walker, J. R. L. (1979). *Chem. N. Z.* **43,** 94.
Muir, A. D., Cole, A. L. J., and Walker, J. R. L. (1979). *Aust. J. Pharm. Sci.* **8,** 28.
Mukherjee, S., and Bose, S. K. (1978). *J. Antibiot.* **31,** 147.
Muller, J. W., Fuhrer, H., Gruner, J., and Voser, W. (1976). *Helv. Chim. Acta* **59,** 2506.
Murai, A., Taketsuru, H., Yagihashi, F., Katsui, N., and Masamune, T. (1980a). *Bull. Chem. Soc. Jpn.* **53,** 1045.
Murai, A., Taketsuru, H., and Masamune, T. (1980b). *Bull. Chem. Soc. Jpn.* **53,** 1049.
Muroi, M., Haibara, K., Asai, M., and Kishi, T. (1980a). *Tetrahedron Lett.* **21,** 309.
Muroi, M., Izawa, M., Kosai, Y., and Asai, M. (1980b). *J. Antibiot.* **33,** 205.
Murthy, A. K., Rao, K. S. R., Krishna, M., and Rao, N. V. S. (1973). *J. Indian Chem. Soc.* **50,** 213.
Murthy, A. K., Rao, K. S. R., and Rao, N. V. S. (1976). *J. Indian Chem. Soc.* **53,** 1047.
Nagano, H., Poyser, J. P., Cheng, K. P., Bang, L., Ourisson, G., and Beck, J. P. (1977). *J. Chem. Res.* **(S)** 218; **(M)** 2522.
Nakakita, Y., Nakagawa, M., and Sakai, H. (1980). *J. Antibiot.* **33,** 514.
Nandi, J., and Bose, S. K. (1976). *J. Antibiot.* **29,** 50.
Nandi, J., De Kumar, B., and Bose, S. K. (1975). *J. Antibiot.* **28,** 988.

Nawata, Y., Ando, K., Tamura, G., Arima, K., and Iitaka, Y. (1969). *J. Antibiot.* **22,** 511.
Newbold, G. T., and Spring, F. S. (1948). *J. Chem. Soc.* 1864.
Nishimura, T., Yoshii, S., Toku, H., and Mochizuki, H. (1973a). *J. Pharm. Soc. Jpn.* **93,** 1236.
Nishimura, T., Yoshii, S., Toku, H., and Morishige, M. (1973b). *J. Pharm. Soc. Jpn.* **93,** 1242.
Nishimura, T., Yoshii, S., Toku, H., and Watanabe, M. (1973c). *J. Pharm. Soc. Jpn.* **93,** 1247.
Noto, T., Sawada, M., Ando, K., and Koyama, K. (1969). *J. Antibiot.* **22,** 165.
Novinson, T., Robins, R. K., and Matthews, T. R. (1977). *J. Med. Chem.* **20,** 296.
Odds, F. C. (1979a). *Postgrad. Med. J.* **55,** 677.
Odds, F. C. (1979b). "Candida and Candidosis." Leicester Univ. Press, England.
Ohmori, T., Hagiwara, S., Ueda, A., Minoda, Y., and Yamada, K. (1978). *Agric. Biol. Chem.* **42,** 2031.
Ohrui, H., and Emoto, S. (1978). *Tetrahedron Lett.* 2095.
Oimomi, M., Hamada, M., and Hara, T. (1974). *J. Antibiot.* **27,** 987.
Omoto, S., Shomura, T., Suzuki, H., and Inouye, S. (1979). *J. Antibiot.* **32,** 436.
Omura, S., Katagiri, M., Atsumi, K., Hata, T., Jakubowski, A. A., Springs, E. B., and Tishler, M. (1974). *J. Chem. Soc., Perkin Trans.* **I** 1627.
Omura, S., Iwai, Y., Takahashi, Y., Sadakane, N., Nakagawa, A., Oiwa, H., Hasegawa, Y., and Ikai, T. (1979a). *J. Antibiot.* **32,** 255.
Omura, S., Nakagawa, A., and Sadakane, N. (1979b). *Tetrahedron Lett.* 4323.
Omura, S., Iwai, Y., Nakagawa, A., Sadakane, N., Oiwa, H., Matsumoto, S., Takahashi, M., Ikai, T., and Ochiai, Y. (1980a). *Annu. Meet. Pharm. Soc. Jpn., 100th, Tokyo* Abstr. 4P, 1–13.
Omura, S., Iwai, Y., Masuma, R., Hayashi, M., Furusato, T., and Takagaki, T. (1980b). *J. Antibiot.* **33,** 758.
Ondrus, T. A., and Kraus, E. E. (1979). *Can. J. Pharm. Sci.* **14,** 55.
Osumi, J. (1972). *Shikoku Igaku Zasshi* **28,** 245 (*Chem. Abstr.* **81,** 145628t, 1974).
Otani, T., Arai, S., Sakano, K., Kawakami, Y., Ishimaru, K., Kondo, H., and Nakamura, S. (1977). *J. Antibiot.* **30,** 182.
Pal, S., and Gupta, I. (1979). *Indian Vet. J.* **56,** 367.
Pandey, R. C., Cook, J. C., Jr., and Rinehart, K. L., Jr. (1977). *J. Am. Chem. Soc.* **99,** 8469.
Parrini, V., Bossio, R., Pepino, R., and De Carneri, I. (1973). *Chim. Ind. (Milan)* **55,** 542.
Patterson, J., Holland, J., and Bieber, L. L. (1979). *J. Antibiot.* **32,** 646.
Pawlak, J., Zielínski, J., Kolodziejczyk, P., Golik, J., Gumieniak, J., Jereczek, E., and Borowski, E. (1979). *Tetrahedron Lett.* 1533.
Pedrazzoli, A., Dall'Asta, L., and Maffi, G. (1973). *Chim. Ther.* **8,** 65.
Pelletier, S. W., Mody, N. V., Bhattacharyya, J., and Miles, D. H. (1978). *Tetrahedron Lett.* 425.
Perlman, D. (1978). *In* "Medicinal Chemistry VI. Proceedings of the 6th. International Symposium on Medicinal Chemistry, Brighton" (A Simkin, ed.), pp. 409–413. Cotswold Press, Oxford.
Perrin, D. R., and Cruickshank, I. A. M. (1969). *Phytochemistry* **8,** 971.
Pesando, D., Gnassia-Barelli, M., Gueho, E., Rinaudo, M., and Defaye, J. (1980). *I.U.P.A.C. Int. Symp. Marine Nat. Prod., 3rd, Brussels* Abstr. P12.
Peypoux, F., Besson, F., Michel, G., and Delcambe, L. (1979). *J. Antibiot.* **32,** 136.
Pietraszkiewicz, M., and Sinaÿ, P. (1979). *Tetrahedron Lett.* 4741.
Plempel, M., Bartmann, K., Buchel, K. H., and Regel, E. (1969). *Dtsch. Med. Wochenschr.* **94,** 1356.

Plociennik, Z., Kowszyk-Gindifer, Z., Horodecka, M., Lewczuk-Mrozek, Z., and Bojarska-Dahlig, H. (1978). *Acta Pol. Pharm.* **35,** 125 (*Chem. Abstr.* **90,** 55195f, 1979).
Poplawski, J., Wrobel, J. T., and Glinka, T. (1980). *Phytochemistry* **19,** 1539.
Poulton, G. A., and Cyr, T. D. (1980). *Can. J. Chem.* **58,** 2158.
Pougny, J. R., and Sinaÿ, P. (1978). *Tetrahedron Lett.* 3301.
Poyser, J. P., Reinach Hirtzbach, F., de, and Ourisson, G. (1974). *Tetrahedron* **30,** 977.
Pryce, R. J., and Langcake, P. (1977). *Phytochemistry* **16,** 1452.
Pugh, C. S. G., Borchardt, R. T., and Stone, H. O. (1978). *J. Biol. Chem.* **253,** 4075.
Rao, K. V., and Cullen, W. P. (1960). *J. Am. Chem. Soc.* **82,** 1127.
Ravi, B. N., Perzanowski, H. P., Ross, R. A., Erdman, T. R., Scheuer, P. J., Finer, J., and Clardy, J. (1979). *Pure Appl. Chem.* **51,** 1893.
Rees, G. D., and Sugden, J. (1973). *Pharm. Acta Helv.* **48,** 157.
Reich, H. J., Gold, P. M., and Chow, F. (1979). *Tetrahedron Lett.* 4433.
Revankar, G. R., Matthews, T. R., and Robins, R. K. (1975). *J. Med. Chem.* **18,** 1253.
Richards, M., Bird, A. E., and Munden, J. E. (1969). *J. Antibiot.* **22,** 388.
Rickards, R. W. (1971). *J. Antibiot.* **24,** 715.
Riganti, V., and Spini, G. (1973). *Farmaco Ed. Sci.* **28,** 243.
Rinehart, K. L., Jr., and Shield, L. S. (1976). *Fortschr. Chem. Org. Naturst.* **33,** 231.
Rinehart, K. L., Jr., Antosz, F. J., Deshmukh, P. V., Kakinuma, K., Martin, P. K., Milavetz, B. I., Sasaki, K., Witty, T. R., Li, L. H., and Reusser, F. (1976). *J. Antibiot.* **29,** 201.
Ringel, S. M. (1978). *Antimicrob. Ag. Chemother.* **13,** 762.
Ringel, S. M., Greenough, R. C., Roemer, S., Connor, D., Gutt, A. L., Blair, B., Kanter, G., and Strandtmann, M., von (1977). *J. Antibiot.* **30,** 371.
Robeson, D. J., and Ingham, J. L. (1979). *Phytochemistry* **18,** 1715.
Roobol, A., Gull, K., and Pogson, C. I. (1976). *FEBS Lett.* **67,** 248.
Roobol, A., Gull, K., and Pogson, C. I. (1977). *FEBS Lett.* **75,** 149.
Sacchi, F. T., Clivio, A., Ferrari, F. A., Pagani, A., Ruozi, P., and Siccardi, A. G. (1979). *J. Med. Microbiol.* **12,** 143.
Sakano, K.-I., Ishimaru, K., and Nakamura, S. (1980). *J. Antibiot.* **33,** 683.
Sakata, K., Sakurai, A., and Tamura, S. (1977a). *Agric. Biol. Chem.* **41,** 2033.
Sakata, K., Uzawa, J., and Sakurai, A. (1977b). *Org. Magn. Reson.* **10,** 230.
Satoi, S., Yagi, A., Asano, K., Mizuno, K., and Watanabe, T. (1977). *J. Antibiot.* **30,** 303.
Saubolle, M. A., and Hoeprich, P. D. (1978). *Antimicrob. Ag. Chemother.* **14,** 517.
Schauer, P., Japelj, M., Povse, A., and Likar, M. (1972). *Proc. Int. Congr. Chemother., 7th, Prague, 1971* 329.
Schindler, F., and Zähner, H. (1971). *Arch. Mikrobiol.* **79,** 187.
Scholer, H. J. (1960). *Pathol. Microbiol.* **23,** 62.
Scholer, H. J. (1980). *In* "Antifungal Chemotherapy" (D. C. E. Speller, ed.), pp. 35–106. Wiley, New York.
Schramm, G., and Steglich, W. (1980). *I.U.P.A.C. Symp. Chem. Nat. Prod., 12th, Tenerife*
Schramm, G., Steglich, W., Anke, T., and Oberwinkler, F. (1978). *Chem. Ber.* **111,** 2779.
Schroder, E. (1970). *Arzneim. Forsch.* **20,** 737.
Schroeder, G., Rohmer, M., Beck, J. P., and Anton, R. (1980). *Phytochemistry* **19,** 2213.
Schwan, T. J., Gray, J. E., and Wright, G. C. (1979). *J. Pharm. Sci.* **68,** 529.
Schwochau, M. E., and Hadwiger, L. A. (1972). *Rec. Adv. Phytochem.* **3,** 181.
Sekhon, A. S., and Funk, A. (1977). *J. Antimicrob. Chemother.* **3,** 95.
Sekhon, A. S., and Hargesheimer, E. (1975). *J. Clin. Pathol.* **28,** 547.

Serafin, B., Modzdewski, M., Kurnatowska, A., and Kadlubowski, R. (1977). *Eur. J. Med. Chem.* **12,** 325.
Seto, H., and Yonehara, H. (1977a). *J. Antibiot.* **30,** 1019.
Seto, H., and Yonehara, H. (1977b). *J. Antibiot.* **30,** 1022.
Severinets, L. Y., Krasilnikova, M. M., Vekshina, N. A., and Sukharevich, V. I. (1977). *Antibiotiki* **22,** 492. (*Chem. Abstr.* **87,** 100614t, 1977).
Shadomy, S. (1969). *Appl. Microbiol.* **17,** 871.
Shadomy, S., and Espinel-Ingroff, A. (1974). *In* "Manual of Clinical Microbiology" (E. H. Lennette, E. H. Spaulding, and J. P. Truant, eds.), 2nd. Ed., pp. 569–574. American Society for Microbiology, Washington D.C.
Shadomy, S., Paxton, L., Espinel-Ingroff, A., and Shadomy, H. J. (1977a). *J. Antimicrob. Chemother.* **3,** 147.
Shadomy, S., Shadomy, H. J., and Wagner, G. E. (1977b). *In* "Antifungal Compounds" (M. R. Siegel and H. D. Sisler, eds.), Vol. 1, pp. 437–461. Dekker, New York.
Shadomy, S., Utz, C. J., and White, S. (1978). *Antimicrob. Ag. Chemother.* **14,** 95.
Sharma, G. M., Michaels, L., and Burkholder, P. R. (1968). *J. Antibiot.* **21,** 659.
Shenin, Y. D., Omelchenko, V. N., and Onoprienko, V. V. (1978). *Antibiotiki* **23,** 582. (*Chem. Abstr.* **89,** 144941t, 1978).
Shibata, M., Uyeda, K., and Mori, K. (1980). *J. Antibiot.* **33,** 679.
Shimi, I. R., Abedallah, N., and Fathy, S. (1977). *Antimicrob. Ag. Chemother.* **11,** 373.
Shoji, J. (1978). *Adv. Appl. Microbiol.* **24,** 187.
Singh, H., and Yadav, L. D. S. (1976). *Agric. Biol. Chem.* **40,** 759.
Singh, H., and Yadav, L. D. S. (1977). *J. Indian Chem. Soc.* **54,** 1143.
Singh, K., Sun, S., and Vézina, C. (1979). *J. Antibiot.* **32,** 630.
Singh, N. B., Singh, H., and Singh, S. (1975). *J. Indian Chem. Soc.* **52,** 1200.
Sinha, S. K., and Basuchaudhary, K. C. (1977). *Curr. Sci.* **46,** 784.
Smith, D. A., Van Etten, H. D., and Bateman, D. F. (1973). *Physiol. Plant Pathol.* **3,** 179.
Smith, D. A., Kuhn, P. J., Bailey, J. A., and Burden, R. S. (1980). *Phytochemistry* **19,** 1673.
Smith, R. M. (1979). *Tetrahedron* **35,** 437.
Speller, D. C. E. (1980). "Antifungal Chemotherapy." Wiley, New York.
Stillwell, M. A., Magasi, L. P., and Strunz, G. M. (1974). *Can. J. Microbiol.* **20,** 759.
Stoessl, A. (1972). *Rec. Adv. Phytochem.* **3,** 143.
Strehlke, P. (1979). *Eur. J. Med. Chem.* **14,** 227.
Strehlke, P., and Kessler, H. J. (1979). *Eur. J. Med. Chem.* **14,** 238.
Strehlke, P., and Schroeder, E. (1974). *Eur. J. Med. Chem.* **9,** 35, 41.
Strehlke, P., Hoyer, G. A., and Schroeder, E. (1975). *Arch. Pharm.* (*Weinheim, Ger.*) **308,** 94.
Suami, T., Ogawa, S., and Chida, N. (1980). *J. Antibiot.* **33,** 98.
Sud, I. J., Chou, D. L., and Feingold, D. S. (1979). *Antimicrob. Ag. Chemother.* **16,** 660.
Sueda, N., Ohrui, H., and Kuzuhara, H. (1979). *Tetrahedron Lett.* 2039.
Sugawara, R. (1963). *J. Antibiot.* **A16,** 115.
Suman, S. P., and Bahel, S. C. (1979). *Agric. Biol. Chem.* **43,** 1339.
Suzuki, S., Nakamura, G., Okuma, K., and Tomiyama, Y. (1958). *J. Antibiot.* **A11,** 81.
Swindells, D. C. N., White, P. S., and Findlay, J. A. (1978). *Can. J. Chem.* **56,** 2491.
Takahashi, N., Suzuki, A., and Tamura, S. (1965). *J. Am. Chem. Soc.* **87,** 2066.
Takasugi, M., Shigemitsu, N., Masamune, T., Shirata, A., and Takahashi, K. (1978). *Tetrahedron Lett.* 797.
Takasugi, M., Nagao, S., Muñoz, L., Ishikawa, S., Masamune, T., Shirata, A., and Takahashi, K. (1979). *Koen Yoshishu-Tennen Yuki Kagobutsu Toronka* 257 (*Chem. Abstr.* **92,** 160540d, 1980).

Takasugi, M., Anetai, M., Masamune, T., Shirata, A., and Takahashi, K. (1980). *Chem. Lett.* 339.

Takatsuki, A., Kawamura, K., Okina, M., Kodama, Y., Ito, T., and Tamura, G. (1977). *Agric. Biol. Chem.* **41,** 2307.

Takeuchi, S., Yonehara, H., and Shoji, H. (1964). *J. Antibiot.* **A17,** 267.

Tanida, S., Hasegawa, T., Hatano, K., Higashide, E., and Yoneda, M. (1980a). *J. Antibiot.* **33,** 192.

Tanida, S., Hasegawa, T., and Higashide, E. (1980b). *J. Antibiot.* **33,** 199.

Taylor, E. P., and D'Arcy, P. F. (1961). *Prog. Med. Chem.* **1,** 220.

Thakar, K. A., and Ghawal, B. M. (1977). *J. Indian Chem. Soc.* **15b,** 1056.

Tin-Wa, M., Farnsworth, N. R., Fong, H. H. S., and Trojanek, J. (1970). *Lloydia* **33,** 267.

Tkacz, J. S. (1980). *Fed. Proc. Fed. Am. Soc. Exp. Biol.* **39,** 1830, Abstr. 1166.

Traber, R., Keller-Juslén, C., Loosli, H. R., Kuhn, M., and Wartburg, A. von (1979). *Helv. Chim. Acta* **62,** 1252.

Traxler, P., Fritz, H., and Richter, W. J. (1977a). *Helv. Chim. Acta* **60,** 578.

Traxler, P., Gruner, J., and Auden, J. A. L. (1977b). *J. Antibiot.* **30,** 289.

Tripathi, R. K., and Gottlieb, D. (1969). *J. Bacteriol.* **100,** 310.

Tsuda, K., Kihara, T., Nishii, M., Nakamura, G., Isono, K., and Suzuki, S. (1980). *J. Antibiot.* **33,** 247.

Tsuji, N., and Kobayashi, M. (1978). *J. Antibiot.* **31,** 939.

Tunac, J. B., McDaniel, L. E., Patel, M., and Schaffner, C. P. (1979). *J. Antibiot.* **32,** 1230.

Turner, J. B., Butler, T. F., Gordee, R. S., and Thakkar, A. L. (1978). *J. Antibiot.* **31,** 33.

Uegaki, R., Fujimori, T., Kaneko, H., Kubo, S., and Kato, K. (1980a). *Phytochemistry* **19,** 1229.

Uegaki, R., Fujimori, T., Kaneko, H., Kubo, S., and Kato, K. (1980b). *Phytochemistry* **19,** 1543.

Ueno, A., Shiraishi, Y., Yamamoto, T., and Mokoki, Y. (1973). *J. Pharm. Soc. Jpn.* **94,** 276.

Umio, S., Kariyone, K., Tanaka, K., Kishimoto, T., Nakamura, H., and Nishida, M. (1970). *Chem. Pharm. Bull.* **18,** 1414.

Uramoto, M., Uzawa, J., Suzuki, S., Isono, K., Liehr, J. G., and McCloskey, J. A. (1978). *Nucleic Acids Res.* **5,** 327.

Uri, J. V., and Actor, P. (1979). *J. Antibiot.* **32,** 1207.

Uri, J. V., Actor, P., Phillips, L., and Weisbach, J. A. (1978). *J. Antibiot.* **31,** 580.

Utz, J. P., Garriques, I. L., Sande, M. A., Warner, J. F., Mandell, G. L., McGehee, R. F., Duma, R. J., and Shadomy, S. (1975). *J. Infect. Dis.* **132,** 368.

Van den Bossche, H. (1974). *Biochem. Pharmacol.* **23,** 887.

Van den Bossche, H., Willemsens, G., Cools, W., Lauwers, W. F. J., and LeJeune, L. (1978). *Proc. Int. Congr. Chemother., 10th, Zurich 1977* Vol. 1, p. 228.

Van Etten, H. D. (1976). *Phytochemistry* **15,** 655.

Vedel, M., Lawrence, F., Robert-Gero, M., and Lederer, E. (1978). *Biochem. Biophys. Res. Commun.* **85,** 371.

Vichkanova, S. A., and Adgina, V. V. (1973). *Antibiotiki* **18,** 902 (*Chem. Abstr.* **80,** 44048c, 1974).

Vigneron, J. P., and Blanchard, J. M. (1980). *Tetrahedron Lett.* **21,** 1739.

Vitali, T., Mossini, F., and Plazzi, P. V. (1974). *Farmaco Ed. Sci.* **29,** 27.

Walker, K. A. M., Braemer, A. C., Hitt, S., Jones, R. E., and Matthews, T. R. (1978a). *J. Med. Chem.* **21,** 840.

Walker, K. A. M., Hirschfeld, D. R., and Marx, M. (1978b). *J. Med. Chem.* **21,** 1335.

Wat, C. K., McInnes, A. G., Smith, D. G., Wright, J. L. C., and Vining, L. C. (1977). *Can. J. Chem.* **55,** 4090.

Wat, C. K., Biswas, R. K., Graham, E. A., Boha, L., Towers, G. H. N., and Waygood, E. R. (1979). *J. Nat. Prod.* **42,** 103.

Whitehead, C. W., and Whitesitt, C. A. (1974). *J. Med. Chem.* **17,** 1298.

Wildfeuer, A. (1974). *Arzneim. Forsch.* **24,** 937.

Winkelmann, G., Lupp, R., and Jung, G. (1980). *J. Antibiot.* **33,** 353.

Winters, G., Mola, N., Berti, M., and Arioli, V. (1979). *Farmaco Ed. Sci.* **34,** 507.

Woodward, M. D. (1979a). *Phytochemistry* **18,** 363.

Woodward, M. D. (1979b). *Phytochemistry* **18,** 2007.

Woodward, M. D. (1980). *Phytochemistry* **19,** 921.

Wratten, S. J., Wolfe, M. S., Andersen, R. J., and Faulkner, D. J. (1977). *Antimicrob. Ag. Chemother.* **11,** 411.

Wratten, S. J., Faulkner, D. J., Hirotsu, K., and Clardy, J. (1978). *Tetrahedron Lett.* 4345.

Wright, G. C., Gray, J. E., and Yu, C-N. (1974). *J. Med. Chem.* **17,** 244.

Wright, J. J., Albarella, J., Krepski, L. R., and Loebenberg, D. (1980). *Intersci. Conf. Antimicrob. Ag. Chemother., 20th, New Orleans* Abstr. 472.

Yale, H. R., and Spitzmiller, E. R. (1977). *Arzneim. Forsch.* **27,** 1396.

Yamada, Y., and Azuma, K. (1977). *Antimicrob. Ag. Chemother.* **11,** 743.

Yamada, Y., Yanagi, H., and Okada, H. (1974). *Agric. Biol. Chem.* **38,** 381.

Yamaguchi, H. (1977). *Antimicrob. Ag. Chemother.* **12,** 16.

Yamaguchi, H. (1978). *Antimicrob. Ag. Chemother.* **13,** 423.

Yano, K. (1980). *Phytochemistry* **19,** 1864.

Yokota, M., Zenda, H., Kosuge, T., and Yamamoto, T. (1978). *Yakugaku Zasshi* **98,** 1508 (*Chem. Abstr.* **90,** 51428m, 1979).

Yoneda, F., Sakuma, Y., Ueno, M., and Nishigaki, S. (1973). *Chem. Pharm. Bull.* **21,** 926.

Yoneyama, K., Sekido, S., and Misato, T. (1978). *J. Antibiot.* **31,** 1065.

Yoshida, S., Yoneyama, K., Shiraishi, S., Watanabe, A., and Takahashi, N. (1977). *Agric. Biol. Chem.* **41,** 849, 855.

Yoshikawa, M. (1978). *Nature* (*London*) **275,** 546.

Zdorenko, V. A., Vladzimirskaya, E. V., and Steblyuk, P. N. (1978). *Farm. Zh.* (*Kiev*) **3,** 58 (*Chem. Abstr.* **89,** 179904k, 1978).

Zhikhareva, G. D., Pronina, E. V., Golovanova, E. A., Pershin, G. N., Novitskaya, N. A., Zykova, T. N., Guskova, T. A., and Yakhontov, L. N. (1976). *Khim.-Farm. Zh.* **10,** 62 (*Chem. Abstr.* **85,** 123848v, 1976).

Zieliński, J., Jereczek, E., Sowinski, P., Falkowski, L., Rudowski, A., and Borowski, E. (1979). *J. Antibiot.* **32,** 565.

ADVANCES IN PHARMACOLOGY AND CHEMOTHERAPY, VOL. 18

Intercalating Drugs: DNA Binding and Molecular Pharmacology

W. DAVID WILSON AND ROBERT L. JONES

Department of Chemistry
and
Laboratory for Microbial and Biochemical Sciences
Georgia State University
Atlanta, Georgia

I. Introduction

There are many drug molecules containing planar aromatic ring systems which can be inserted between base pairs of DNA in a process called intercalation. This interaction can lead to inhibition of DNA and/or RNA polymerase reactions and can, thus, cause metabolic changes and death in organisms or cells treated with intercalating drugs. There is evidence that many intercalating compounds, such as those shown in Fig. 1, which have activity against microbial organisms and neoplastic cells exert their activity through a binding process of this type with DNA. There are several questions which arise concerning the relationship between intercalation and medicinal activity: (1) How do the conformational changes which the drugs induce in DNA relate to the medicinal activity? (2) Are the thermodynamics or the kinetics of the intercalation reaction of more importance in affecting activity? (3) How does intercalation influence the selec-

ISBN 0-12-032918-2

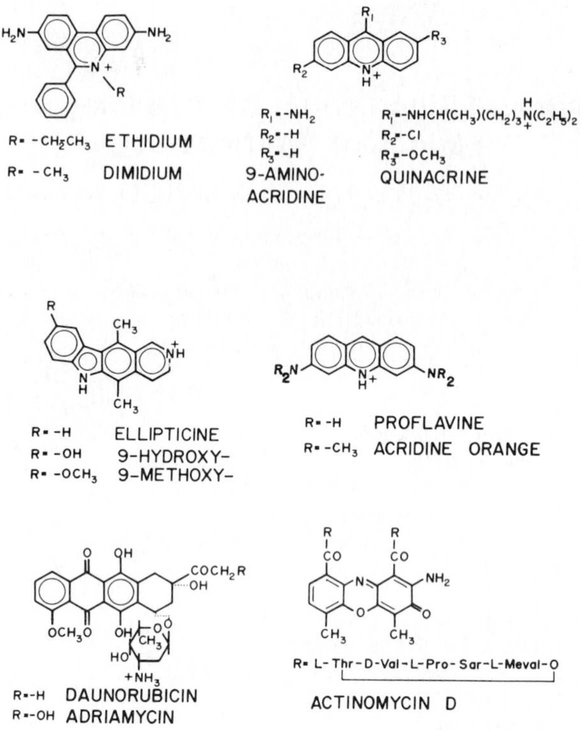

FIG. 1. The structures of some common intercalating drugs, whose interaction with DNA has been thoroughly studied, are shown.

tivity of the drug for the target cell? (4) How could the drug structure be modified to increase DNA binding and would this affect activity? (5) How do the toxic effects of the drugs relate to intercalation? There are obviously considerations, not directly related to intercalation, such as transport through membranes and metabolic transformation of the drugs, which also affect activity. All of these factors will be discussed in this article when results are available to allow conclusions to be made. Unfortunately, although there have been numerous studies of the binding of drugs to DNA and many analyses of membrane transport or partitioning, these have rarely been combined into a systematic study with a broad enough range of drugs to provide conclusive results.

Several general reviews of intercalation and intercalating drugs have been published (Blake and Peacocke, 1968; Newton, 1970; Waring, 1972; Bloomfield *et al.*, 1974; Kersten and Kersten, 1974; Corcoran and Hahn, 1975; Neidle, 1979; Wilson and Jones, 1981) and it is hoped that the present article will update and prove complementary to this previous coverage of the field. In addition, thousands of papers on intercalating drugs and reviews on specific intercalating drugs or classes of drugs have been published and there will be no effort here to provide summaries of all these findings. We will attempt to establish any principles which underlie the medicinal activity of intercalating drugs in general.

In Section II of this article we provide a background description of the intercalation model with particular emphasis on recent developments in the knowledge of this binding process. We then discuss, in Section III, what is known with some certainty about how this model relates to the medicinal activity of intercalating drugs. In Section IV we discuss specific drugs which have been used successfully in the treatment of various diseases and for which detailed studies have been conducted on the interaction of the drugs with DNA.

II. Current Concepts of Intercalation

A. The Classical Model

Over the years preceding the Watson–Crick (1953) model for DNA, it was realized that many planar aromatic cations had biological activity. These compounds had established uses in chemotherapy and many were also known to be mutagenic. The growing realization that DNA was the genetic material and the interest in DNA generated by publication of the Watson–Crick model for the double helix led to studies on the interaction of these planar cations with DNA. One of the early attempts to quantitate this type of interaction was conducted by Peacocke and Skerrett (1956). They measured the amount of proflavine bound to DNA at different concentrations using spectral shifts induced in proflavine on interaction with DNA and using equilibrium dialysis. The Scatchard plots (Scatchard, 1949) obtained from these results were curved and Peacocke and Skerrett proposed that the curvature was the result of two classes of independent, noninteracting binding sites for proflavine on DNA. The first class of sites (Type I) saturated at one ligand molecule for every four to five DNA nucleotides and had a much greater binding constant than for the second class of sites (Type II) which reached saturation at approximately one ligand per nucleotide. Peacocke and Skerrett (1956) did not feel that either interaction caused any significant structural change in the DNA double helix. They felt the ligand spectral shifts which resulted from Type I binding could be accounted for through interaction of the proflavine ring system with the DNA bases in the grooves of the double helix. The weaker (Type II) binding was considered to be primarily an electrostatic interaction between the polyanions of the DNA sugar–phosphate chain and a self associated stack of the planar cations. Because of the cooperative stacking of the cations in Type II binding, this interaction was found to decrease dramatically with increasing ionic strength and to be unimportant at physiological conditions. Experimental evidence of this type indicates that Type I binding accounts for the biological effects of proflavine and similar intercalating compounds on nucleic acid metabolism *in vivo.* Characterization of the Type I complex, thus, became of utmost importance for development of this field.

In an effort to elucidate the structure of the biologically important Type I complex, Lerman (1961, 1963, 1964a,b) conducted systematic structural studies on the DNA complexes of several acridines including proflavine. He found that the viscosity of a DNA solution was markedly increased by all the acridine derivatives while simple inorganic cations and nonplanar organic cations, similar in composition to the acridines, caused slight viscosity decreases in agreement with previous results (Cavalieri *et al.*, 1956). The sedimentation coefficient of DNA, on the other hand, decreased on interaction with the acridines while it increased with the nonplanar cations which bound to DNA. In the region of Type II binding of proflavine the sedimentation coefficient began to increase suggesting that Type I and Type II complexes have markedly different structures with Type II binding being more analogous to the binding of nonplanar cations. The X-ray diffraction of DNA–proflavine fibers retained the characteristic 3.4 Å meridional spots while losing the standard layer-line pattern of B-form DNA and no new spots were found (Lerman, 1961). The combined results of these experiments suggested that as a result of binding of acridine derivatives, the DNA double helix: (1) became longer or some combination of longer and stiffer; (2) had a decreased mass per unit length; (3) approximately retained its 3.4 Å spacing with the base pairs essentially perpendicular to the helix axis; and (4) lost the regular repeating nature of the phosphates in the double helix.

In addition to investigating the DNA structure in the Type I complex, Lerman, using flow dichroism, flow polarized fluorescence, and ligand reaction rates, began to look at the properties of the bound acridine molecule. He found that the plane of the bound acridine molecules was essentially parallel to the DNA base pairs and perpendicular to the axes of the double helix. Given all of these experimental findings, Lerman proposed that an intercalation model best described the acridine–DNA complex. Other structures such as surface attachment of the ligand or insertion of the ligand into the double helix with displacement of a base pair agreed with some but not all of the experimental results. Model building studies indicated that the B-form double helix could be extended, with simple single bond rotation, to create a space for insertion of a planar aromatic molecule of approximately 3.4 Å in thickness (Lerman, 1964a). This classical intercalation model has the following features: (1) the rod-like structure, hydrogen bonding, and covalent bonding of B-form DNA is retained; (2) two adjacent base pairs are separated by approximately 3.4 Å to create a planar space for intercalation of an aromatic ring; (3) an unwinding of the double helix is required (this unwinding could not be measured and was simply a best guess based on model building; Lerman's initial estimate was 45° for unwinding) leaving the adjacent base pairs positioned more directly over each other; and (4) the aromatic ring is inserted between and essentially parallel to the base pairs in a manner to fill the space created by extension of the double helix as fully as possible. The size of the space created was close to that required to insert the acridine ring with its long axis oriented in a similar manner to the long axes of the two adjacent base pairs. The proposal of this model sparked a tremendous research effort to determine how the model applied to other planar aromatic drugs, aromatic amino acid groups of peptides, carcinogens, and similar compounds. In this research the features of the intercalation model have undergone considerable development but the general concepts originally postulated by Lerman have been retained.

B. Development of the Intercalation Model

One of the characteristics of intercalation is the length increase which it produces in the double helix and the resulting changes in the hydrodynamic properties of DNA such as intrinsic viscosity and sedimentation coefficient. Lerman (1961, 1964a) had some difficulty treating his original viscosity and sedimentation results because of the complexity of the tertiary structure of high-molecular-weight DNA in solution (Bloomfield *et al.*, 1974). Intercalation could affect both the local secondary structure of the double helix and the long range coiling of the molecule. Cohen and Eisenberg (1969) reasoned that this problem could be greatly simplified if shorter molecules, near or less than the persistence length of DNA in solution, were used in analyzing intercalation. With these short rod-like segments of double helical DNA the tertiary effect due to long range structural changes could be largely eliminated. Assuming rod-like behavior of these short DNA segments, they derived equations to relate the viscosity and sedimentation changes which occur on intercalation to length changes in the double helix (Cohen and Eisenberg, 1969). They found that the average length increase produced by proflavine binding to DNA was approximately 80% of that predicted for a theoretical length increase of 3.4 Å per bound proflavine molecule. This was the first quantitative hydrodynamic experiment to test the structural predictions of the intercalation model and the results agreed well with predicted values.

Saucier *et al.* (1971), also using sonicated calf thymus DNA and other experimental and theoretical methods developed by Cohen and Eisenberg (1969), analyzed the DNA viscosity enhancement of several additional planar aromatic cations. They found that daunorubicin and 9-methoxyellipticine gave the predicted increase in viscosity. Ethidium bromide, on the other hand, gave a length increase of only about 70% of the expected value and quinacrine and proflavine also gave less than the theoretically predicted increase. This result and similar experiments with other ligands (Gabbay *et al.*, 1973a; Davidson *et al.*, 1977a; Jones *et al.*, 1979) indicated that the DNA length increase produced on intercalation could vary significantly with ligand structure and was generally less than the predicted value. The reasons for the variation are still not completely clear, but some modification of the classical intercalation model to include these effects was clearly necessary.

Gabbay and co-workers (1973a), working with a series of methylated phenanthroline derivatives, found that the viscosity enhancement produced on binding of these compounds to DNA depended upon the number and position of the methyl substituents. They found that two pentamethyl compounds (including a quaternary *N*-methyl group) with the methyl groups spread around the ring gave the largest increase in viscosity on complex formation of any compound in this series. The viscosity increases for these methylated compounds are considerably larger than the increase for the unsubstituted compound. Gabbay *et al.* (1973a) attributed this effect to the increased effective thickness of the ring system when extensively methylated. They found with several trimethyl derivatives, however, that the position of substitution of the methyl groups dramatically affected the viscosity increase on complex formation. A symmetrically substituted trimethyl compound gave a viscosity increase almost as large as the pentamethyl derivative while an asymmetrically substituted trimethyl compound gave the smallest increase of all derivatives studied (even smaller than the unsubstituted compound). It was suggested that these results could best be explained by a nonclassical intercalation binding mechanism as follows: (1) the unsubstituted compound binds in a classical manner; (2) symmetrically substituted compounds bind in a more or less classical manner but cause larger length increases than the unsubstituted compound because of the greater effective thickness of their methylated intercalating ring systems; (3) the asymmetrically substituted compounds bind by intercalation but can cause both lengthening and bending of the double helix. The net result of this latter binding mode is a smaller increase in viscosity than is produced in a classical binding mechanism. This type of binding model is shown in Fig. 2 where various combinations of helix length changes are illustrated.

The concept of Gabbay and co-workers that insertion of an aromatic

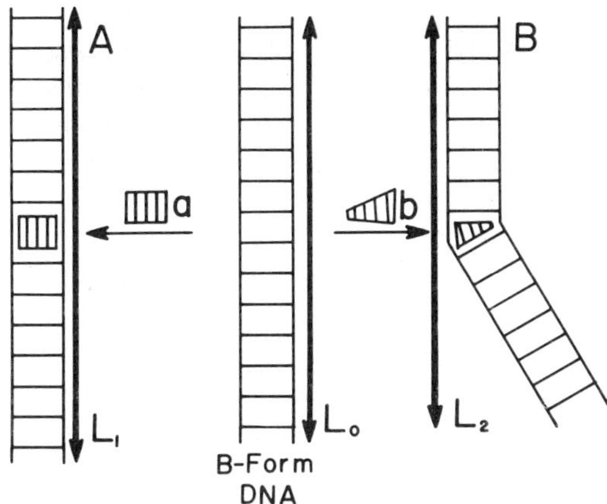

FIG. 2. Both classical (A) and nonclassical (B) intercalation models are illustrated for ligand–DNA interactions: L_0 is the length of a section of B-form DNA, L_1 is the length of the same section of DNA after binding an intercalating molecule such as those shown in Fig. 1, and L_2 is the length of the same section of DNA after binding a nonclassical intercalating molecule (e.g., a small or nonplanar aromatic ring system or a larger aromatic ring system with an asymmetrical distribution of bulky substituents).

group between DNA base pairs can cause bending of the double helix has received support from X-ray analysis of intercalating drugs crystallized with complementary dinucleoside monophosphates (reviewed by Sobell *et al.*, 1977). With ethidium bromide, for example, the phenyl and ethyl substitutents are located in the minor groove of the miniature double helix and the helix is bent toward the major groove at the intercalation point (Sobell *et al.*, 1977). The possibility of bending the helix with larger ring systems and the steric restrictions on intercalation have also been supported by viscosity studies using the berberinium ion (Davidson *et al.*, 1977a) and using several quinoline methanol derivatives with different numbers of bulky substituents (Davidson *et al.*, 1977b). Small aromatic ring systems and the aromatic amino acids of peptides also cause pronounced DNA viscosity decreases which suggests that these compounds can cause significant bending of the DNA double helix (reviewed by Gabbay, 1977).

Another characteristic of intercalation as proposed by Lerman is the unwinding which it produces in the DNA double helix. In the B-form double helix with 10 base pairs per turn (360°) each base pair is rotated +36° with respect to the base pair immediately below it (Arnott and Hukins, 1973). If these neighboring base pairs are separated to create a space for intercalation, this rotation is reduced and the amount of the reduction in degrees is termed the intercalation unwinding angle. In the development of the intercalation model, Lerman (1964a) revised his original postulate of 45° unwinding (a net reversed or left-handed rotation of 9°) to 36° unwinding (no net rotation). Fuller and Waring (1964) conducted extensive model building studies on ethidium bromide and concluded that a 12° unwinding angle allowed maximum separation of anionic phosphate groups, and allowed the optimum interaction of the ethidium molecule with the double helix (hydrogen bonding of ethidium amino groups with the phosphate oxygens of DNA and optimum overlap of the drug and base pair aromatic ring systems). The 12° value for ethidium became somewhat of a standard for intercalation until the early 1970s (Waring, 1972).

The discovery of closed circular superhelical DNA has now allowed unwinding angles on intercalation to be quantitatively determined and much of the controversy concerning these unwinding angles has been removed. As intercalating molecules are added to superhelical DNA, the double helix is unwound and initially the natural right handed superhelical turns are removed until the DNA has no remaining superhelical structure at which time it is hydrodynamically equivalent to nicked circular DNA (Waring, 1972; Bauer, 1978). If more of the intercalating drug is added, the double helix continues to unwind with the formation of a left-handed superhelical structure. These changes in superhelix density and viscosity are shown schematically in Fig. 3. The maximum in the viscometric titration shown in Fig. 3 (or the minimum in a sedimentation experiment) corresponds to closed circular DNA with no remaining superhelical turns. It is obvious that if both the initial number of superhelical turns is known and if the amount of bound drug required to completely remove these turns is determined (the amount of bound drug required to reach the maximum in the curve in Fig. 3), the unwinding angle of the drug can be calculated. Vinograd and co-workers developed an especially accurate experimental technique for measuring unwinding angles using a 26° unwinding angle for ethidium bromide as a standard value (Révet *et al.*, 1971). The 26° unwinding angle for ethidium has resulted from several different experiments with superhelical DNA and has now replaced Waring's earlier estimate of 12° as the standard for intercalation unwinding angles (Wang, 1974; Pulleyblank and Morgan, 1975; Bauer and Vinograd, 1974).

Few molecules have been quantitatively analyzed for unwinding at this time and the influence of the various structural features which determine a ligand's unwinding angle is still largely unknown. The 26° unwinding angle for ethidium and some related phenanthridines (Wakelin and Waring, 1974) is the largest unwinding angle found to date for any intercalating monomer ligand. The classical acridine drugs originally studied by Ler-

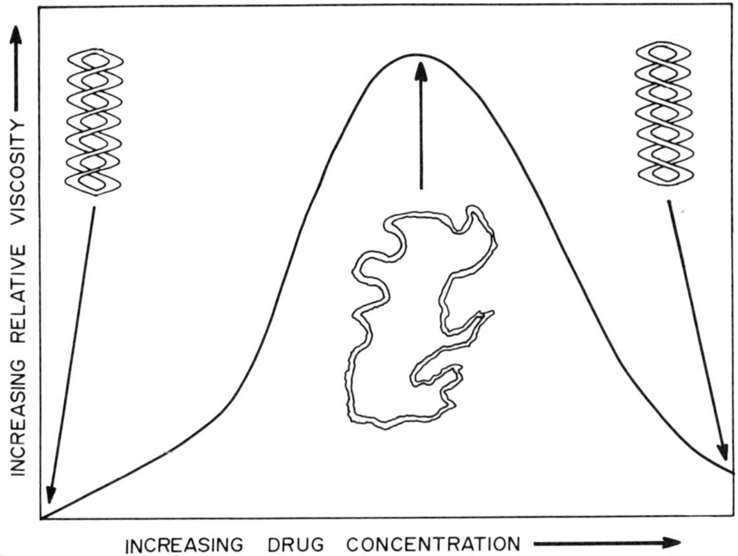

FIG. 3. Schematic representation of the effects of an intercalating drug upon the solution viscosity of closed circular superhelical DNA. The diagram illustrates the three main stages of binding: (1) on the left, the DNA molecule has not bound enough drug to remove the natural right-handed superhelical turns, thus the relative viscosity is low; (2) in the center, enough drug has been added to exactly remove the superhelical turns and a maximum is obtained in the relative viscosity; (3) on the right, enough intercalating drug has been added to reverse the DNA supercoiling, producing left-handed superhelical turns, and again reducing the relative viscosity.

man seem to give lower unwinding angles which cluster between 17 and 20° (Jones *et al.,* 1980). The anthracycline drugs, daunorubicin and adriamycin, have been reported to have lower unwinding angles, between 10 and 12°, relative to ethidium bromide (Waring, 1971). It is interesting to note that a large number of intercalating molecules seem to have unwinding angles near 18°. The phenanthridines which have a very specific hydrogen bonding interaction with DNA (Fuller and Waring, 1964; Tsai *et al.,* 1977; Jain *et al.,* 1977) unwind by 8° more than this 18° value. It has also been proposed that the anthracyclines have a very specific hydrogen bonding interaction with DNA (Pigram *et al.,* 1972; Henry, 1976; Quigley *et al.,* 1980) and they unwind approximately 8° less than this common 18° value. The 26° phenanthridine value is the highest unwinding angle that has been found for monointercalators and the 10° anthracycline value is the lowest. It seems possible that an unwinding angle of approximately 18° may be optimum for intercalators in general and that this value may be increased or decreased by specific drug–DNA interactions.

In developing a model for the intercalation complex of a drug, it is essential to know what the orientation of the aromatic ring is with respect to the helix axis. Lerman (1964a) used flow dichroism in his original characterization of the interaction of acridine drugs with DNA and was able to determine that the acridine plane of these drugs is roughly perpendicular to the helix axis. These studies were extended using electric dichroism, but because the DNA is incompletely oriented, even at high field, and because of the uncertainty concerning exactly what the orientation mechanism is in electric dichroism, this technique was not widely used. Recent advances in instrumentation (adaptation of temperature-jump instruments for electric dichroism measurements), and theory (Crothers *et al.*, 1978; Dattagupta *et al.*, 1978; Hogan *et al.*, 1979) for this method as well as techniques for preparing homogeneous DNA (Hogan *et al.*, 1978) have increased the potential of electric dichroism for providing information about the structure of DNA and its complexes with small molecules.

Crothers and co-workers have applied this electric dichroism technique to intercalating drugs (Hogan *et al.*, 1979) and they were able to determine the orientation of two nonparallel transition vectors in ethidium bromide, proflavine, and 9-aminoacridine. The results with ethidium and 9-aminoacridine are quite similar and suggest a considerable variation from perpendicularity of both the long and short axes of the drugs. Ethidium's long axis (the tilt) is 23° from perpendicular and the short axis (the twist) is 10° from perpendicular. With proflavine these values are 14 and 2° for the long and short axes, respectively. These values indicate that intercalating drugs are much less nearly perpendicular to the helix axis than in Lerman's model for intercalation. Crothers and co-workers (Hogan *et al.,* 1979) analyzed numerous possible experimental and theoretical artifacts as possible explanations for these somewhat unusual findings, and were able to eliminate most of the possible errors based on various control experiments. Using their experimental DNA orientation from electric dichroism, they also analyzed earlier qualitative results from both flow and electric dichroism and concluded that all of these experimental findings predict a tilt and twist for intercalated ligands which is consistent with their more quantitative results. Starting with the Levitt (1978) modified B-DNA structure, which they prefer from previous dichroism studies (Hogan *et al.,* 1978), they use these tilt and twist angles to prepare a modified intercalation model which is consistent with the electric dichroism results. Their model does not involve any bending of the helix axis but does have both base pairs and the intercalated ligand oriented at an angle significantly different from 90° in contrast to most other intercalation models. This model is extremely interesting and should generate ideas for its experimental testing and refinement, but it must be viewed as Levitt's (1978) model for B-DNA, as hypothetical until additional confirmatory results are available. Sokerov and Weill (1979), for example, have criticized the extrapolation methods of Hogan *et al.* (1979) and using a different theoretical treatment, have calculated a different, more traditional, orientation for intercalating ring systems with respect to the base pairs of DNA.

Development of the original general intercalation model to specific structures for various intercalating drug molecules has been significantly advanced by high resolution nuclear magnetic resonance and X-ray crystallographic studies on the complexes of intercalating drugs with small complementary nucleotide segments. These techniques are not readily applied to high-molecular-weight DNA because of the broadening of signals which occurs in NMR and the difficulty of obtaining crystals for X-ray diffraction studies. Most work in the NMR area has been conducted by Krugh, Patel, and their co-workers (reviewed by Krugh and Nuss, 1979). The most fruitful experiments to date have been analyses of chemical shifts in ^{1}H NMR. These results coupled with a theoretical treatment of predicted ring current induced chemical shifts strongly support the formation of intercalation complexes for both ethidium and actinomycin (Krugh and Nuss, 1979). Based on chemical shift calculations with plausible intercalated models, these experiments also allow prediction of specific complex structures in solution. An additional finding of interest with these short nucleotide segments is the sequence specificity exhibited by ethidium (Reinhardt and Krugh, 1977) and propidium iodide (Davidson *et al.*, 1977c). Ethidium shows only a slight preference for binding to G · C base pairs in native DNA (Müller and Crothers, 1975) but with the short complementary nucleotides it has a strong preference for pyrimidine (3′-5′) purine sequences. Considering adjacent base pairs, DNA contains 10 different intercalation sites (Waring, 1972), but it is impossible to systematically analyze independent binding to each of these using heterogeneous natural DNA. With synthetic dinucleotide monophosphates and longer complementary nucleotide segments, however, this type study can be done. As mentioned above, ethidium has a marked preference for pyrimidine (3′-5′) purine sequences in both ribo- and deoxyribodinucleoside monophosphates (for example, CpG and UpA). Extrapolating these results to heterogeneous DNA does not imply any net G · C or A · T binding specificity since the ethidium binding preference holds for all sequences analyzed. With the potential additional influence from solvent interactions in dinucleotides, one is uncertain as to how far to extrapolate these results to natural DNA. It does seem, however, that similar results are obtained with ethidium and tetranucleotides that have been analyzed thus far (Krugh and Nuss, 1979).

The application of NMR to DNA has been facilitated by the development of ^{31}P techniques and their application to studies of the double helix (Shindo, 1980; Shindo and McGhee, 1980; Wilson and Jones, 1980; Mariam and Wilson, 1979; Bolton and James, 1979; Klevan *et al.*, 1979; Kallenbach *et al.*, 1978; Hogan and Jardetzky, 1979, 1980a, and references contained therein). These experiments have shown that the sugar–phosphate backbone of the double helix has considerable internal motion which leads to narrowing of the ^{31}P NMR lines for DNA. The mobility of the double helix largely continues even when DNA is complexed with histones to form nucleosomes. Shindo, Cohen, and co-workers (Shindo *et al.*, 1979, 1980; Simpson and Shindo, 1979) have analyzed ^{31}P NMR spectra of synthetic polydeoxynucleotide double helices and of synthetic nucleosomes prepared from natural histones and the synthetic polymers. These studies have suggested that the sugar–phosphate chain of DNA has different conformations along its length and that the local conformation will be some variation of the B form double helix. The exact conformation will depend on the local sequence of base pairs. These local conformational differences have been dramatically illustrated by Rich and co-workers with their novel Z-form structure for poly(dG · dC) (Wang *et al.*, 1979). It is not known at present how these local conformational differences along the double helix affect the specificity of binding of intercalating drugs, but it seems possible that when these conformations are better understood, they may suggest the syntheses of drugs of higher binding specificity. Hogan and Jardetsky (1980b) have suggested that when ethidium binds to DNA much of the mobility of the chains of the double helix is lost. This reduction in the dynamic motion of the double helix could be quite important in the inhibition of polymerase enzymes in the medicinal action of intercalating drugs. Wilson and Jones (1980) have determined the ^{31}P chemical shift changes induced in DNA by a series of intercalating drugs and find that these changes correlate well with the DNA unwinding angles of these drugs.

Lerman's original experiments with X-ray diffraction of DNA–acridine fibers have been extended by more recent X-ray crystallographic studies on complexes of complementary nucleotide segments with intercalating drugs and dyes. Sobell and co-workers have been especially active in this area (see Sobell *et al.*, 1977, for a review of this work). The most detailed work to date has been with iodinated derivatives of ribodinucleoside monophosphates. The structures obtained with ethidium bromide and iodo CpG and iodo UpA are especially informative and interesting and have the following features: (1) the sugar puckering at the intercalation sites is C3′ endo (3′-5′) C2′ endo; (2) changes in backbone torsional angles occur; (3) the helix axis is displaced by approximately 1.0 Å at the base pairs above and below the intercalated molecule; (4) a total unwinding angle of 26° (10° winding) is obtained; and (5) the base pair above the intercalated ligand is tilted approximately 8° with respect to the base pair immediately below the intercalated drug resulting in a bend or kink in the double helix. The 26° unwinding angle agrees with results obtained from superhelical DNA (Wang, 1974; Pulleyblank and Morgan, 1975) and the mixed sugar puckering at the intercalation site can explain neighbor exclusion binding (Section II,C). Crystal studies of 5-iodo CpG with acridine orange (Reddy *et al.*, 1979), 9-aminoacridine (Sakore *et al.*, 1977), and ellipticine and a phenanthrolinium derivative (Jain *et al.*, 1979) have provided supporting evidence for the above structural findings. Sobell and co-workers have used these results to provide a general possible model for intercalated complexes as described above, and to postulate models for DNA in chromatin based on the bending obtained in the crystal structures (Sobell *et al.*, 1977). Neidle and co-workers [reviewed by Neidle (1979)] have also obtained crystals of complementary dinucleoside monophosphates with intercalating drugs and have found some significant differences in their structures as compared to those of Sobell. Neidle (1979) does not observe symmetrical sugar pucker changes and finds very small unwinding angles in his crystal studies. The differences will probably be resolved when intercalating drugs are crystallized with longer complementary nucleotide segments.

C. Quantitative Analysis of Intercalation

As discussed above, the early binding experiments of Peacocke and Skerrett identified two binding modes of proflavine to DNA and this behavior seems quite general for intercalating drugs. The weaker binding, Type II, is due to a nonspecific self association (stacking) of the planar cationic drug molecules along the polyanionic DNA sugar–phosphate chains. Because of the multiple charge and the cooperativity of the stacking interactions involved in Type II binding, it can be eliminated by increasing concentrations of simple salts more easily than Type I binding can be eliminated (Jones *et al.*, 1980).

As more intercalating molecules were analyzed quantitatively, it became apparent that (1) even when Type II binding was eliminated, Scatchard plots for intercalation still indicated some curvature and (2) no intercalating molecules ever bound at a saturation ratio higher than one drug per two DNA base pairs. This has lead to the concept of "neighbor exclusion" binding for intercalating drugs (Crothers, 1968; Bauer and Vinograd, 1970; Bloomfield *et al.*, 1974). In this model each base pair in DNA is a potential binding site but when a drug is bound, a neighboring

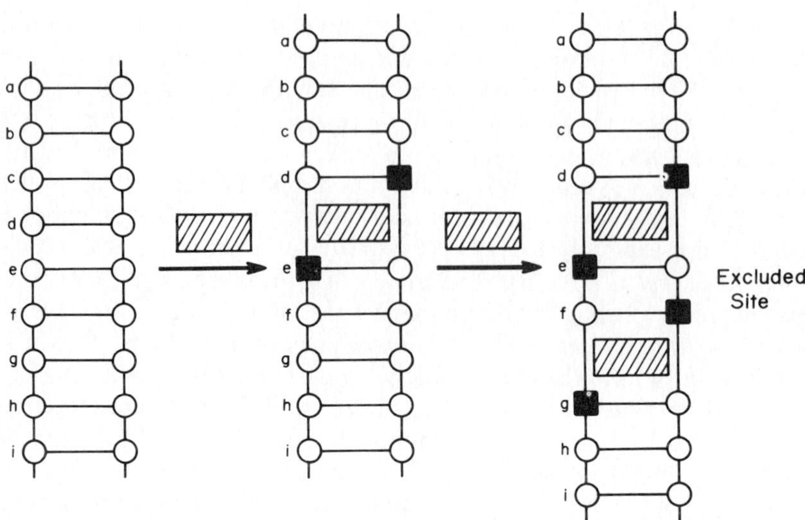

FIG. 4. A possible conformational explanation (Sobell *et al.*, 1977) for neighbor exclusion in the binding of intercalating drugs is schematically illustrated. In the left drawing a native double helical DNA (C2′ endo sugar conformation) or RNA (C3′ endo sugar conformation) is shown. On binding an intercalating ligand, as shown in the center drawing, a symmetrical conformational change occurs in the base pairs adjacent to the intercalation binding site (d and e). In B-form DNA, for example, this would involve altering the normal C2′ endo deoxyribose ring puckering to a mixed sugar puckering of the type C3′ endo (3′-5′) C2′ endo. The result of these sugar conformational changes is to create sites at neighboring base pairs where other intercalating ligands cannot bind (for example the site at base pairs e and f). Excluded sites are illustrated in the drawing on the right of the figure.

binding site is eliminated or in some manner becomes unable to bind a drug. Thus at saturation there will be only one drug bound for every two base pairs. In addition to binding studies, other types of experimental results have supported the neighbor exclusion model. As discussed in Section II,B, Sobell and co-workers (1977) in their X-ray analysis of crystals of intercalating ligands with dinucleosides have found that the sugar pucker can vary from C2′-endo to C3′-endo at alternating sugars as a result of intercalation. They point out that if this is true in DNA it would restrict binding to alternating sites and would automatically lead to neighbor exclusion binding. This type of conformational change and the resulting excluded site are shown schematically in Fig. 4. Studies with synthetic bisintercalating molecules, two intercalating aromatic rings connected by a variable length linking chain, have shown that when the chain was long enough to allow intercalation at every other base pair, both rings intercalated in agreement with the neighbor exclusion model, however, when the chains were shorter, and could allow intercalation only at adjacent base

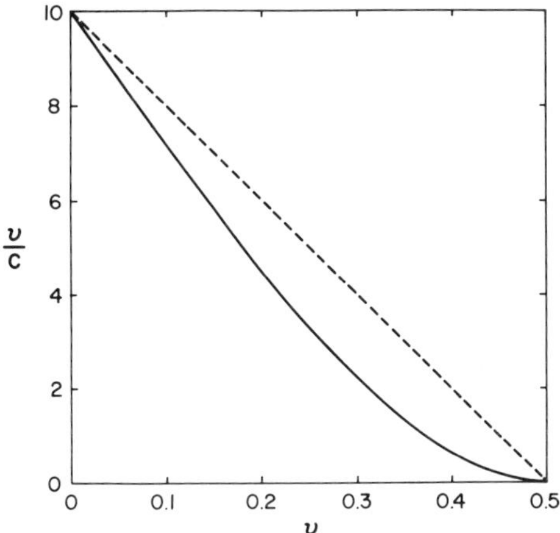

FIG. 5. Idealized Scatchard plots are shown for an intercalating drug binding to DNA by an independent, noninteracting binding site model (Scatchard model, broken line) and by the neighbor exclusion model (solid line). In both cases the number of base pairs per binding site at saturation is two ($\nu_{max} = 0.5$). Using these plots, the observed equilibrium constant from the neighbor exclusion model would be 10 while from the independent site model an equilibrium constant of 20 would be obtained. This illustrates the importance of careful definition of binding models when comparing relative DNA binding constants for different intercalating drugs. Note also that linear extrapolation of the neighbor exclusion curve (solid line) from results at low ν values ($\nu = 0$ to 0.2) would result in an intercept on the ν axis of between 0.3 and 0.4 or between 2.5 and three base pairs per binding site. Since the neighbor exclusion curve is fairly linear at low ν values, many workers have incorrectly treated this binding by the Scatchard Model and have thus obtained incorrect equilibrium constant and binding site size results.

pairs, only one ring at a time intercalated (LePecq *et al.*, 1975). Experiments with other bisintercalating ring systems of diverse structure have supported these findings (Waring, 1977; Dervan and Becker, 1978; Capelle *et al.*, 1979; Becker and Dervan, 1979; Kuhlmann *et al.*, 1978, 1980, and references contained therein). Lippard and co-workers (Bond *et al.*, 1975), using X-ray fiber diffraction studies of a DNA fiber with an intercalated platinum metallointercalation reagent, have also found that their results were best explained by a model with the platinum scattering center regularly intercalated at every other base pair leaving neighboring sites empty.

Neighbor exclusion is a type of negative cooperativity and can thus explain the curved Scatchard plots obtained in careful binding studies of intercalating drugs as can be seen in Fig. 5. Several investigators have derived equivalent quantitative expressions for the neighbor exclusion model (Bauer and Vinograd, 1970; Gurskii *et al.*, 1972; McGhee and von

Hipple, 1974). For the intercalating drugs analyzed to this point the fit has been quite good. Wilson and Lopp (1979) have pointed out, however, that with dicationic intercalating drugs such as quinacrine, an additional negative cooperativity term may be required in the binding analysis due to electrostatic repulsion of the bound dications.

The Scatchard equation has been quite successful in treating protein–ligand intercalations, such as enzyme–inhibitor binding, where discrete binding sites are involved. With a linear duplex repeating polymer such as DNA, however, this type model is incorrect. Although much work remains to be done in the development of the fine points of the neighbor exclusion model, its general validity for monointercalating drugs seems to be well established by structural and thermodynamic experiments. The Scatchard equation has been applied many times to the equilibria of intercalating drugs with DNA but it can now be seen that this model can lead to significant errors in the analysis of the DNA–drug reactions and it should, in general, be replaced by the excluded site treatment.

Recent quantitative studies with complex bisintercalating molecules (Wakelin *et al.*, 1976, 1978; Gaugain *et al.*, 1978; Lown *et al.*, 1978) have suggested that the restraints which lead to neighbor exclusion binding may be relaxed in some cases. Bisintercalators with long linking chains bind by neighbor exclusion in all cases analyzed to this point. Molecules with short linking chains intercalate only one of the two ring systems. Some molecules with linking chains of intermediate length, long enough to allow intercalation at adjacent sites but not long enough to allow intercalation with an empty intervening site, seem to be able to bind with both rings intercalated. This has raised questions about whether neighbor exclusion arises from a structural basis as suggested by Sobell *et al.* (1977) or from a thermodynamic basis (Gaugain *et al.*, 1978) which could be violated by molecules with very high binding constants such as bisintercalators (Wakelin *et al.*, 1978). These results do not invalidate neighbor exclusion effects for monointercalators but they do indicate that binding of bisintercalators may be much more complex than for the simpler monocompounds. This of course also means that these compounds could be used to exert very different effects on DNA and, in particular, on chromatin. These effects, when they are better understood, may prove to be quite useful in the design of drug molecules with very high binding specificity.

Another factor which must be considered in quantitating intercalation binding is the fact that apparent binding constants measured for drug–DNA interactions are quite ionic strength dependent (Wilson and Lopp, 1979). It now appears, however, that the ion-condensation theory, developed by Manning (1978) and by Record and co-workers (Record *et al.*, 1978; Lohman *et al.,* 1980), can explain ionic effects for the binding of intercalating drugs to DNA. Basically the ion-condensation theory says that B-form DNA is unstable due to its excessively high charge density. This instability is overcome in electrolyte solutions by "condensation" (a loose association of mobile counterions) of enough cations to stabilize the structure. The remaining charges on DNA are treated in a Debye-Hückel manner. The number of cations associated in the thermodynamic sense per phosphate, Ψ, in DNA is calculated to be 0.88. When a cation such as an intercalating drug binds to DNA, some of the counterion (such as sodium ions) is released and this accounts for the ionic strength dependence of the binding of such drugs. The theory quantitatively predicts the following dependence of the observed equilibrium constant for intercalation K_{obs}, on counterion concentration, $[M^+]$:

$$\frac{\partial \log K_{obs}}{\partial \log [M^+]} = - m'\Psi \tag{1}$$

where m' is related to the number of ion pairs formed between the drug and DNA and is generally equal to the number of cationic charges on the drug. All intercalating drugs analyzed so far exhibit linear plots of $\log K_{obs}$ versus $-\log[M^+]$ in agreement with the condensation theory. The slopes of these plots have been reasonably close to values predicted by Eq. (1).

As can be seen in Fig. 6 and as predicted by the condensation theory in Eq. (1), the dication and monocation intercalating ligand equilibrium constants are affected to different extents by salt. This has perhaps led to some confusion in the literature when comparing relative DNA binding affinities for intercalating drugs of different charge. Even less justified but perhaps more common is the comparison of binding results of drugs which have been determined at different ionic strengths. This can obviously lead to large errors and any conclusions made from binding data at different salt concentrations will have little meaning and may be totally misleading. As a standard procedure when analyzing drug–DNA interactions, observed equilibrium constants should be determined at several ionic strengths and plotted as in Fig. 6. Comparison with other compounds at any ionic strength can then be made using these plots. Two precautions are necessary when using this type of analysis: (1) the plot in Fig. 6 is for monovalent counterions such as Na^+ and will be different for dicationic counterions such as Mg^{2+}; and (2) the dimerization of intercalating ligands is also ionic strength dependent and this must be corrected for in quantitative work, especially at high ionic strengths (Wilson and Lopp, 1979). Because of possible conformational changes when other cationic ligands and macromolecules such as proteins bind to DNA, a detailed analysis of the interdependence of conformational and ionic effects on binding should also be conducted. It should also be emphasized that much of the ob-

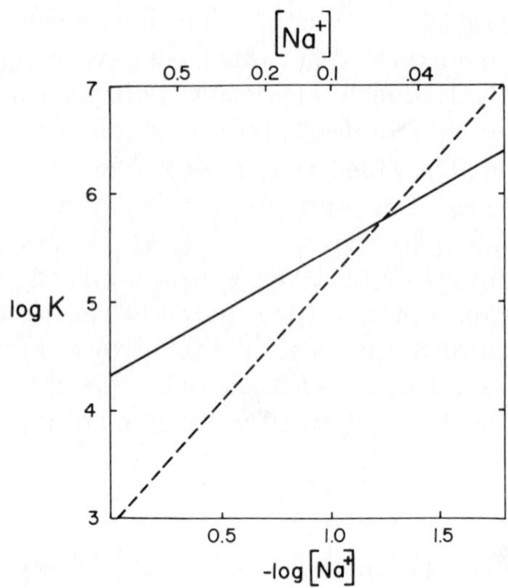

FIG. 6. The logarithms for the observed equilibrium constants (K) for intercalating drugs binding to DNA at different sodium ion concentrations are plotted versus the logarithm of the sodium ion concentration for a monocation, ethidium (solid line), and a dication, quinacrine (broken line). The slopes of these plots allow a determination of m', the number of ion pairs formed in the drug–DNA complex, as shown in Eq. (1). Note that quinacrine binds more strongly to DNA at low ionic strength but because its plot has a steeper slope, it binds more weakly at physiological ionic strength. Much of the binding free energy for both compounds at low ionic strength comes from release of sodium ions when the intercalating drug binds to DNA. Actual sodium ion concentrations ($[Na^+]$) are shown at the top of the figure for reference.

served free energy of intercalation (calculated from K_{obs}) determined from experiments at low ionic strength is due to sodium ion release and not to any especially favorable interaction between the intercalating drug and DNA. These findings illustrate the importance of analyzing drugs at several ionic strengths and evaluating the binding results through a plot such as Fig. 6. The ionic strength dependence of intercalation may be the most frequently misinterpreted concept in this area of research. The application of the ion condensation theory to intercalation reactions and to drug–DNA interactions in general should eliminate this problem.

III. Factors Which Relate Intercalation and Medicinal Activity

The binding of an intercalating drug to DNA can dramatically affect the metabolic reactions of the macromolecule. Intercalation of specific drugs can inhibit replication, or transcription, and frequently inhibits both. This inhibition can be detected either with purified DNA and enzymes *in vitro* or by an *in vivo* assay of nucleic acid synthesis. The inhibition can either lead directly to cell death or can weaken the target cell sufficiently that it is more susceptible to the normal defense mechanisms of the host organism. In this section the various factors which characterize the intercalation reaction will be related to the medicinal activity which results from intercalation. In spite of the considerable detail, described in Section II, with which intercalation has now been characterized, the relationship of the various factors which characterize this interaction to biological effects are not as clear cut. This is, no doubt, partially due to other important pharmacological factors such as drug transport and metabolism which also affect the activity of intercalating drugs. It has also been shown that very lipophilic derivatives of intercalators such as fatty acid esters of adriamycin (Israel *et al.*, 1975; Blum *et al.*, 1979) and bisintercalators containing aliphatic connecting chains (Fico *et al.*, 1977; Chen *et al.*, 1978) can have excellent medicinal properties which are not directly related to DNA binding. This suggests that intercalators themselves may have multiple modes of action which could vary in effect with substituent changes and which could complicate attempted correlations between intercalation and activity.

A. Binding Constant

In order for a drug to exert its medicinal action through intercalation with DNA it must obviously bind significantly to DNA under conditions which exist *in vivo.* Exactly what minimum value of the equilibrium constant is necessary for activity is open to some question and obviously depends on secondary factors such as what drug concentration is obtained within the target cell, competitive metabolic inactivation of the drug, and other similar factors. As discussed in Section II,C, the apparent equilibrium constant for intercalation is quite dependent on the ionic strength of the medium and there is no uniform set of conditions for reporting these constants. The best solution for comparative purposes would be to measure K at several ionic strengths and construct a $\log K$ versus $-\log [Na^+]$ plot as discussed in Section II,C. Unfortunately, this method is time consuming and has been applied to very few drugs at present. At a sodium ion concentration of near 0.1 M, intercalating drugs such as ethidium, daunorubicin, and quinacrine have binding constants of near 10^5 (Wilson and Jones, 1981) and it seems reasonable to propose that if a drug exerts its medicinal action by intercalation with DNA, it should have a binding constant near or above this value.

Drug–DNA binding constants can also vary greatly simply due to the manner in which the experimental data are treated (Bloomfield *et al.*, 1974; Wilson and Lopp, 1979; Howe-Grant and Lippard, 1979). For example, analysis of binding data using the Scatchard equation will give a different equilibrium binding constant than analysis of the same data using a neighbor exclusion binding model as can be seen in Fig. 5. Since it is often difficult, due to solubility, dimerization, or other experimental difficulties, to obtain data on intercalating compounds over a broad range of binding through site saturation, Howe-Grant and Lippard (1979) have recommended plotting binding data in a Scatchard type plot and extrapolating to the ν/C intercept (see Fig. 5) to obtain a relative binding affinity. If the extrapolation is done empirically, it eliminates the need for fitting of the binding results to a specific equation or model. Whatever method is used, it should be clearly stated along with experimental conditions so that comparison with other drugs is possible.

It is well known that there is an optimum in the medicinal activity of many drugs when plotted against a partition coefficient which is related to membrane transport (Hansch, 1969). It is not known whether there is also an optimum in the activity of intercalating drugs as a function of their binding constant. There must obviously be some minimum value for the binding constant if DNA is to be the bioreceptor for a drug. Although there is a generally accepted view that the higher the binding constant for the bioreceptor (at constant partitioning and metabolism) the higher the activity, it seems possible, that if very high binding constants are achieved, nonspecific binding to RNA and perhaps host cell DNA may cause loss of drug or increases in toxicity which outweigh any gains due to increased binding to target DNA. Compounds to test this hypothesis are not yet available and techniques for increasing DNA binding (without significantly affecting partitioning) are still uncertain. Adding substituents with varying electronic character to the intercalating ring system seems to be a method that may allow significant alterations in the binding constant with minimal changes in partitioning and metabolic transformations of the drug (Panter *et al.*, 1973), but this concept has not been rigorously tested.

Although nonspecific increases in binding constants may not always increase activity, as discussed above, if specificity for target DNA can also be increased, dramatic increases in activity could be achieved. This has been a goal in the synthesis of bisintercalators (see Section IIC). These compounds show dramatically enhanced binding constants for DNA and there is some indication of increased specificity. Most of these compounds have been tested for antineoplastic activity. One of the problems with these inherently large and complex intercalating molecules is to maintain appropriate membrane partitioning so that the advantages of bisintercalation are not lost due to lower drug uptake (Kuhlmann *et al.*, 1978).

B. Kinetics

Studies of the kinetics of the interaction of intercalating molecules with DNA have been much less frequently conducted than have thermodynamic analyses of the reaction. For most intercalators the reaction with DNA is so fast as to require measurement by rapid kinetics techniques (Crothers, 1971; Bloomfield *et al.*, 1974). This area has been further complicated by the suggestion that temperature jump techniques with DNA are subject to some error due to partial orientation of DNA in the electric field applied to produce the temperature jump (Dourlent and Hogrel, 1976). Stopped-flow techniques are not limited by this potential artifact, but are generally not fast enough to allow experimental analysis of the association reaction.

Müller and Crothers (1968) analyzed the kinetics of the interaction of actinomycin D with DNA and suggested that the slow dissociation of this molecule from DNA was important to its biological activity. They found a multistep process for the association and dissociation of this compound with DNA. The dissociation of actinomycin from DNA could be described by a three step process. Müller and Crothers (1968) attributed this multistep behavior to sequential conformational changes in the peptide groups of actinomycin which are coupled to binding of the peptides to DNA. Recently, however, Krugh and co-workers (Hook *et al.*, 1979; Krugh *et al.*, 1979) have obtained evidence using synthetic duplex deoxypolynucleotides that the three step binding is due to binding site heterogeneity in DNA and is not due to actinomycin or to DNA conformational changes.

With poly(dG · dC) these authors find that the kinetics of actinomycin D dissociation, at all ratios of drug to nucleotide, can be described by a single first order reaction but that the rate constant for the reaction depends on the drug to nucleotide ratio. One possible explanation for this behavior is an actinomycin-induced conformational change in the polydeoxynucleotide double helix which reequilibrates more slowly than the actinomycin dissociation reaction. Spectral analysis of the dissociation reaction by circular dichroism, however, did not reveal any conformational changes which could account for this behavior (Krugh *et al.*, 1979). These authors (Krugh *et al.*, 1979) have also found that the anthracycline drugs when complexed to poly(dA · dT), induce the binding of actinomycin to this polymer. Since actinomycin does not normally bind to DNA samples which do not contain guanine, Krugh *et al.* (1979) suggest that anthracycline-induced conformational changes in the double helix are responsible for the cooperative binding of actinomycin. It is not clear at present as to how common this type of drug binding cooperativity is, but it does suggest that intercalating drugs given in combination may be able to exert specific medicinal effects which neither alone is able to do.

Shafer *et al.* (1980) have measured dissociation of several actinomycin derivatives from DNA and have concluded that the 3′ amino acid position of the peptide rings (which is occupied by L-proline in actinomycin D) is of critical importance in the slow dissociation of actinomycins from DNA. Their results with natural DNA agreed with those of Müller and Crothers (1968), but Shafer *et al.* (1980) did not attempt to determine the mechanism for the multistep dissociation reaction.

In spite of these studies, the importance of kinetics versus thermodynamics in determining the medicinal activity of intercalators is an extremely important point which is not yet resolved. The question arises as to whether activity of existing drugs could be significantly enhanced by slowing their dissociation from DNA. Gabbay and co-workers (1973a,b) have shown that addition of bulky groups, which must slide between base pairs during intercalation, can significantly slow dissociation of intercalating molecules from DNA. This method of adding bulky groups could perhaps be used to decrease dissociation rates of existing drugs and it would be of interest to determine whether this increases activity if other factors are held constant. Although actinomycin D is a slowly dissociating intercalating molecule which is highly active, other active drugs such as ethidium bromide (Bresloff and Crothers, 1975; Garland *et al.*, 1980), daunorubicin (Gabbay *et al.*, 1976), and proflavine (Li and Crothers, 1969) dissociate quite rapidly from DNA. All of these compounds bind strongly to DNA by intercalation and cause the expected inhibition of replication and/or transcription. Müller and Crothers (1968) pointed out that actinomine which has the peptide rings of actinomycin replaced by simple alkyl amino groups binds strongly to DNA but dissociates rapidly and is devoid of activity. Unfortunately, the loss of activity of this compound could also be related to other factors such as membrane permeability (actinomine is a dication while actinomycin is neutral) or changes in metabolic degradation of the molecules. The binding of actinomine to DNA also has a large electrostatic component due to its positive charges while the binding of actinomycin is much less ionic strength dependent than other intercalators. The conclusion then must be that all known active intercalating molecules bind strongly but most also have very fast association and dissociation reactions with DNA. Actinomycin is a striking example of an active drug with slow and complex association and dissociation reactions with DNA, but the importance of these slow reactions is not clear at present. For most intercalating drugs, slow dissociation from DNA is not a necessary condition for activity. Actinomycin specifically inhibits RNA polymerase while many other intercalators inhibit DNA and RNA polymerases more equally and this distinction may be related to the dissociation kinetics of the various compounds. Synthesis of additional drugs which dissociate slowly from DNA would help resolve these questions.

C. Structural Effects and Activity

As discussed in Section II, depending on the structure of the intercalating drug, intercalation can cause a lengthening and unwinding of DNA which can be accompanied by other structural distortions of the double helix such as bending. Unwinding of DNA gives intercalating drugs a binding advantage to closed circular superhelical DNA which could be important in selective action against trypanosomal kinetoplast DNA (Newton, 1974; Hajduk, 1978), viruses, bacterial plasmids (Bauer, 1978), and other sources containing superhelical DNA (Waring, 1972). The question also arises as to whether there is a correlation between unwinding angles and medicinal activities or between unwinding angles and the type of activity (antitrypanosomal, antimalarial, antineoplastic, etc.) exhibited by an intercalating drug. Although there have been only a limited number of experiments with a series of closely related derivatives, the present results suggest that no such correlations exist. For example, dimidium and ethidium are phenanthridine derivatives which differ markedly in antitrypanosomal activity yet have very similar unwinding angles (Waring, 1970). In the same manner, antineoplastic drugs of the acridinylmethanesulfonanilide series (Waring, 1976) and anthracycline series (Lanier *et al.*, 1980), which differ markedly in activity within each set of derivatives, have quite similar unwinding angles within the specific series.

There are, however, large differences in the magnitude of the unwinding angles among the different classes of drugs. Of the drugs discussed above, for example, the phenanthridines have unwinding angles near 26° (Wang, 1974; Pulleyblank and Morgan, 1975), the acridine series near 20° (Jones *et al.*, 1980), and the anthracyclines near 10° (Lanier *et al.*, 1980). The antimalarial acridine quinacrine has an unwinding angle near 18° (Jones *et al.*, 1980) while the antitumor acridinylmethanesulfonanilides have unwinding angles near 20° Waring, 1976). These results suggest that the unwinding angle depends strongly on the drug structure and is not closely correlated with the total activity or with the type activity of the drug. Waring (1970, 1972) has shown that when large changes are made in the intercalating part of a drug molecule, the unwinding angle can be affected. The exact factors which influence the unwinding angle for a particular intercalating ring system are still not clear and will probably require considerably more study on a broad range of compounds before any general principles become apparent.

Wu *et al.* (1980) have shown that ethidium binding to the nucleosome subunits of chromatin induces dramatic conformational changes in these particles. The conformational change is evidently the result of intercalation of ethidium into the nucleosome DNA. The unwinding of DNA produced by ethidium binding leads to the conformational changes in the nucleosome and results in an increased binding constant for the first molecules of ethidium which bind. This strong binding could lead to a direct inhibiting of replication and transcription. The conformational changes in the nucleosome could lead to large scale disruption of chromosomal structure and control of gene expression (McGhee and Felsenfeld, 1980). The disruption of chromosome structure may occur at much lower drug levels than is required for a direct inhibition of polymerases for purified DNA. Certain cells may also be more sensitive to the disruption which could be a cause of selective drug action. Although the purified DNAs from organisms such as trypanosomes and humans are quite similar, their nucleosomal structure and arrangement are no doubt quite different. Drugs such as ethidium do not show any pronounced differences in their effects on purified DNAs but they may show pronounced differences in their effects on nucleosomes from humans and trypanosomes. Enhancing specific differences in effects on nucleohistone complexes seems to be the most promising direction for development and modification of intercalating drugs to increase selectivity and activity.

As discussed in Section II, intercalation also causes a separation of the base pairs and a resulting increase in the double helix contour length. This length increase, measured by techniques such as viscosity, should be quite sensitive to any bending of the double helix which can also occur at the point of intercalation (see Fig. 2). Although energetic considerations would suggest that any bending per drug molecule should be slight, the overall effect on a DNA molecule could be large and this may be important in inhibiting enzyme action and, therefore, in affecting medicinal activity. At present so little is known about bending of DNA by intercalating drugs that no definite statements can be made about how bending correlates with activity.

D. Intercalation and Selective Drug Action

Since the original proposal by Watson and Crick (1953) of the B-form double helical structure of DNA, it has generally been accepted that DNA from most organisms largely adopts this conformation (McGhee and Felsenfeld, 1980). Since intercalating drugs are usually in contact with only two or three base pairs in a long DNA molecule, it is not clear as to how these type drugs select their specific target cells for medicinal action. There are several possible mechanisms for this selectivity and these mechanisms may act singly or in combination. It should be mentioned, however, that most intercalating compounds are toxic at doses not greatly above their therapeutic level and this suggests that their selectivity is, in general, quite limited.

One possibility for selectivity is modification of the DNA structure in specific cells or organisms, by protein interactions (McGhee and Felsenfeld, 1980; Wu *et al.*, 1980) or by supercoiling through covalently closed circular DNA (Bauer, 1978) both of which can enhance the binding of intercalating drugs to DNA. The DNA of eukaryotic organisms is extensively folded into compact nucleosomes which are further integrated into highly organized chromatin (McGhee and Felsenfeld, 1980). This DNA is then much less exposed and less available for binding of intercalating drugs than the DNA of prokaryotic microorganisms (Gabbay and Wilson, 1978). In the same manner the DNA of neoplastic cells might be more exposed than that of normal cells due to either a modification of the DNA in these cells which leads to a partial disruption of the nucleosome structure (LePecq *et al.*, 1974a) or due to the high metabolic rate of the malignant cells. These diseased cells would, thus, tend to concentrate drugs which bind to more exposed regions of DNA. This high relative concentration of absorbed drug could lead to severe metabolic perturbations in the neoplastic cells and could directly kill the diseased cells or make them more susceptible to normal host defense mechanisms. As discussed in Section III,C, it is known that ethidium bromide has a very strong specific binding to the nucleosomal subunits of chromatin which disrupts their structure (Wu *et al.*, 1980). It is not known how this binding can vary among cells but it is known that the binding is very sensitive to factors such as protein cross-linking and magnesium ion concentration. Similarly *in vivo* factors may also selectively influence the sensitivity of the nucleosomes of a particular cell to interactions with intercalating drugs.

Selectivity can also arise due to differences between chromosomal DNA and closed circular superhelical DNA which exists, for example, in mitochondria, bacterial plasmids, viruses, and trypanosomal kinetoplasts (Bauer, 1978). Because intercalating drugs can relieve some of the supercoiling strain in closed circular superhelical DNA, their binding free energy, in the region where superhelical turns are removed, is greater for this DNA than for nonsuperhelical DNA (Bauer and Vinograd, 1970; Waring, 1972). Intercalating drugs, thus, selectively bind to closed circular superhelical DNA and this could account for some of their specific biological effects.

Effects not directly connected with intercalation can also lead to selective drug action. The drug may, for example, selectively penetrate membranes of the target cell through passive or active means. One technique that has been used to enhance this type of specificity with intercalating drugs is to complex the drugs with DNA and administer them as a complex (Trouet *et al.*, 1972). It has been speculated that the more metabolically active tumor cells will absorb by pinocytosis more of the DNA–drug complex and when this is digested in the cellular lysosomes, the active drug should be released at a relatively high intracellular concentration. Studies of this technique with anthracyclines (Trouet *et al.*, 1972, 1974; Atassi *et al.*, 1975; Trouet, 1978; and Trouet and Sokal, 1979), with actinomycin (Marks and Venditti, 1976), and with ethidium bromide (Heinen *et al.*, 1974; Avila *et al.*, 1979) have shown some promise. There have been similar attempts to target intercalating drugs to specific cells by attaching them to antibodies against those cells (Hurwitz *et al.*, 1975). Although there are still some questions about the mechanism by which anthracycline–DNA complexes enter cells, the equal or increased activity and lower toxicity of these complexes make them an attractive area for future development (Henry, 1976). The idea of enhancing specific cellular recognition by intercalating drugs is of such importance that research in this area should continue to be quite active.

One promising development for increasing the selectivity and activity of intercalating drugs is the synthesis of bisintercalating molecules as discussed in Section II,C. This approach can obviously be extended to three or more connected intercalating ring systems. Monomer intercalators may have specificity for a particular base pair or for two adjacent base pairs (Müller *et al.*, 1973; Müller and Crothers, 1975), but because of their small size this binding specificity must be limited. By joining covalently two or more units of this type specificity for specific sequences in DNA can be generated and concurrently the DNA binding constant for the drug can be increased by orders of magnitude. Drugs can be synthesized in this manner which bind to specific critical sequences in target cell DNA resulting in very selective attack on the metabolism of these cells. If reactive chemical groups are attached to the connecting segments of the multiintercalating drugs, specific chemical reactions, such as hydrolysis, or crosslinking, can be performed on the target cell DNA. Potential problems in this research are synthetic difficulties, reduced membrane transport of the multiintercalators, and the necessity for identification of the specific target cell DNA sequence to use as the binding receptor.

There is no obvious correlation between the base pair specificity of monointercalators and their medicinal activity. Müller and Crothers (1975) devised a method for accurately measuring base pair specificity and have found that most monointercalators have from slight to quite pronounced specificity for G · C base pairs. Diverse intercalating drugs such as proflavine, ethidium, and quinacrine have only slight G · C specificity

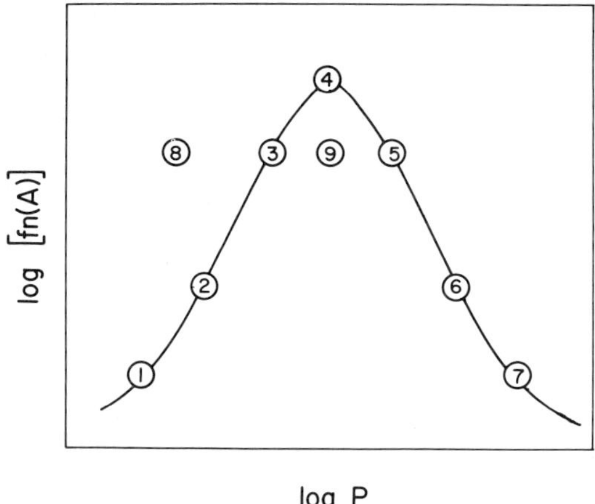

FIG. 7. The logarithm of some function of the activity of a drug (log[fn(A)]) such as the percentage increase in lifetime of treated versus control animals, is plotted versus the logarithm of the octanol–aqueous buffer partition function (log P) for that drug. Compounds 1–7 represent a standard series of hypothetical intercalating drugs with a constant intercalating ring system and a substituent that has varying alkane groups. The different alkane substituents yield the observed variations in partition function. Compounds 8 and 9 have substituted ring systems which affect their activity. The usefulness of the substitution can be judged by comparing the activity of a substituted compound with the standard curve at the same log P value (isolipophilic comparison). The substitution producing compound 8 can immediately be seen to be advantageous while the substitution to give compound 9 is detrimental to activity.

while actinomycin has pronounced G · C specificity (Müller *et al.*, 1973). High G · C specificity is not a necessity for antitumor activity since the anthracyclines seem to have no pronounced base pair specificity and are active antitumor drugs (Henry, 1976; Neidle, 1978).

Cain and co-workers (Cain *et al.*, 1974; Cain, 1975) following the method of Hansch (1969) have emphasized the importance of considering drug partition coefficients or hydrophilic–lipophilic balance when evaluating the selective action of intercalating drugs against a particular type cell or when evaluating activity differences for a series of drugs which have been tested against a particular disease. Intercalating drugs which bind quite strongly to DNA can be completely inactive because of poor membrane transport. If partitioning is not evaluated, erroneous conclusions about the importance of DNA (or any other biopolymer) interactions may be reached. Cain *et al.* (1974) have suggested preparing a reference curve of activity versus partitioning for a series of intercalating compounds and using this as a standard for evaluating the activity of new derivatives. They used a series of acridinylalkanesulfonanilide antitumor drugs with varying alkane groups on the sulfonanilide group to construct a standard curve. It is important that within the standard series of compounds, groups added to change the hydrophilic–lipophilic balance do not cause significant changes in the binding equilibrium of the drugs with the bioreceptor. This method of comparing derivatives is shown schematically in Fig. 7 where the logarithm of some function of medicinal activity for a series of hypothetical drugs is plotted against the logarithm of their partition coefficient. Points 1–7 represent a series of intercalating drugs with varying alkane substituents. It is assumed that compounds 1–7 have essentially equivalent binding constants for their bioreceptor, DNA, but have systematic changes in their log P values. The activity of substituted derivatives such as 8 and 9 can now be evaluated versus the predicted activity from the standard curve at the same log P value (isolipophilic comparisons). The modification to make compound 8, for example, has increased DNA binding and created greater than the predicted activity while compound 9 has lower DNA binding and less activity than predicted. Compounds 3, 5, 8, and 9 all have the same activity but their DNA binding constants vary considerably. In a routine comparison of derivatives this might create some confusion about the importance of DNA binding in the mode of action of this series of drugs but when membrane effects are also considered, the results can be understood. From the results in Fig. 7 a curve can be generated that plots the log of the activity function versus a function that includes contributions from partitioning and from DNA binding. This should suggest modifications of existing drugs and should allow selection of new derivatives for synthesis which have significantly increased activity. In addition compounds that do not fit this second curve can be examined for other competing effects such as metabolic activation or inactivation which were not considered in the original analysis.

IV. Specific Drugs Which Bind to DNA by Intercalation

There will be no attempt in this section to summarize all intercalating drugs which have been discussed. Emphasis will be placed on drugs whose activity is well established and whose intercalation with DNA has been studied in some detail. The drugs are grouped by their pharmacological activity although some compounds appear in more than one section. Most of these compounds also display antibacterial properties which can be traced largely to their interaction with DNA (cf. Corcoran and Hahn, 1975). The antibacterial effects are not presented as a separate section since most of the intercalating drugs are too toxic to be widely used as antibacterials.

A. ANTITRYPANOSOMAL DRUGS

The most active member of the phenanthridine antitrypanosomal drugs is ethidium bromide (Newton, 1974) and this compound has been used extensively to characterize the intercalation reaction (Waring, 1972,1975; Sobell *et al.*, 1977). Ethidium causes the expected length increase and unwinds the double helix by 26° on intercalation (Wang, 1974; Pulleyblank and Morgan, 1975). X-Ray studies with complementary nucleotide segments indicate that the phenyl and ethyl substituents protrude into the minor groove while the amino groups are in a position to hydrogen bond to oxygens of the DNA sugar–phosphate chain on opposite sides of the intercalation site. The bulk of the phenyl group seems to induce some bending of the double helix toward the major groove (Tsai *et at.*, 1977). Sobell *et al.* (1977) have analyzed this conformational change as a model for folding processes of the double helix in general such as packing of DNA into the nucleosome particles of chromatin and the dynamics of DNA breathing (Lozansky *et al.*, 1979). Garland *et al.* (1980) have studied the interaction of ethidium, its monoazide (at the 8 amino position), and diazide derivatives with DNA using fluorescence and stopped flow kinetics techniques. Ethidium and the monoazide bind to DNA in a quite similar manner but the monoazide has higher antitrypanosomal activity. They propose that the monoazide has higher activity due to its potential for covalent bond formation with DNA. The diazide binds quite differently to DNA than ethidium and this compound, thus, has reduced activity even though it has enhanced potential for covalent bond formation. Garland *et al.* (1980) point out that the ethidium monoazide should prove to be an ideal probe for the *in vivo* sites of action of ethidium.

Because of the extensive use of ethidium to characterize intercalation and its long history as an antitrypanosomal drug, the probable relationships between DNA binding of this compound and its antitrypanosomal activity have been extensively discussed (Hajduk, 1978; Waring, 1972, 1975; Newton, 1970, 1974, and references quoted therein). Other intercalating drugs such as acriflavine and 9-methoxyellipticine also have antitrypanosomal activity and seem to act preferentially on the DNA of the kinetoplast as ethidium does. These drugs seem to have very little base pair binding specificity and bind essentially equally well to linear DNA from all types of organisms (Müller *et al.*, 1973; Newton, 1974; Hajduk, 1978). Because of the unwinding produced by intercalation, the initial binding of these drugs is more favorable to superhelical DNA than to linear DNA (Waring, 1972; Bauer, 1978). This may partially account for the selectivity of intercalating drugs for the kinetoplast DNA of trypanosomes, although protein–DNA interactions *in vivo* are also no doubt important in these selectivity considerations (Newton, 1974; Hajduk, 1978;

Benard *et al.*, 1979). Ethidium selectivity for the trypanosomes may also be partially due to a selective uptake of the drug by trypanosomes due to differences between the trypanosomal cellular membranes and those of the host cells. This selectivity may be enhanced by the ability of ethidium to form an uncharged pseudo-base species (Newton, 1974; Waring, 1975). At sufficiently high levels, ethidium can enter essentially all cells and produce toxic effects.

Studies on the development of resistance to intercalating drugs, to be discussed in Section IV,C, suggest that resistance and perhaps selectivity for target over host cells arise due to differences in membrane transport of the drugs plus other factors which are not yet clear. These other factors may be related to differential inhibition of RNA and/or DNA polymerases between normal and diseased cells or between sensitive and resistant cells. The selective uptake of intercalating drugs by trypanosomes may also be due in part to the fact that the kinetoplast DNA is the initial site of action of these compounds. Since this DNA is not extensively complexed with proteins or folded into nucleosomes as nuclear DNA, it contains more exposed DNA for binding intercalating drugs which enter the trypanosome (Hajduk, 1978; Bernard *et al.*, 1979). For drugs which can be transported through the membrane of the trypanosome quickly enough, this factor alone could account for their selective action against this parasite.

B. Antimalarial Drugs

Many antimalarials have planar aromatic ring systems and one or more cationic groups in their structure (Steck, 1972). These compounds, including the classical antimalarial quinine, quinacrine (the drug of choice through World War II), and the currently more widely used chloroquine, have been shown to bind to DNA by intercalation (Hahn *et al.*, 1966). Mefloquine, a related quinoline methanol derivative with excellent antimalarial properties, was synthesized as part of the Vietnam War effort to develop new antimalarials (Ohnmacht *et al.*, 1971; Trenholme *et al.*, 1975; Rozman and Canfield, 1979). This compound binds quite weakly to DNA and it seems highly unlikely that DNA is its biological receptor (Davidson *et al.*, 1975). The weak binding of this quinoline derivative prompted the reexamination of the interaction of other quinolines with DNA (Davidson *et al.*, 1977b). A study of the compounds shown in Fig. 8 indicated that compound **1** and quinine could bind to DNA through an intercalation complex. Mefloquine, however, has bulky groups at positions 2, 4, and 8 while compound **2** has bulky groups at positions 2 and 4 and these bulky groups effectively prevent stacking of the quinoline ring system of these

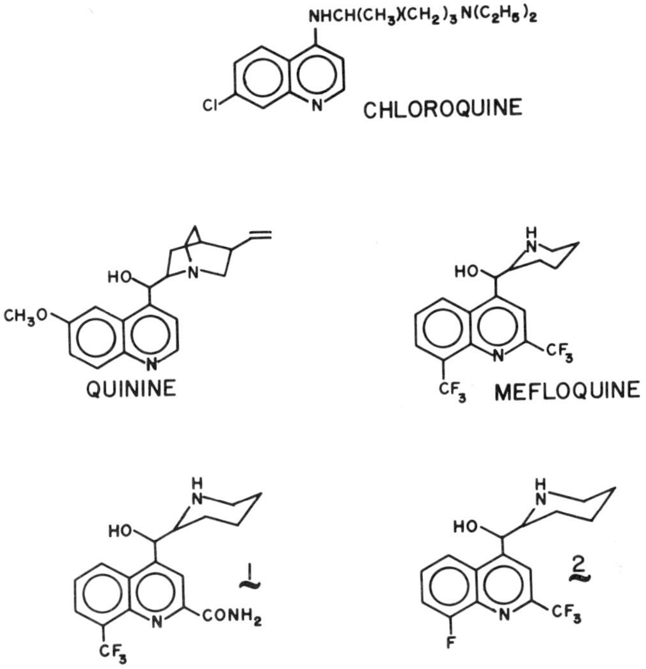

FIG. 8. The structures of the antimalarial quinoline methanol drugs quinine and mefloquine are shown along with control compounds **1** and **2**. The structure of the antimalarial chloroquine is included for reference.

compounds with the base pairs of the double helix. The binding of mefloquine and **2** to DNA is, therefore, quite weak and not by intercalation (Davidson *et al.*, 1977b). In Fig. 9, viscometric titrations of closed circular superhelical DNA with the compounds of Fig. 8 are shown. As can be seen, quinine and **1** unwind the DNA, although the binding is quite weak relative to quinacrine. Mefloquine and **2** do not unwind superhelical DNA. In the same manner quinine and **1** caused viscosity increases for sonicated DNA, as expected for intercalation, while mefloquine and **2** do not cause these increases. These results indicate that the ability of quinolinemethanol amines to intercalate with DNA is strongly dependent on the location and type of substituent placed on the quinoline ring. We refer to a bulky substituent as one which extends significantly beyond the 3.4 Å thickness of a typical fused aromatic ring system and which can interfere with the stacking of the aromatic ring system of a drug with the DNA base pairs in an intercalated complex. CPK space-filling models indicate that the methoxy group of quinine and the carboxamide group of **1** can be rotated into the plane of the quinoline ring forming a planar

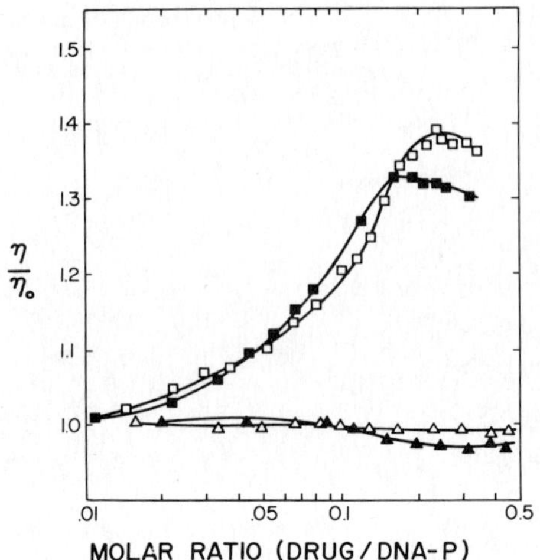

FIG. 9. Viscometric titrations of closed circular superhelical DNA with the quinoline methanol compounds of Fig. 8 are shown: quinine, □; mefloquine, △; compound **1**, ■; and compound **2**, ▲. The ratio of the reduced specific viscosity of the DNA–drug complex, η, to the reduced specific viscosity of DNA alone, η_0, is plotted versus the molar ratio of drug added per DNA phosphate group (nucleotide).

system which is capable of intercalation. All compounds of Fig. 8 contain a bulky group on position 4, the cationic group. Mefloquine and **2** do not intercalate and both have an additional bulky group at position two. Quinine and **1** intercalate and neither contains a bulky substituent at position two, although **1** does have an additional bulky substituent at position eight. A study of possible interactions of all four compounds with DNA using CPK space-filling molecular models indicated that the trifluoromethyl substituent of **1** can project into one groove of the DNA double helix leaving the cationic group in the opposite groove. An intercalation complex of this type allows stacking of the quinoline ring system and the carboxamide substituent with the DNA base pairs. A similar complex can be obtained with quinine since it contains only one bulky substituent, the side chain (Davidson *et al.*, 1977b).

Evidently, the cationic group and the additional bulky substituent at position two in mefloquine and **2** are too close on the ring system for the two substituents to lie in opposite grooves of the double helix. Thus, for intercalation of these compounds one bulky substituent would have to be partially pulled between the base pairs of DNA resulting in a severe disruption of stacking. Alternately, both bulky substituents could lie in the same groove allowing at least partial insertion of the quinoline ring system. This, however, would lead to a large decrease in sonicated DNA viscosity in contrast to the results obtained. Viscometric studies suggest that both mefloquine and **2** simply interact with DNA through weak external electrostatic attraction (Davidson *et al.*, 1977b).

It has been shown with naphthothiopheneethanol amine antimalarial drugs that addition of a trifluoromethyl substituent to a planar aromatic ring system can actually enhance DNA binding (Panter *et al.*, 1973). In this case, however, model building studies indicated that the cationic group can lie in one groove of the DNA double helix and the trifluoromethyl substituent in the other as with compound **1**. Addition of bulky substituents to small molecules can, thus, lead either to increases or to decreases in DNA binding depending on their relative position with respect to other bulky substituents, the electronic characteristics of the substituent, and the structure of the DNA–drug complex.

These results also called attention to the fact that even though quinolines such as quinine and chloroquine can intercalate, they bind to DNA quite weakly under physiological ionic strength (Davidson *et al.*, 1977b). This fact makes it highly unlikely that DNA is the primary bioreceptor for the quinoline antimalarials, although DNA binding may have some secondary importance in the final disruption of the metabolism of the parasite.

Acridines such as quinacrine do bind quite strongly to DNA under physiological conditions and this binding may be important to their antimalarial action. Carter and Van Dyke (1972) have shown that quinacrine and similar intercalating drugs which bind strongly to DNA inhibit polymerization of nucleic acids in *Plasmodium berghei* growing in cell culture. Chloroquine and quinine did not cause such an inhibition at normal drug dosages. Carter and Van Dyke (1972) concluded that the quinoline derivatives must exert their antimalarial effects through some other binding mechanism.

The selectivity of quinacrine for the malaria parasite seems to be enhanced by making the compound more hydrophilic such as by replacing one of the carbons of the acridine ring with a nitrogen. The selectivity of quinacrine derivatives as antimalarials is decreased by making them more lipophilic and, in fact, this can change their specificity entirely (Albert, 1972). This illustrates the point that these type compounds and intercalators in general have a cytotoxic action which is fairly nonspecific and in most cases results from inhibition of replication and transcription. The selectivity of these compounds then arises due to their enhanced transport into target cells and/or specific sensitivity of the target cells to the drug. This is discussed in more detail in the following section.

C. ANTITUMOR DRUGS

Antitumor drugs represent one of the most thoroughly studied classes of intercalating compounds. Of these drugs the actinomycins, anthracyclines, and some acridine and ellipticine derivatives have shown promising activity, including clinical trials, and in addition have had their DNA binding interactions thoroughly characterized. Actinomycin derivatives have been known for some time and their interaction with DNA, which causes a specific inhibition of RNA polymerase, seems to be responsible for their antibiotic and antitumor activity (Meienhofer and Atherton, 1977; Remers, 1979). The interaction of actinomycin with DNA is somewhat different than for other common intercalating drugs (cf. Müller and Crothers, 1968). Early investigations (Cerami *et al.*, 1967; Hamilton *et al.*, 1963) suggested that actinomycin did not form an intercalation complex with DNA. Müller and Crothers (1968) found, however, that when they used low-molecular-weight sonicated DNA, they obtained viscosity increases and Waring (1970) found that actinomycin unwinds superhelical DNA as expected for intercalation. More recent investigations with high resolution NMR spectroscopy (Krugh and Nuss, 1979) and X-ray crystallographic analysis of actinomycin–nucleotide crystals (Jain and Sobell, 1972) have also supported intercalation as the binding mode for this drug. Actinomycin seems to give around the typical 3.4 Å length increase for sonicated DNA (Müller and Crothers, 1968) and has an unwinding angle similar to that of ethidium (Waring, 1972) which is now known to be 26° (Wang, 1974; Pulleyblank and Morgan, 1975). Perhaps the most interesting aspect of the actinomycin–DNA complex is that the association and dissociation kinetics of the complex are much slower than for other intercalating drugs (Müller and Crothers, 1968; Crothers, 1971). As discussed in Section III,B, the biological significance of this effect is not yet clear. It is interesting that actinomycin inhibits RNA polymerase more than DNA polymerase while many other intercalating drugs seem to inhibit both polymerases more equally. Actinomycin does inhibit DNA-dependent RNA polymerases at very low levels of the drug per DNA base pair and it is possible that this very specific inhibition depends on the slow kinetics of the drug dissociation to block the progression of the enzyme along the DNA molecule (Müller and Crothers, 1968; Krugh *et al.*, 1979). The more general inhibition by drugs with faster dissociation rates may be primarily due to other factors such as inhibition of DNA strand separation so that access of the enzyme to the bases of DNA is blocked or to specific conformational changes induced in nucleosomes by drug binding. The actinomycin inhibition of DNA polymerase at higher drug levels (Meienhofer and Atherton, 1977) could result from a similar mechanism.

Other aspects of the actinomycin–DNA complex have also been thoroughly investigated. Both peptide rings of actinomycin are located in the minor groove of DNA when the ring system of the drug is intercalated (Jain and Sobell, 1972). Actinomycin exhibits pronounced specificity for G · C base pairs (Wells, 1971), and Sobell (1973) has proposed that this is due to specific hydrogen bonding between the peptide rings of actinomycin and guanine. Müller and Crothers (1975) have pointed out, however, that a G · C specificity, equally as high as that for actinomycin, can be generated through stacking interactions of the aromatic rings of the intercalated drug and the DNA base pairs. It seems possible that with actinomycin both type effects may be partially responsible for the observed specificity.

There is little doubt that actinomycin derivatives exert their antibiotic and antitumor effects through a DNA complex (Meienhofer and Atherton, 1977). These drugs accumulate selectively in cell nuclei where they are bound to DNA. This binding leads to rapid inhibition of RNA synthesis, and protein synthesis stops as preexisting messenger RNA disappears. As with *in vitro* experiments, DNA synthesis *in vivo* is not as sensitive to actinomycin as RNA synthesis. The rather high toxicity of actinomycin is probably due to a similar binding to the DNA of normal cells. The general selectivity of these drugs for target cells seems to be fairly low. The specificity of actinomycin for sensitive over resistant tumor cells seems to reside partially in altered membrane transport and partially in some as yet unspecified mechanism which may be associated with altered actinomycin association with nuclear DNA or nucleosomes (Papahadjopoulos *et al.*, 1976).

The anthracyclines, specifically daunorubicin and adriamycin, have been the most promising intercalating antitumor compounds to come from recent efforts to discover new antitumor drugs. There have been numerous reviews of the properties, structure–activity relationships, and DNA binding of these drugs (cf. DiMarco, *et al.*, 1975; DiMarco and Arcamone, 1975; Henry, 1976; Gabbay, 1976; Von Hoff *et al.*, 1978; Arcamone, 1978; Neidle, 1978; and Remers, 1979). As discussed in these reviews, the anthracyclines penetrate cells *in vivo* and are found primarily localized in the nucleus where they cause pronounced changes in morphology and biochemical reactions of chromatin. These changes can be largely correlated with DNA interactions of these compounds suggesting that at least a large part of the medicinal action of the anthracyclines must be due to an *in vivo* complex with DNA. These compounds dissociate from DNA much faster than actinomycin (Gabbay, 1976) and it seems likely that their inhibition of RNA and DNA polymerases results more from a thermodynamic stabilization of the double helical structure of DNA than from a kinetic effect (see Section III). An alternative explanation is that anthracyclines disrupt nucleosome structure, as has been found for ethidium (Wu *et al.*, 1980), and exert their effects on nucleic acid metabolism in this manner.

The anthracyclines unwind superhelical DNA and increase the viscosity of sonicated DNA as expected for intercalating compounds (Waring, 1971; Saucier *et al.*, 1971; Lanier *et al.*, 1980). Waring (1971) found an unusually low unwinding angle for daunorubicin (less than one-half the unwinding angle for ethidium) and proposed that approximately half of the bound drug was intercalated with the other half bound in a complex that did not cause DNA unwinding. Other studies (Saucier *et al.*, 1971; Lanier *et al.*, 1980), however, have indicated that essentially all of the anthracycline is intercalated but that these compounds unwind the double helix much less than ethidium and other classical intercalating drugs. Based on physical evidence of this type and on X-ray diffraction experiments with DNA–daunorubicin fibers, Pigram *et al.* (1972) proposed a model for the DNA–anthracycline complex which has been modified by others (Henry, 1976; Neidle, 1978). This model has aroused considerable interest since it correctly predicts the low unwinding angle of the anthracyclines and in addition proposes that the bulky amino sugar substituent of the anthracyclines lies in the major groove of DNA in the intercalated complex. Most other intercalating drugs which have bulky nonintercalated substituents seem to have these groups located in the minor groove (Wilson and Jones, 1980). Recently this model has come under criticism due to the finding from NMR experiments that daunorubicin actually seems to bind better to synthetic polydeoxynucleotide double helices with bulky groups in the major groove than to samples without the bulky substituents (Patel and Canuel, 1978). If the amino sugar of the anthracyclines is in the major groove, these bulky groups on the polydeoxnucleotide helices would be expected to inhibit binding. Rich and co-workers (Quigley *et al.*, 1980) have also obtained a crystal containing two intercalated daunorubicin molecules complexed with a complementary hexanucleotide. X-Ray diffraction analysis of this crystalline complex has indicated that the amino sugar group of the anthracycline is in the minor groove of the miniature double helix formed by the complementary hexanucleotides. Although considerable evidence has been accumulated which correlates the model of Pigram *et al.* (1972) with the medicinal properties of the anthracyclines (Henry, 1976; Neidle, 1978), the current uncertain state of the model leaves the significance of such correlations in doubt. If the amino sugar of the anthracyclines is in the minor groove, this means that all well-characterized intercalating molecules which have bulky cationic substituents have them in the minor groove in the intercalation complex (Wilson and Jones, 1981). More detailed studies on the medicinal activity of the diimides of Gabbay *et al.* (1973b) should then be of interest since it would appear that these compounds must have a cationic substituent in both the major and minor grooves in the intercalation complex.

The origin of the specificity of anthracyclines for tumor as opposed to normal cells is not yet clearly established. The specificity could arise, as with the other drugs discussed above, through differential transport through cellular membranes or through differential effects on the DNA or nucleosomes of normal and tumor cells. Danø *et al.* (1972) compared the effects of daunorubicin on sensitive and resistant Ehrlich tumor cells grown in culture. It took about five times more drug to inhibit RNA and DNA synthesis in the resistant cells than in the sensitive cell line. The mechanism of daunorubicin action in both sensitive and resistant cells appeared to be very similar but to require much higher concentrations for the effects to be apparent in the resistant cells. The resistance arose due to both decreased cellular uptake of daunorubicin and a decreased inhibition of polymerase reactions at constant intracellular drug levels in the resistant cells. A similar effect has been observed by Papahadjopoulos *et al.* (1976) for actinomycin D. These authors were actually able to partially overcome resistance to actinomycin in a Chinese hamster tumor cell line by incorporating the drug in lipid vesicles. These vesicles become integrated into the plasma membrane and dramatically increase the intracellular concentration of actinomycin in the resistant cells. As with daunorubicin (Danø *et al.*, 1972), however, Papahadjopoulos *et al.* (1976) find that even at equivalent intracellular drug concentrations, nucleic acid synthesis is inhibited more in sensitive than in resistant cells. As discussed above, these additional effects may be due to specific effects of drugs on nucleosomes in sensitive cells. Selectivity of drugs for target over normal cells, no doubt, also involves factors such as these.

Cain and co-workers (cf. Cain *et al.*, 1974, 1978; Cain, 1975; Denny *et al.*, 1979; Ferguson and Denny, 1980, and references contained therein) have developed a technique for resolving the overall lipophilic–hydrophilic properties of a drug molecule from other factors which affect activity such as receptor interactions and metabolic changes in the drug (see Fig. 7). Using this approach, they have designed and synthesized a series of 4′-(9-acridinylamino)alkanesulfonanilide antitumor drugs which bind to DNA by intercalation (Waring, 1976). Cain *et al.* (1974) constructed a plot of the logarithm of the increase in median life span of L1210 cells at the optimum drug dose versus a chromatographically determined partition coefficient for a series of alkane derivatives of their antitumor acridines. They used this plot as a standard curve for evaluating other derivatives in the same series. The activity of substituted derivatives could be compared to the activity of a standard compound with the same lipophilic–hydrophilic character (isolipophilic comparison) as is illustrated in Fig. 7. The difference between predicted activity from the standard curve and the observed activity for a derivative gives a quantitative measure of substituent effects such as electronic, hydrophobic, and steric contributions to drug–bioreceptor interactions. Cain *et al.* (1974) then compared substituent effects to those predicted from a DNA intercalation model since they feel that DNA is the probable bioreceptor for their acridine antitumor derivatives. They noted the similarity between the structures of their derivatives and ethidium bromide and proposed a binding model for the acridine compounds based on the structural information available on ethidium–DNA complexes (Sobell *et al.*, 1977). In the Cain *et al.* (1974) model the alkanesulfonanilide group, which is essentially perpendicular to the acridine ring, lies in the minor groove in analogy with the perpendicular phenyl substituent of ethidium. Substituent effects, deduced by the methods described above, can then be evaluated with respect to this binding model. As shown in the above references, Cain and co-workers have had considerable success with this approach both for intercalating and nonintercalating DNA binding drugs.

Cain *et al.* (1978) have expanded this series of 4′-(9-acridinylamino)alkanesulfonanilide antitumor compounds to include potential bisintercalating compounds. They point out that bisintercalating compounds will have especially strong interactions with closed circular superhelical DNA and that these type compounds can greatly enhance the specificity of intercalating drugs. These authors have also developed a qualitative measure of drug interactions with DNA, using changes in ethidium fluorescence as drugs are added to an ethidium–DNA complex, as an indicator of relative binding affinity. The ethidium competition experiments with the bisintercalators did not correlate well with antitumor activity and Cain *et al.* (1978) speculated that this was due to the complexity of, and precise orientation required for, bisintercalator–DNA complexes. Fico *et al.* (1977) have also had difficulty correlating DNA interactions with antitumor activity of bisintercalators.

The general method of Cain (1975), which involves making quantitative comparisons for a series of derivatives at isolipophilicity, is obviously the logical method for comparison of drugs of this type. It would be interesting to fit the activity of series of antitumor or antiparasitic intercalating drugs to an equation containing terms for lipophilic–hydrophilic balance and for DNA binding. Such an equation would provide a much better evaluation of the importance of DNA interactions to the activity of these compounds than binding studies alone and would also provide a rational basis for synthesis of new derivatives. Unfortunately, partitioning measurements and binding experiments have rarely been coupled in a concerted study on a series of intercalating drugs.

The DNA binding properties and antitumor activity of ellipticine and some of its derivatives at the 9 position (Fig. 1) have been thoroughly investigated (Festy *et al.*, 1971; LePecq *et al.*, 1974a,b; Kohn *et al.*, 1975; Juret *et al.*, 1978; Sorace and Sheid, 1978; Paoletti *et al.*, 1979; Jain *et al.*, 1979). The binding mode of ellipticine and its derivatives has been identified as intercalation (LePecq *et al.*, 1974a,b; Kohn *et al.*, 1975). Jain *et al.* (1979) using X-ray diffraction studies of ellipticine crystals with complementary dinucleoside monophosphates have found that this molecule intercalates in much the same manner as ethidium, proflavine, and other similar DNA binding drugs (Sobell *et al.*, 1977). LePecq and co-workers (1974a,b) discovered that a hydroxy group at the 9 position significantly increased the DNA binding constant and also enhanced the antitumor activity of ellipticine. They pointed out that within a series of compounds, such as the ellipticines, which have DNA as their bioreceptor, an initial investigation of the strength of binding to DNA is an excellent method to search for more active drugs. Although enhanced binding does not automatically ensure increased activity, compounds with lower binding constants can be eliminated and compounds with increased binding constants can undergo more thorough testing for membrane partitioning and metabolic inactivation. This is the method that led to the discovery of the highly active 9-hydroxyellipticine derivative. The advantage of this method is that as more knowledge of the factors responsible for intercalation is available, more strongly binding derivatives can be predicted before synthesis and this should dramatically enhance the probability of finding improved drugs.

Paoletti *et al.* (1979) have pointed out that, in general, the concentration of ellipticine derivatives required to produce significant toxicity for L1210 cells is much lower than would be expected based on the DNA binding constants of these drugs. As Wu *et al.* (1980) have pointed out, however, nucleosomes have higher affinities for intercalating drugs than purified DNA at low levels of saturation. These compounds could then exert toxic effects on cells at much lower concentrations than predicted by purified DNA binding constants if nucleosome binding and conformational changes are responsible for the toxic effects of the drugs. Selective accumulation of active drugs by sensitive cells can also affect the dosage of the drugs required to exert toxicity.

This section on antitumor drugs is larger than the preceding two sections. This is in part due to the fact that recently more funds have been available for developing and studying antitumor drugs than for drugs active against other diseases and in part because intercalating drugs of diverse structure and properties have shown high activity against tumor cells. There is significant overlap in activities, of course, with compounds such as ethidium and 9-methoxyellipticine having both antitumor and antitrypanosomal activity.

V. Conclusions

We have summarized the current model for the interaction of intercalating drugs with DNA and have related this model to the *in vivo* effects of intercalating drugs. There are two particular problems in evaluating activity from an analysis of intercalation. First, as has been pointed out by Cain and co-workers (Cain, 1975; Cain *et al.*, 1974) and as is illustrated in Fig. 7, comparison of compounds must be made at isolipophilicity to allow evaluation of the importance of various intercalation factors to activity. Second, a study of the binding of intercalating drugs to purified DNA may not accurately reflect the effect that these drugs have on chromatin (Gabbay and Wilson, 1978). Wu *et al.* (1980) have pointed out that at low saturation levels, ethidium binds more strongly to nucleosomes than to purified DNA and causes a pronounced disruption in nucleosome structure. Many intercalating drugs may exert their biological effects at this level and display activity at concentrations lower than would be predicted based on their DNA binding constants. It should also be emphasized that binding constants for intercalating drugs are, in general, quite ionic strength dependent (see Fig. 6) and a high binding constant obtained at low salt concentration does not ensure that a drug will bind significantly to DNA under physiological conditions. Future progress in structure–activity determinations for intercalating drugs requires that a standard method be developed for comparing various compounds. Plots such as the one shown in Fig. 7 are becoming more common for drugs which bind to DNA and currently this seems to be the best method for standardization of comparative studies.

One problem with the medicinal use of intercalating drugs is their relatively high toxicity for all cells. One of the goals of research in this area has to be to increase the selectivity of these compounds for target cells. Current research on nucleosome and chromatin structure (McGhee and Felsenfeld, 1980) may describe differences between the chromosomal and/or nucleosomal structure of host and parasitic cells, for example, which can be exploited in the design of specific drugs. This research area is still quite new and should provide significant findings and ideas in the near future.

Another possibility for increasing selectivity is the design of intercalating drugs which bind to specific DNA sequences which occur only in target cells or which are particularly important for gene expression or metabolic control in target cells. It is difficult to design monointercalators which have this high level of binding specificity. The development of bis or multiintercalating drugs, however, does have the promise of allowing design of drugs which bind strongly to specific DNA sequences. These type drugs have very high binding constants (see Capelle *et al.*, 1979 and references therein) and with the appropriate choice of monointercalating units can exhibit high specificity for DNA sequences. These molecules are quite complex and depending on the hydrophobic nature of their linking groups may exert additional types of activity (Fico *et al.*, 1977).

As can be seen from Section IV, there seems no doubt that a wide range of drugs active against diverse diseases exert their biological effects through an intercalation complex with DNA and a resulting perturbation of nucleic acid metabolism. Intercalating compounds are particularly common in the list of drugs being tested clinically as antitumor agents. Current research in chromatin structure and the quantitative requirements for intercalation indicate that the design of compounds with greatly increased selectivity and activity should be possible. If this occurs, the clinical use of intercalating drugs against a wider range of diseases should become more common.

Acknowledgments

The work from our laboratory which is discussed in this article has been supported in large part by grant CA 24454 from the National Cancer Institute of The National Institutes of Health. Continued discussions of this work with Professor David Boykin have helped form our ideas expressed in this article and have made our research in this area more enjoyable and productive. We thank Ms. Pricilla Phillips for her friendly and thoughtful assistance in the preparation of this manuscript.

References

Albert, A. (1972). *In* "Drug Design" (E. J. Ariëns, ed.), Vol. III, pp. 229–243. Academic Press, New York.

Arcamone, F. (1978). *In* "Topics in Antibiotic Chemistry" (P. G. Sammes, ed.), Vol. 2, pp. 89–239. Wiley, New York.

Arnott, S., and Hukins, D. W. L. (1973). *J. Mol. Biol.* **81,** 93.

Atassi, G., Duarte-Karim, M., and Tagnon, H. J. (1975). *Eurp. J. Cancer* **11,** 309.

Avila, J. L., Bretana, A., and Avila, A. (1979). *Am. J. Trop. Med. Hyg.* **28,** 456.

Bauer, W. R. (1978). *In* "Annual Review of Biophysics and Bioengineering" (L. J. Mullins, ed.), Vol. 7, pp. 287–313. Annual Reviews, Palo Alto, California.

Bauer, W., and Vinograd, J. (1970). *J. Mol. Biol.* **47,** 419.

Bauer, W., and Vinograd, J. (1974). *In* "Basic Principles in Nucleic Acid Chemistry", (P.O.P. Ts'o, ed.), pp. 265–303. Academic Press, New York.

Becker, M. M., and Dervan, P. B. (1979). *J. Am. Chem. Soc.* **101,** 3664.

Bernard, J., Riou, G., and Saucier, J. (1979). *Nucleic Acids Res.* **6,** 1941.

Blake, A., and Peacocke, A. R. (1968). *Biopolymers* **6,** 1225.

Bloomfield, V. A., Crothers, D. M., and Tinoco, I., Jr. (1974). *In* "Physical Chemistry of Nucleic Acids," Ch. 7. Harper, New York.

Blum, R. H., Garnick, M. B., Israel, M., Cannellos, G. P., Henderson, I. C., and Frei, E., III (1979). *Cancer Treat. Rep.* **63,** 919.

Bolton, P. H., and James, T. L. (1979). *J. Phys. Chem.* **83,** 3359.

Bond, P. J., Langridge, R., Jennette, K. W., and Lippard, S. J. (1975). *Proc. Natl. Acad. Sci. U.S.A.* **72,** 4825.

Bresloff, J. L., and Crothers, D. M. (1975). *J. Mol. Biol.* **95,** 103.

Cain, B. F. (1975). *Cancer Chemother. Rep.* **59,** 679.

Cain, B. F., Seelye, R. N., and Atwell, G. J. (1974). *J. Med. Chem.* **17,** 922.

Cain, B. F., Atwell, G. J., and Denny, W. A. (1977). *J. Med. Chem.* **20,** 987.

Cain, B. F., Baguley, B. C., and Denny, W. A. (1978). *J. Med. Chem.* **21,** 658.

Canellakis, E. S., Shaw, Y. H., Hanners, W. E., and Schwartz, R. A. (1976). *Biochim. Biophys. Acta* **418,** 227.

Capelle, N., Barbet, J., Dessen, P., Blanquet, S., Roques, B. P., and LePecq, J. B. (1979). *Biochemistry* **15,** 3354.

Carter, G., and Van Dyke, K. (1972). *In* "Basic Research in Malaria" (E. H. Sadun, ed.), pp. 240–249. Walter Reed Army Inst. of Research, Washington, D.C.

Cavalieri, L. F., Rosoff, M., and Rosenberg, B. H. (1956). *J. Am. Chem. Soc.* **78,** 5239.

Cerami, A., Reich, E., Ward, D. C., and Goldberg, I. H. (1967). *Proc. Natl. Acad. Sci. U.S.A.* **57,** 1036.

Chen, T. K., Fico, R., and Canellakis, E. S. (1978). *J. Med. Chem.* **21,** 868.

Cohen G., and Eisenberg, H. (1969). *Biopolymers* **8,** 45.

Corcoran, J. W., and Hahn, F. E. (1975). "Antibiotics." Springer-Verlag, Berlin and New York.

Crothers, D. M. (1968). *Biopolymers* **6,** 575.

Crothers, D. M. (1971). *In* "Progress in Molecular and Subcellular Biology" (F. E. Hahn, ed.), Vol. II, pp. 10–20. Springer-Verlag, Berlin and New York.

Crothers, D. M., Dattagupta, N., Hogan, M., Klevan, M., and Lee, K. S. (1978). *Biochemistry* **17,** 4525.

Danø, K., Frederiksen, S., and Hellung-Larsen, P. (1972). *Cancer Res.* **32,** 1307.

Dattagupta, N., Hogan, M., and Crothers, D. M. (1978). *Proc. Natl. Acad. Sci. U.S.A.* **75,** 4286.

Davidson, M. W., Griggs B. G., Jr., Boykin, D. W., and Wilson, W. D. (1975). *Nature (London)* **254,** 632.

Davidson, M. W., Lopp, I., Alexander, S., and Wilson, W. D. (1977a). *Nucleic Acids Res.* **4,** 2696.

Davidson, M. W., Griggs, B. G., Boykin, D. W., and Wilson, W. D. (1977b). *J. Med. Chem.* **20,** 1117.

Davidson, M. W., Griggs, B. G., Lopp, I.G., and Wilson, W. D. (1977c). *Biochim. Biophys. Acta* **479,** 378.

Denny, W. A., Atwell, G. J., and Cain, B. F. (1979). *J. Med. Chem.* **22,** 1453.

Dervan, P. B., and Becker, M. N. (1978). *J. Am. Chem. Soc.* **100,** 1968.

DiMarco, A., and Arcamone, F. (1975). *Arzneim. Forsch.* **25,** 368.

DiMarco, A., Arcamone, F., and Zunino, F. (1975). *In* "Antibiotics" (J. W. Corcoran and F. E. Hahn, eds.), Vol. III, pp. 101–128. Springer-Verlag, Berlin and New York.

Dourlent, M., and Hogrel, J. F. (1976). *Biochemistry* **15,** 430.

Ferguson, L. R., and Denny, W. A. (1980). *J. Med. Chem.* **23,** 269.

Festy, B., Poisson, J., and Paoletti, C. (1971). *FEBS Lett.* **197,** 321.
Fico, R. M., Chen, T. K., and Canellakis, E. S. (1977). *Science* **198,** 53.
Fuller, W., and Waring, M. J. (1964). *Ber. Bunsenges. Phys. Chem.* **68,** 805.
Gabbay, E. J. (1976). *Int. J. Quantum Chem. Quantum Biol. Symp.* **3,** 217.
Gabbay, E. J. (1977). *In* "Bioorganic Chemistry" (E. E. Van Tamelen, ed.), Vol. III, pp. 33–70. Academic Press, New York.
Gabbay, E. J., and Wilson, W. D. (1978). *In* "Methods in Cell Biology" (G. Stein, J. Stein, and L. Kleinsmith, eds.), pp. 351–384. Academic Press, New York.
Gabbay, E. J., Scofield, R., and Baxter, C. S. (1973a). *J. Am. Chem. Soc.* **95,** 7850.
Gabbay, E. J., De Stefano, R., and Baxter, C. S. (1973b). *Biochem. Biophys. Res. Commun.* **51,** 1083.
Gabbay, E., Grier, D., Fingerle, R., Reimer, R., Levy, R., Pearce, S. W., and Wilson, W. D. (1976). *Biochemistry* **15,** 2062.
Garland, F., Graves, D. E., Tielding, L. W., and Cheung, H. C. (1980). *Biochemistry* **19,** 3221.
Gaugain, B., Barbet, J., Capelle, N., Roques, B. P., and LePecq, J. B. (1978). *Biochemistry* **17,** 5078.
Gurskii, G. V., Zasendatelev, A. S., and Volkenshtein, M. V. (1972). *Mol. Biol.* **6,** 385.
Hahn, F. E., O'Brien, R. L., Ciak, J., Allison, J. L., and Olenick, J. G. (1966). *Mil. Med.* **131,** 1071.
Hajduk, S. L. (1978). *In* "Progress in Molecular and Subcellular Biology" (F. E. Hahn, H. Kersten, W. Kersten, and W. Szybalski, eds.), pp. 158–200. Springer-Verlag, Berlin and New York.
Hamilton, L., Fuller, W., and Reich, E. (1963). *Nature (London)* **198,** 538.
Hansch, C. (1969). *Acc. Chem. Res.* **2,** 232.
Heinen, E., Bassler, R., Calberg-Bacq, C. M., Desaive, C., and Lepoint, A. (1974). *Biochem. Pharmacol.* **23,** 1549.
Henry, D. W. (1976). *In* "Cancer Chemotherapy" (A. C. Sartorelli, ed.), pp. 15–57. American Chemical Society, Washington, D.C.
Hogan, M. E., and Jardetzky, O. (1979). *Proc. Natl. Acad. Sci. U.S.A.* **76,** 6341.
Hogan, M. E., and Jardetzky, O. (1980a). *Biochemistry* **19,** 3460.
Hogan, M. E., and Jardetzky, O. (1980b). *Biochemistry* **19,** 2079.
Hogan, M., Dattagupta, N., and Crothers, D. M. (1978). *Proc. Natl. Acad. Sci. U.S.A.* **75,** 195.
Hogan, M., Dattagupta, N., and Crothers, D. M. (1979). *Biochemistry* **18,** 280.
Hook, J. W., Petersheim, M., Lin, S., and Krugh, T. R. (1979). *Biophys. J.* **25,** 6a.
Howe-Grant, M., and Lippard, S. J. (1979). *Biochemistry* **18,** 5762.
Hurwitz, E., Levy, R., Mason, R., Wilchek, M., Arnon, R., and Sela, M. (1975). *Cancer Res.* **35,** 1175.
Israel, M., Modest, E. J., and Frei, E., III (1975). *Cancer Res.* **35,** 1365–1368.
Jain, S. C., and Sobell, H. M. (1972). *J. Mol. Biol.* **68,** 1.
Jain, S. C., Tsai, C., and Sobell, H. M. (1977). *J. Mol. Biol.* **114,** 317.
Jain, S. C., Bhandary, K. K., and Sobell, H. M. (1979). *J. Mol. Biol.* **135,** 813.
Jones, R. L., Davidson, M. W., and Wilson, W. D. (1979). *Biochim. Biophys. Acta* **561,** 77.
Jones, R. L., Lanier, A. L., Keel, R. A., and Wilson, W. D. (1980). *Nucleic Acids Res.* **8,** 1613.
Juret, P., Tanguy, A., LeTalaer, J. Y., Abbatucci, J. S., Xuong, N. D., LePecq, J. B., and Paoletti, C. (1978). *Eur. J. Cancer* 205.
Kallenbach, N. R., Appleby, D. W., and Bradley, C. H. (1978). *Nature (London)* **272,** 134.

Kersten, H., and Kersten, W. (1974) "Inhibitors of Nucleic Acid Synthesis." Springer-Verlag, Berlin and New York.

Klevan, L., Armitage, I. M., and Crothers, D. M. (1979). *Nucleic Acids Res.* **6,** 1607.

Kohn, K. W., Waring, M. J., Glaubiger, D., and Friedman, C. A. (1975). *Cancer Res.* **35,** 71.

Krugh, T. R., and Nuss, M. E. (1979). *In* "Biological Applications of Magnetic Resonance" (R. G. Shulman, ed.), pp. 113–175. Academic Press, New York.

Krugh, T. R., Hook, J. W., III, Lin, S., and Chen, F-M. (1979). *In* "Stereodynamics of Molecular Systems" (R. H. Sarma, ed.), pp. 423–435. Pergamon, New York.

Kuhlmann, K. F., Charbeneau, N. J., and Mosher, C. W. (1978). *Nucleic Acids Res.* **5,** 2629.

Kuhlmann, K. F., Mosher, L. W., and Hammen, R. F. (1980). *Biochem. Biophys. Res. Commun.* **92,** 1172.

Lanier, A., Jones, R. L., and Wilson, W. D. (1980). In preparation.

LePecq, J. B., Le Bret, M., Gosse, C., Paoletti, C., Chalvet, O., and Xuong, N. D. (1974a). *In* "Molecular and Quantum Pharmacology" (E. Bergmann and B. Pullman, eds.), pp. 515–535. Reidel Publ., Dordrecht.

LePecq, J. B., Xuong, N. D., Gosse, C., and Paoletti, C. (1974b). *Proc. Natl. Acad. Sci. U.S.A.* **71,** 5078.

LePecq, J. B., Le Bret, M., Barbet, J., and Roques, B. (1975). *Proc. Natl. Acad. Sci. U.S.A.* **72,** 2915.

Lerman, L. S. (1961). *J. Mol. Biol.* **3,** 18.

Lerman, L. S. (1963). *Proc. Natl. Acad. Sci. U.S.A.* **49,** 94.

Lerman, L. S. (1964a). *J. Cell. Comp. Physiol.* **64** (1), 1.

Lerman, L. S. (1964b). *J. Mol. Biol.* **10,** 367.

Levitt, M. (1978). *Proc. Natl. Acad. Sci. U.S.A.* **75,** 640.

Li, J. H., and Crothers, D. M. (1969). *J. Mol. Biol.* **39,** 461.

Lohman, T. M., DeHaseth, P., and Record, M. T., Jr. (1980). *Biochemistry* **19,** 3522.

Lown, J. W., Gunn, B. C., Chang, R. Y., Majumdar, K. C., and Lee, J. S. (1978). *Can. J. Biochem.* **56,** 1006.

Lozansky, E. D., Sobell, H. M., and Lessen, M. (1979). *In* "Stereodynamics of Molecular Systems" (R. H. Sarma, ed.), pp. 265–270. Pergammon, New York.

McGhee, J. D., and Felsenfeld, G. (1980). *In* "Annual Review of Biochemistry" (E. E. Snell, ed.), Vol. 49, pp. 1115–1156. Annual Reviews, Palo Alto, California.

McGhee, J. D., and von Hipple, P. H. (1974). *J. Mol. Biol.* **86,** 469.

Manning, G. S. (1978). *Q. Rev. Biophys.* **2,** 179.

Mariam, Y. H., and Wilson, W. D. (1979). *Biochem. Biophys. Res. Commun.* **88,** 861.

Marks, T. A., and Venditti, J. M. (1976). *Cancer Res.* **36,** 496.

Meienhofer, J., and Atherton, E. (1977). *In* "Structure-Activity Relationships Among the Semisynthetic Antibiotics" (D. Perlman, ed.), pp. 427–529. Academic Press, New York.

Müller, W., and Crothers, D. M. (1968). *J. Mol. Biol.* **35,** 251.

Müller, W., and Crothers, D. M. (1975). *Eur. J. Biochem.* **54,** 267.

Müller, W., Crothers, D. M., and Waring, M. J. (1973). *Eur. J. Biochem.* **39,** 223.

Neidle, S. (1978). *In* "Topics in Antibiotic Chemistry" (P. G. Sammes, ed.), Vol. 2, pp. 240–278. Wiley, New York.

Neidle, S. (1979). *In* "Progress in Medicinal Chemistry" (G. P. Ellis and G. B. West, eds.), Vol. 16, pp. 151–221. Elsevier, Amsterdam.

Newton, B. A. (1970). *In* "Advances in Pharmacology and Chemotherapy" (S. Garattini, A. Goldin, F. Hawking, and I. J. Kopin, eds.), Vol. 8, pp. 150–184. Academic Press, New York.

Newton, B. A. (1974). *In* "Trypanosomiasis and Leishmaniasis," Ciba Foundation Symposium 20, pp. 285–308. Elsevier, Amsterdam.

Ohnmacht, C. J., Patel, A. R., and Lutz, R. E. (1971). *J. Med. Chem.* **14,** 926.
Panter, J. W., Boykin, D. W., and Wilson, W. D. (1973). *J. Med. Chem.* **16,** 1366.
Paoletti, C., Cros, S., Xuong, N. D., Lecointe, P., and Moisand, A. (1979). *Chem. Biol. Interact.* **25,** 45.
Papahadjopoulos, D., Poste, G., Vail, W. T., and Biedler, J. L. (1976). *Cancer Res.* **36,** 2988.
Patel, D. J., and Canuel, L. L. (1978). *Eur. J. Biochem.* **90,** 247.
Peacocke, A. R., and Skerrett, J. H. N. (1956). *Trans. Faraday Soc.* **52,** 261.
Pigram, W. J., Fuller, W., and Hamilton, L. D. (1972). *Nature (London) New Biol.* **235,** 17.
Pulleyblank, D. E., and Morgan, A. R. (1975). *J. Mol. Biol.* **91,** 1.
Quigley, G., Wang, A., Ughetto, G., Marel, G., van Brom, J., and Rich, A. (1980). *Proc. Natl. Acad. Sci. U.S.A.* **77,** 7204.
Record, M. T., Jr., Anderson, L. F., and Lohman, T. M. (1978). *Q. Rev. Biophys.* **2,** 103.
Reddy, B. S., Seshadri, T. P., Sakore, T. D., and Sobell, H. M. (1979). *J. Mol. Biol.* **135,** 787.
Reinhardt, C. G., and Krugh, T. R. (1977). *Biochemistry* **16,** 2890.
Remers, W. A. (1979). "The Chemistry of Antitumor Antibiotics." Wiley, New York.
Révet, B. M. J., Schmir, M., and Vinograd, J. (1971). *Nature (London) New Biology* **229,** 10.
Rozman, R. S., and Canfield, C. J. (1979). *In* "Advances in Pharmacology and Chemotherapy" (S. Garattini, A. Goldin, F. Hawking, and I. J. Kopin, eds.), Vol. 16, pp. 1–44. Academic Press, New York.
Sakore, T. D., Jain, S. C., Tsai, C., and Sobell, H. M. (1977). *Proc. Natl. Acad. Sci. U.S.A.* **74,** 188.
Sakore, T. D., Reddy, B. S., and Sobell, H. M. (1979). *J. Mol. Biol.* **135,** 763.
Saucier, J. M., Festy, B., and Le Pecq, J. B. (1971). *Biochimie* **53,** 973.
Scatchard, G. (1949). *Ann. N. Y. Acad. Sci.* **51,** 660.
Shafer, R. H., Burnette, R. R., and Mirau, P. A. (1980). *Nucleic Acids Res.* **8,** 1121.
Shindo, H. (1980). *Biopolymers* **19,** 509.
Shindo, H., and McGhee, J. D. (1980). *Biopolymers* **19,** 523.
Shindo, H., Simpson, R. T., and Cohen, J. S. (1979). *J. Biol. Chem.* **254,** 8125.
Shindo, H., Wooten, J. B., Pheiffer, B. H., and Zimmerman, S. B. (1980). *Biochemistry* **19,** 518.
Simpson, R. T., and Shindo, H. (1979). *Nucleic Acids Res.* **7,** 481.
Sobell, H. M. (1973). *In* "Progress in Nucleic Acid Research and Molecular Biology" (J. N. Davidson and W. E. Cohn, eds.), pp. 153–190. Academic Press, New York.
Sobell, H. M., Reddy, B. S., Bhandray, K. K., Jain, S. C., Sakore, T. D., and Seshadri, T. P. (1977). *In* "Cold Spring Harbor Symposia on Quantitative Biology," pp. 87–102. Cold Spring Harbor Lab., Cold Spring Harbor, New York.
Sokerov, S., and Weill, G. (1979). *Biophys. Chem.* **10,** 161.
Sorace, R. A., and Sheid, B. (1978). *Chem. Biol. Interact.* **23,** 379.
Steck, E. A. (1972). *In* "The Chemotherapy of Protozoan Diseases," pp. 23, 77, 177. U.S. Gov. Printing Office, Washington, D.C.
Trenholme, G. M., Williams, R. L., Desjardins, R. E., Frischer, H., Carson, P. E., Rieckmann, K. H., and Canfield, C. J. (1975). *Science* **190,** 792.
Trouet, A. (1978). *Eur. J. Cancer* **14,** 105.
Trouet, A., and Sokal, G. (1979). *Cancer Treat. Rep.* **63,** 895.
Trouet, A., Campeneere, D. D., and de Duve, C. (1972). *Nature (London) New Biol.* **239,** 110.
Trouet, A., Campeneere, D. D., de Smedt-Malengreaux, M., and Attassi, G. (1974). *Eur. J. Cancer* **10,** 405.
Tsai, C., Jain, S. C., and Sobell, H. M. (1977). *J. Mol. Biol.* **114,** 301.
Von Hoff, D. D., Rozencweig, M., and Slavik, M. (1978). *In* "Advances in Pharmacology

and Chemotherapy" (S. Garatti, A. Goldin, F. Hawking, and I. J. Kopin, eds.), pp. 2–50. Academic Press, New York.

Wakelin, L. P. G., and Waring, M. J. (1974). *Mol. Pharmacol.* **10,** 544.

Wakelin, L. P. G., Romanos, M., Canellakis, E. S., and Waring, M. J. (1976). *Stud. Biophys.* **60,** 111.

Wakelin, L. P. G., Romanos, M., Chen, T. K., Glaubiger, D., Canellakis, E. S., and Waring, M. J. (1978). *Biochemistry* **17,** 5057.

Wang, J. C. (1974). *J. Mol. Biol.* **89,** 783.

Wang, A. H-J., Quigley, G. J., Kolpak, F. J., Crawford, J. L., van Boom, J. H., van der Marcel, G., and Rich, A. (1979). *Nature (London)* **282,** 680.

Waring, M. J. (1970). *J. Mol. Biol.* **54,** 247.

Waring, M. J. (1971). *In* "Progress in Molecular and Subcellular Biology" (F. Hahn, ed.), pp. 216–231. Springer-Verlag, Berlin and New York.

Waring, M. J. (1972). *In* "The Molecular Basis of Antibiotic Action" (E. F. Gale, E. Cundliffe, P. E. Reynolds, M. H. Richmond, and Waring, M. J., eds.), pp. 173–277. Wiley, New York.

Waring, M. J. (1975). *In* "Antibiotics" (J. W. Corcoran and F. E. Hahn, eds.), Vol. III, pp. 141–165. Springer-Verlag, Berlin and New York.

Waring, M. J. (1976). *Eur. J. Cancer* **12,** 995.

Waring, M. J. (1977). *In* "Drug Action at the Molecular Level" (G. C. K. Roberts, ed.), pp. 167–189. Univ. Park Press, London.

Watson, J. D., and Crick, F. H. C. (1953). *Nature (London)* **171,** 737.

Wells, R. D. (1971). *In* "Progress in Molecular and Subcellular Biology" (F. E. Hahn, ed.), Vol. II, pp. 21–32. Springer-Verlag, Berlin and New York.

Wilson, W. D., and Jones, R. L. (1980). *J. Am. Chem. Soc.* **102,** 7776–7778.

Wilson, W. D., and Jones, R. L. (1981). *In* "Intercalation Chemistry" (M. S. Whittingham and A. J. Jacobson, eds.). Academic Press, New York, in press.

Wilson, W. D., and Lopp, I. G. (1979). *Biopolymers* **18,** 3025.

Wu, H-M., Dattagupta, N., Hogan, M., and Crothers, D. M. (1980). *Biochemistry* **19,** 626.

The Action of Metronidazole on Anaerobic Bacilli and Similar Organisms

E. J. BAINES AND J. A. MCFADZEAN

Pharmaceutical Division
May & Baker Ltd.
Dagenham, Essex, England

ISBN 0-12-032918-2

I. Introduction

Metronidazole, which was introduced into chemotherapy in 1960 as the first clinically effective systemic antitrichomonal agent, has subsequently proved to be remarkable for the breadth, intensity, and consistency of its antiinfective activity.

Its outstanding value as an antitrichomonal agent was duly recognized in an article in this publication by Michaels (1968), as was the extension of its antiprotozoal activity against *Giardia lamblia* to the treatment of amebiasis (Powell, 1972).

Comprehensive discussions of developments with metronidazole from 1960 to 1978 have been provided by Baines (1977, 1978). The first of these was presented at the International Metronidazole Conference in Montreal, May 26–28, 1976, when the available evidence on the product's chemical, biochemical, and biological properties was reviewed together with communications on its established therapeutic uses and its safety evaluation.

Among potential new therapeutic uses, that of radiosensitization was discussed; but we shall leave it to better qualified observers to elaborate on this interesting development, for which misonidazole, a 2-nitroimidazole derivative, is more potent but more toxic.

Although single communications to the Montreal Conference were made on clinical trials of metronidazole in the management of Crohn's disease (Ursing, 1977) and in chronic proctitis (Davies *et al.*, 1977), a substantial part of the Conference was devoted to anaerobic bacteria, their role in disease, and to the use of metronidazole in the treatment and prevention of anaerobic infections in man.

New evidence obtained by British workers on this use of the product was presented at a symposium on "The Management of Non-clostridial Anaerobic Infections," held at the Luton and Dunstable Hospital, May 20, 1977; the proceedings were published in Supplement C to Volume 4 of the *J. Antimicrob. Chemother.*, September 1978.

By April 1979, investigators from Canada, India, New Zealand, South Africa, Sweden, Switzerland, and the United States were able to join their British confrères in reporting their experiences to the Second International Symposium on Anaerobic Infections in Geneva. The proceedings, which covered the microbiology of anaerobic infection, the pharmacokinetics of metronidazole, its therapeutic application, its use in chemoprophylaxis, and its toxicological aspects, were published in The Royal Society of Medicine International Congress and Symposium Series No. 18, 1979.

The evidence presented at these meetings and that contained in scores of published articles and reviews clearly establishes metronidazole's value in the treatment and prevention of anaerobic bacterial infections and justifies the suggestion that it represents a major advance in antimicrobial chemotherapy.

As was pointed out in an editorial on "The Nitroimidazole Family of Drugs" (1978), the first analog of metronidazole to be marketed, nimorazole, appeared in Britain in 1970, when the therapeutic indications for the former had already been extended from urogenital trichomoniasis and giardiasis to include amebiasis. This was followed, about 2 years later, by tinidazole and, more recently, by ornidazole. Both products were introduced as trichomonacides and amebicides but, as was to be expected, they also share with metronidazole bactericidal activity against obligate anaerobes. Some favorable clinical reports on their use in the treatment and prevention of anaerobic infections have been published, but the evidence available to us at present is insufficient to warrant detailed discussion.

II. The Relevant Properties of Metronidazole

A. Chemical and Physical

Metronidazole, with a molecular weight of 171, is soluble in water at 20°C to the extent of 1% w/v and is essentially nonionized at physiological pH, rapidly permeating cell membranes.

B. Absorption

In humans the substance is rapidly and completely absorbed after oral administration, giving peak and minimum plasma metronidazole concentrations at steady-state, after 8-hourly 500 mg doses, which are of the same order as those provided by 500 mg intravenous doses; viz. mean values of 26 and 14 μg/ml, respectively, with oral medication and 26 and 12 μg/ml with iv medication (G. W. Houghton, J. Smith, and P. S. Thorne, unpublished results). These are higher than the minimum bactericidal concentrations (MBC) for most anaerobic bacterial pathogens (Houghton *et al.*, 1979).

Metronidazole is less rapidly absorbed from rectal suppositories, the first 1 gm dose taking several hours to provide a mean peak plasma concentration of 7.3 μg/ml. Thereafter, with 8-hourly administration, an average steady-state concentration of 16–29 μg/ml can be expected; but for maximum chemoprophylactic activity during surgery, the preoperative rectal suppository should be given as early as possible.

Metronidazole in the form of an aqueous solution/suspension given as a retention enema appears to be rapidly absorbed, producing peak blood levels after 2 hours.

C. Distribution

Metronidazole is distributed in virtually all tissues and body fluids in concentrations which do not differ markedly from the corresponding serum levels except in the case of urine, in which it is concentrated and of feces, in which it is largely inactivated by the gut microflora.

Thus anaerobicidal concentrations are readily achieved after therapeutic doses in blood, saliva, cerebrospinal fluid, ventricular fluid, brain abscess contents, middle ear discharges, gums, alveolar bone, empyema fluid, human breast milk, bile, liver abscess contents, myometrium, Fallopian tubes, amniotic fluid, cord blood, placenta, embryonic tissues, and seminal fluid.

Metronidazole is secreted into the lumen of the large bowel where it is inactivated by the aerobic and facultatively anaerobic microflora by a process which appears to involve little more than absorption; when the product has been administered orally with nonabsorbed antiaerobic agents such as kanamycin, phthalylsulfathiazole, or neomycin for preoperative bowel preparation of patients for colorectal surgery, the numbers of both anaerobes and aerobes have been greatly reduced.

D. Metabolism in Animals and Man

Ings *et al.* (1966) showed that metronidazole exhibited identical metabolic patterns in dogs and in humans.

Houghton *et al.* (1979) found that 30% of the metronidazole and metabolites detected in the urine of healthy female volunteers was unchanged drug. This was equivalent to about 10% of the administered dose.

The major metabolic pathway involved oxidation of the hydroxy group of the side chain in the 1-position to give the 1-acetic acid (II). A conjugate with glucuronic acid was also formed and this was thought to be the ether conjugate of metronidazole (III) (Ings *et al.*, 1966).

No evidence was found of reduction of the nitro group.

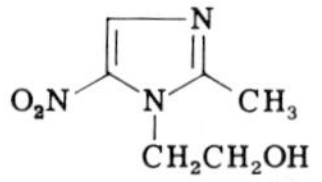

Metronidazole	(II)	(III)
O_2N, N, CH_3; CH_2CH_2OH	O_2N, N, CH_3; CH_2COOH	O_2N, N, CH_3; $CH_2CH_2O \cdot C_6H_9O_6$

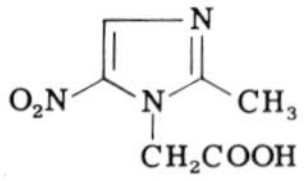

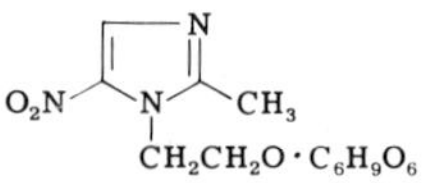

Stambaugh *et al.* (1968) made an analogous study in mice and humans which partly confirmed the findings of Ings *et al.* However, they claimed that the 2-methyl group was oxidized more than the 1-β-hydroxyethyl group, giving five metabolites as follows:

(II) O_2N–imidazole–CH_3, N–CH_2COOH ← (I) O_2N–imidazole–CH_3, N–CH_2CH_2OH → (III) O_2N–imidazole–CH_3, N–$CH_2CH_2O \cdot C_6H_9O_6$

(I) ↓

(V) O_2N–imidazole–$COOH$, N–CH_2CH_2OH ← (IV) O_2N–imidazole–CH_2OH, N–CH_2CH_2OH → (VI) O_2N–imidazole–CH_2OH, N–$CH_2CH_2O \cdot C_6H_9O_6$

They estimated the urinary contents in man to be: I + III, 30–40%; II, 15–20%; IV + VI, 40–50%; and V, 8–12%.

These workers, like Ings *et al*. (1966), saw no evidence of reduction of the 5-nitro group of metronidazole.

The unconjugated metabolites identified in significant concentrations in blood and/or urine are: II, which has only slight antimicrobial activity (Ralph and Kirby, 1975; Lindmark and Müller, 1976) and is nonmutagenic for aerobic and facultatively anaerobic test organisms; and IV, which has one-third of the activity of metronidazole against *Bacteroides fragilis* (Ralph and Kirby, 1975) and one-fifth of its activity against *Trichomonas vaginalis,* and is also less mutagenic than the parent compound against *Salmonella typhimurium* auxotroph TA 100 (Lindmark and Muller, 1976).

Although Connor *et al.* (1977) have claimed that with auxotroph RA 1535, metabolite IV was 10 times more mutagenic than metronidazole, conversion of the data to absolute values resolves the apparent contradiction of the findings of Lindmark and Müller (1976).

The implications of the mutagenicity of this metabolite are discussed later. It is, however, important to note that there is no scientific justification for the sweeping and alarming suggestions of Connor *et al.* (1977) or of Speck *et al.* (1976) that in man the liver metabolizes metronidazole to produce substances having increased mutagenic activity.

Gabriel *et al.* (1979), in a study of the pharmacokinetics of single doses of metronidazole administered intravenously before and after dialysis to patients in chronic renal failure, found that the unchanged substance and metabolite IV were dialyzed from the plasma up to three times more rapidly than their clearance in normal subjects. Metabolite II was not detected in the plasma. During the days after dialysis, the plasma metronidazole concentration decreased at a rate similar to that in normal subjects, metabolite IV was removed less rapidly, and the level of II remained high.

After Koch and Goldman (1978) had shown that *N*-(2-hydroxyethyl)-oxamic acid was found when metronidazole was incubated anaerobically with rat fecal contents, Koch *et al.* (1979) reported that acetamide was also found under the same conditions. These workers then proceeded to show that when a 200 mg/kg dose of radioactively labeled metronidazole was given by gavage to conventional rats, 1.3 to 1.8% of the dose was recovered as acetamide from the urine and 0.9 to 2.4% was recovered from the feces. No such recovery was made with germ-free rats similarly medicated and it was concluded that the intestinal flora of rats had effected reduction of the nitro group and cleavage of the imidazole ring. Koch *et al.* (1979) having noted that acetamide had been shown to be a liver carcinogen for rats, raised the question of a similar metabolism of metronidazole by the human gut microflora.

There appears to be no information about this at present, but the vast difference between the exposure to 6 mg of acetamide per kg to which the metronidazole-medicated rats were subjected and the dosage of about 1875 mg of acetamide per kg/day which was carcinogenic for rats (Jackson and Dessau, 1961) should be borne in mind.

E. Pharmacology

1. *Animal*

In animal experiments metronidazole appeared to exert no significant effect on the cardiovascular, respiratory, and reproductive systems.

High oral dosages in rats reduced pentagastrin-induced gastric secretion and inhibited indomethacin-induced gastric ulcer formation (Banerjee, 1978).

Metronidazole, unlike benzylpenicillin, erythromycin, bacitracin plus neomycin, neomycin, and kanamycin did not increase the bile acid index to that of germ-free rats (Gustafsson *et al.*, 1977).

Some immunosuppressant activity has been reported, e.g., prolongation of rejection and survival times in rats with transplanted hearts (Kostakis and Calne, 1977) and suppression of granuloma formation around *Schistosoma mansoni* eggs injected into the pulmonary vasculature of mice (Grove *et al.*, 1977).

2. *Human*

Therapeutic doses given to healthy men for 10 days decreased bile cholesterol saturation and the proportion of deoxycholate in bile acids with corresponding increases in the proportion of chenodeoxycholate (Low-Beer and Nutter, 1978).

III. Antibacterial Activity in Laboratory Studies

A. *In Vitro* Tests for Bacteriostatic Activity

The first published report of metronidazole's activity against an anaerobic organism, described at that time as *Bacteroides necrophorus*, was that of Davies *et al*. (1964).

Freeman *et al*. (1968) showed that this substance had activities of the same order as tetracycline and benzylpenicillin against *Clostridium tetani* and *Cl. perfringens*.

Prince *et al*. (1969) were the first to draw attention to the intense activity of metronidazole against anaerobic bacteria and the absence of significant activity against aerobes and facultative anaerobes.

Füzi and Csukás (1970) measured the sensitivities of 88 strains of anaerobic bacteria (MICs ranging from 0.03 to 8.0 μg/ml) and of 312 strains of aerobes (MICs > 32 μg/ml). Ten strains of *Bacteroides* species were inhibited by 2.0 μg/ml.

Ueno *et al.* (1971a) determined the sensitivities to metronidazole of 75 strains of anaerobes recently isolated from clinical material and found MICs for *Peptococcus, Veillonella, Bacteroides, Sphaerophorus, Fusobacterium,* and *Clostridium* species within the range of 0.7 to 6.2 μg/ml; the strains of *Peptostreptococcus* species were insensitive.

Tally *et al.* (1972) found that all but 3 of 54 strains of anaerobes were inhibited by concentrations of 6.2 μg/ml or less; one strain of *Bacteroides fragilis* had an MIC of 25 μg/ml, one strain of *Bacteroides oralis* needed 12.5 μg/ml, and one microaerophilic Gram-positive coccus was not inhibited by 100 μg/ml.

Chow *et al.* (1977) determined the susceptibilities to metronidazole of various genera and species of allegedly obligate anaerobes from 1054 clinical isolates and reported more strains requiring concentrations greater than 6.25 μg/ml in genera such as *Fusobacterium, Bacteroides* other than *B. fragilis, Peptococci, Peptostreptococci,* and *Clostridia,* than those reported by Sutter and Finegold (1977).

Sutter and Finegold (1977), having examined 730 strains of anaerobes, reiterated their previous conclusion that metronidazole at achievable tissue concentrations inhibited the majority of anaerobic bacteria found most frequently in anaerobic infection. They suggested that problems of identification and classification might account for the less favorable findings of Chow *et al.* (1977) and support for this suggestion came later from Garcia Sanchez *et al.* (1978), who found that only 1 out of 64 strains of

Bacteroides species had an MIC of 12.5 μg/ml, all of the others having been inhibited by concentrations of 0.1 to 9.6 μg/ml. Similar results were reported by Gnarpe and Lundbäck (1978) in respect to metronidazole, ornidazole, and tinidazole but Appelbaum and Chatterton (1978) claimed that 3 out of 41 strains of *Bacteroides fragilis* had MICs greater than 16.0 μg/ml.

However, no group of workers appears to have sought or obtained independent confirmation of the correctness of their identification and MIC value for allegedly resistant strains of *Bacteroides fragilis.* In this connection the findings of Watt and Jack (1977) on anaerobic cocci, of Sisson *et al.* (1978) on nonhemolytic streptococci, and Milne *et al.* (1978) on *Clostridium perfringens* have served to emphasize the need for strict anaerobiosis in making primary and subcultures and in measuring sensitivity to metronidazole as well as the fact that microaerophilic or carbon dioxide-dependent strains are not obligate anaerobes.

Indeed the only fully authenticated isolations of a metronidazole-resistant strain of *Bacteroides fragilis* so far reported have been: (1) that of Ingham *et al.* (1978a) which, with an MIC of 70 μg/ml metronidazole, was isolated from a patient with Crohn's disease who in spite of surgery had recurring fistulas and who had been kept well by oral metronidazole for 3.5 years; (2) a strain, designated AM24, isolated from a urinary tract infection by Britz and Wilkinson (1979) and found to have an MIC of 150 μg/ml metronidazole. No information was given about the patient's history or treatment; and (3) a strain, identified as *B. fragilis* ss. *distasonis,* isolated from a peritoneal swab taken at laparotomy from a 9-year-old boy with an acute suppurative perforated appendix (Rotimi *et al.*, 1979). The patient had never received metronidazole, and the MIC was 64 μg/ml against this organism.

Present evidence suggests that short-term metronidazole therapy does not cause the emergence of resistant strains of *B. fragilis* (Willis *et al.*, 1978). This consistency of activity against obligate anaerobes has been largely maintained during the 8 years which have elapsed since metronidazole was first used to treat anaerobic sepsis by Tally *et al.* (1972). This is evident from a report by Ahart *et al.* (1979) in a national anaerobic bacteriology reference center for a multicenter clinical trial of intravenous metronidazole in the United States. Four hundred and twenty-five anaerobic isolates were tested for susceptibility to penicillin, tetracyline, chloramphenicol, clindamycin, and metronidazole.

All strains of *B. fragilis* showed some resistance to penicillin; most had intermediate resistance (MIC 4–6 μg/ml) but in 12% the MIC was greater than 128 μg/ml. Intermediate penicillin resistance was found in strains of *B. melaninogenicus,* other *Bacteroides* species, *Clostridium* species, and anaerobic cocci. Most anaerobes were susceptible to 4–16 μg/ml chloramphenicol. No high level resistance to clindamycin was found in *Bacteroides* species but 3–4% of all anaerobes tested had MICs of 4 to 32 μg/ml. Metronidazole was the most active agent against Gram-negative anaerobes, all of which were inhibited by 8 μg/ml and 90% by 2 μg/ml; 2.8% of anaerobic cocci, 1.8% of *Clostridium* species, and 26.8% of the nonsporing Gram-positive bacilli were regarded as metronidazole-resistant.

B. *In Vitro* Tests for Bactericidal Activity

The virtually complete and consistent bacteriostatic activity of metronidazole against the most frequently isolated obligate anaerobes is paralleled by its bactericidal activity, the MBC being equal to or twice the MIC in most cases (Nastro and Finegold, 1972; Whelan and Hale, 1973; Sutter and Finegold, 1975; Churcher and Human, 1977; Jokipii and Jokipii, 1977; Dublanchet *et al.*, 1977; Garcia Rodriguez *et al.*, 1977).

In these respects metronidazole is clearly superior to those antibiotics such as chloramphenicol, lincomycin, clindamycin, and cefoxitin which have been recommended for the treatment of anaerobic infections.

C. *In Vivo* Tests for Antibacterial Activity

The incisive activity of metronidazole against obligate anaerobes has also been evident in experimental infections in animals. Thus, Freeman *et al.* (1968) found that it was superior to tetracycline and benzylpenicillin in curing mice infected with *Clostridium tetani* or *Cl. perfringens;* Ueno *et al.* (1971b) showed that metronidazole prevented abscess formation and caused the disappearance of established abscesses produced by *Sphaerophorus necrophorus* in mice; Takazoe *et al.* (1973) reported that it prevented inguinal abscess formation in guinea pigs inoculated with a mixed cell suspension of *Bacteroides melaninogenicus* (MIC 0.5 μg/ml metronidazole), a heparinase-producing *Bacteroides* (MIC 0.5 μg/ml), and an anaerobic *Corynebacterium* (MIC 7500 μg/ml). Hutchinson *et al.* (1977) demonstrated that metronidazole premedication reduced the severity of peritonitis induced by appendix ligation in rabbits and intravenous metronidazole, given 10 hours after ligation, prevented death whereas six of nine control animals died.

Onderdonk *et al.* (1978) found that metronidazole, but not gentamicin or sulfatrimethoprim, protected guinea pigs against carrageenan-induced experimental ulcerative colitis.

Welkos *et al.* (1977) reported that metronidazole, but not penicillin or kanamycin, selectively decreased the anaerobic microflora and completely decreased vitamin B_{12} malabsorption in rat self-filling blind-loop models.

Bartlett (1978) reviewed the experiences of himself and his colleagues with a technique which involved challenging rats by intraperitoneally inserted capsules containing pooled cecal contents or single or paired cultures of *E. coli* and *B. fragilis*. Unmedicated rats inoculated with cecal contents developed a biphasic infection; initially there were acute peritonitis and *E. coli* bacteremia with 30–40% mortality and all survivors after 5 to 7 days developed intraabdominal abscesses in which *B. fragilis* predominated. Gentamicin therapy, started 4 hours after inoculation and continued 8-hourly for 10 days, reduced the mortality rate to 4% but did not prevent abscess formation in the survivors; clindamycin reduced only abscess formation; but metronidazole not only reduced abscess formation but reduced the early mortality rate to 10%. Inoculation with *E. coli* caused 100% mortality which was not significantly reduced by metronidazole but the mortality rate was only 20% for animals given metronidazole after a lethal inoculation of *E. coli* and *B. fragilis*.

D. Mode of Antimicrobial Action

1. *Anaerobicidal Action*

Ings *et al.* (1974) proposed the following hypothesis for the mode of action of metronidazole on anaerobic protozoa and bacteria.

> The compound penetrates the cell membrane with its nitro group unchanged; once inside the cell the nitro group is reduced in the redox conditions prevalent in the anaerobic cell. A reactive intermediate, possibly a hydroxylamine, is formed which reacts with DNA so that the resultant DNA complex can no longer function as an effective primer for DNA and RNA polymerases; thus all nucleic acid synthesis is stopped.
>
> The parent compound is absorbed preferentially through the cell membrane because of its conversion to the reactive derivative which in turn reacts with cell constituents; thus a favourable gradient for the entry of the parent compound is maintained.
>
> The hypothesis can be considered proved if it can be shown that nucleic acid synthesis is inhibited by the formation of a complex with a metabolite of metronidazole rather than with the parent compound.

Other workers have produced evidence which supports the suggestion of reductive biotransformation and favors a four-electron transfer giving hydroxylamine derivatives (Coombs, 1976; Lindmark and Müller, 1976; Tally *et al.*, 1978; Müller, 1979).

However, until the product or products of reduction can be identified and their properties can be defined, there appear to be unanswered questions about the action of metronidazole on facultative anaerobes, including mutagenicity tester strains, about the possibility that metronidazole can undergo nitro reduction in mammalian tissues other than hypoxic tumor cells or about the possible release *in vivo* of the products of reduction from anaerobic microorganisms in their normal habitats or in tissues.

2. *Activity on Facultative Anaerobes*

Initially, it appeared that metronidazole was active only on obligately anaerobic microorganisms. However, the microaerophilic *Campylobacter fetus* has been found sensitive *in vitro* to concentrations of metronidazole ranging from 0.2 to 12.5 μg/ml (Chow *et al.*, 1978) and from 0.48 to 100 μg/ml (Vanhoof *et al.*, 1978).

In addition, Pheifer *et al.* (1978) reported that the MICs of metronidazole for 20 clinical isolates of *Haemophilus vaginalis* varied from 2 to 8 μg/ml anaerobically and from 8 to 16 μg/ml aerobically: MBCs were from 2 to 12 μg/ml for six isolates and 25 and 50 μg/ml, respectively, for two others. Moreover, metronidazole has been found effective in the treatment of infections caused by this species (see Section V,E,4,d).

Foster and Willson (1976) reported that the growth of strains of *E. coli* was inhibited when they were incubated under conditions of reduced oxygen tension with concentrations of metronidazole many times higher than those provided by therapeutic doses. More recently, Ingham *et al.* (1979) have observed a 1000-fold reduction in the viable counts of nine strains of *E. coli,* three strains of *Klebsiella* species, and seven strains of *Proteus* species when incubated in a reducing medium supplemented with 1% glucose or 1% ascorbic acid, inside an anaerobic jar with cooled catalyst and gassed with 90% hydrogen and 10% carbon dioxide. Ingham *et al.* (1980) also reported that when *B. fragilis* and *E. coli* were incubated in mixed culture in the presence of metronidazole, its bactericidal effect on *E. coli* was impaired because, it was suggested, the preferential reduction of metronidazole by the anaerobe decreased its concentration to levels which are subinhibitory for *E. coli.*

3. *Bacterial "Inactivation" of Metronidazole*

Ralph and Clarke (1978) studied the rate of inactivation of metronidazole *in vitro* while establishing time-kill curves for anaerobic, facultatively anaerobic, and aerobic bacteria in the stationary growth phase in pure and mixed cultures.

A preliminary experiment established that for *Fusobacterium nucleatum, Peptostreptococcus anaerobius, Bacteroides fragilis, Eubacterium lactum,* and *Clostridium perfringens,* MICs were 1 μg/ml or less and MBCs were 3 μg/ml or less. For *Propionibacterium acnes,* however, these values were 1500 μg/ml. The corresponding figures for facultative anaerobes were: *Proteus morgani,* 500 and 750 μg/ml; *E. coli,* 1000 and 1000 μg/ml; *Streptococcus faecalis,* 2000 and 2000 μg/ml; and *Staphylococcus aureus,* 1000 and 2000 μg/ml.

Metronidazole, added to cultures to give a concentration of 10 μg/ml, was rapidly inactivated by and killed all of the anaerobes except *P. acnes.* The facultative anaerobes, with the exception of *Staphylococcus aureus,* reduced the metronidazole concentration to 2 μg/ml or less, but more slowly than the anaerobes. However, metronidazole at 10 μg/ml had no bactericidal effect on the facultative and aerobic organisms.

In experiments with mixed cultures of *B. fragilis* and each of the facultative and aerobic organisms there was no inhibition of the anaerobicidal effect of metronidazole but the investigators remarked on the possibility that, *in vivo,* facultative anaerobes capable of inactivating metronidazole could inhibit its action on anaerobes in mixed infections.

Such an effect had been suggested to explain rare instances of therapeutic failure when metronidazole had been used to treat trichomonal vaginitis (Nicol *et al.*, 1966; McFadzean *et al.*, 1969).

Nicol *et al.* (1966) had demonstrated inactivation by an organism of the genus *Mimae* which had been isolated from the vagina of a patient whose infection did not respond to metronidazole until after tetracycline had been administered per vaginam.

McFadzean and his colleagues reported *in vitro* inactivation of metronidazole by *E. coli, Streptococcus faecalis, Proteus* spp., and *Klebsiella* spp.

Ingham *et al.* (1979) also observed that when metronidazole, under conditions of enhanced anaerobiosis, inhibited the growth of *E. coli, Klebsiella* species, and *Proteus* species, it was inactivated in the process.

The inactivation of metronidazole by obligately and facultatively anaerobic organisms apparently involves both absorption into the cell and biochemical reduction to antibacterial metabolite(s).

In this context it is interesting and important to consider metronidazole's antibacterial spectrum in the lumen of the gastrointestinal tract in the light of what is known about the product's delivery to that site and the effect on the microflora of concurrent administration of agents with antiaerobic activity.

4. *Antibacterial Activity in the Gastrointestinal Tract*

Whelan (unpublished) found that 800 mg metronidazole ingested three times a day for 5 days by healthy volunteers completely eliminated *Clos-*

tridia and *Veillonella* spp. from the feces but caused no change in the concentrations of *Bacteroides* spp. or *Bifidobacteria*. The concentrations of metronidazole in fecal extracts, measured polarographically, were never higher than 2.0 μg/gm.

Lewis *et al.* (1977) gave metronidazole orally in doses of 10–30 mg/kg for 8 days and showed that it had little effect on the anaerobic bowel microflora of healthy volunteers, except on some *Clostridia; Cl. welchii* was eliminated from the stools of some subjects. In a patient with diarrhea oral metronidazole eliminated *Bacteroides* from the stool. In both patients and volunteers, metronidazole caused a reversible increase in the stool concentrations of the *Klebsiella–Enterobacter–Serratia* group of organisms.

Arabi *et al.* (1977) found that oral metronidazole, 200 mg 8-hourly for 5 days, had no effect on the total numbers of anaerobes or aerobes in the feces of four healthy volunteers. In nine other volunteers who received similar metronidazole medication and neomycin 1 gm 8-hourly for 5 days, there was a mean reduction of total aerobes from 10^5 to 10^1 organisms per ml and counts of anaerobes were reduced from 10^7 to 10^1 organisms/ml. Neomycin alone, given to four other subjects, produced a moderate reduction in aerobic counts with no effect on anaerobic counts. As can be seen in Section VI,C,1, several investigators have used oral metronidazole together with nonabsorbed antiaerobic agents such as kanamycin (Goldring *et al.*, 1975), phthalylsulfathiazole (Taylor and Cawdery, 1977), and neomycin for preoperative bowel preparation of patients for colorectal surgery and have reported marked reductions in the numbers of anaerobes and aerobes in the colon or in feces.

Although metronidazole is secreted in the bile, we do not know how much of this is absorbed in the small intestine and it would appear to reach the bowel lumen mainly by secretion through the bowel wall. Using [^{14}C]metronidazole in rats, Ings (1973) demonstrated rapid concentration in the gastrointestinal tract, particularly in the walls of the large intestine. The bile duct was cannulated and the stomach, small intestine, cecum, and large intestine ligated to prevent lumenal passage of radioactivity. The bile contained 7% of the radioactivity but larger proportions were found in the tissues and contents of each ligated section indicating that unchanged metronidazole was being distributed into the gastrointestinal lumen mainly by secretion through the gut wall.

In the healthy small intestine with its scanty microflora and even in the abnormal small bowel with bypass enteropathy and overgrowth from the colonic microflora, the inactivation of metronidazole administered orally in modest dosage does not appear to be significant because bypass enteropathy is quickly relieved.

The phenomenon of inactivation of metronidazole by populations containing aerobic or facultatively anaerobic microorganisms seems relevant to certain clinical situations, e.g., the treatment of massive pleuropulmonary suppurations containing both anaerobes and aerobes, which do not always respond to systemic metronidazole therapy.

5. *The Compatibilities of Metronidazole with Other Antibacterial Agents against Anaerobic and Aerobic Pathogens*

The synergism between metronidazole and spiramycin against anaerobic bacteria was described by Videau (1971), Videau *et al.* (1973), and Laufer *et al.* (1973).

Salem *et al.* (1975) investigated interactions between metronidazole and 14 other antibacterial agents, viz. ampicillin, cephalexin, chloramphenicol, co-trimoxazole, erythromycin, fusidic acid, gentamicin, nalidixic acid, neomycin, nitrofurantoin, novobiocin, rifampicin, spiramycin I, and tetracyline.

Nine of these agents were tested with metronidazole against *B. fragilis* by the chess-board method of determining MICs and fractional inhibitory concentrations (FICs) by making serial dilutions of binary mixtures. Ampicillin, streptomycin, gentamicin, and fusidic acid were each indifferent to metronidazole but spiramycin I, rifampicin, clindamycin, tetracyline, and nalidixic acid interacted favorably with metronidazole.

The MIC values for metronidazole were reduced in the presence of subinhibitory amounts of each of these five agents. The potentiation of metronidazole activity by nalidixic acid was unexpected because *B. fragilis* is insensitive to nalidixic acid alone.

The MICs of all 14 agents were also determined alone and in the presence of 100 μg/ml of metronidazole against representative strains of *Enterobacter, Pseudomonas, Streptococcus,* and *Staphylococcus* with some determinations under anaerobic conditions. In no case did metronidazole increase more than twofold (i.e., one dilution tube) the MIC of any agent against a given organism.

The chess-board dilution method was also used to test the effect of metronidazole on some of these antimicrobial agents against *Staphylococcus aureus, Escherichia coli,* and *Proteus mirabilis.* Metronidazole at concentrations up to 500 μg/ml, which alone had no action against the aerobic or anaerobic growth of these organisms, nevertheless reduced the MIC values of spiramycin against *Staph. aureus* and that of nitrofurantoin against *E. coli* to give at least an additive effect.

These workers also made *in vivo* studies which showed that the CD_{50} values of novobiocin, cephalexin, tetracycline, spiramycin I, and fusidic acid against *Staph. aureus* infections in mice were not significantly affected by simultaneous metronidazole medication. Similar results were obtained from an analogous study with ampicillin, chloramphenicol, rifampicin, nalidixic acid, and co-trimoxazole against *E. coli* infection in mice.

In discussing their results, Salem *et al.* (1975) suggested that the specificity of metronidazole's action against anaerobes is possibly beneficial in that it is unlikely to confer any selective advantage on mutants of aerobes or facultative anaerobes and should not encourage interspecies transmission of drug resistance and that in mixed infections where multiple drug therapy involving metronidazole is required, there is little likelihood that adverse bacteriological interactions will occur.

IV. Safety Evaluation

The substantive available evidence which was relevant to the safety of metronidazole for its approved and potential indications as an antimicrobial agent was discussed at the International Metronidazole Conference in Montreal (1976), the Proceedings of which were published in *Excerpta Medica International Congress Series* No. 438, 1977.

That evidence and more recent findings were reviewed by Roe (1979) who reached the conclusions presented in the following sections.

A. Clinical Toxicology

Metronidazole, given in modest dosage for short periods in the treatment of trichomoniasis, gives rise to only trivial side-effects.

With the extension of the use of the product in higher dosage and for longer periods in the treatment of some anaerobic infections and of patients with Crohn's disease, adverse reactions involving the gastrointestinal tract have tended to become more frequent and, in some cases, more intense; the central and peripheral nervous systems have also been targets for toxicity. This has taken the form of peripheral neuropathy which was usually reversible by dosage reduction or drug withdrawal and a few instances of transient encephalopathy, in cancer patients who received massive doses.

B. Animal Toxicology

Standard tests for acute and chronic toxicity have not revealed any target for metronidazole toxicity which has not already been recognized clinically in man, apart from the reduced testicular weight and spermatogenesis seen in mice and rats which had received very large doses of metronidazole.

C. Embryotoxicity and Teratogenicity

Studies in animals and clinical experience have shown that metronidazole is not embryotoxic or teratogenic; nevertheless it should not normally be administered to women during the first trimester of pregnancy.

D. Mutagenic Potential

1. *Bacterial Tests*

The weak mutagenic effects of metronidazole and its principal human metabolite observed by several investigators using facultative anaerobic bacteria as tester-organisms probably depend on the abilities of these strains to affect some degree of nitro reduction to electrophilic metabolites which are not completely lethal to DNA. They may, therefore, be laboratory artifacts in that the conditions in which they occur never arise *in vivo* except possibly in facultatively anaerobic tumor cells.

2. *Mammalian Tests*

Conventional tests for lethal dominant effects in mice and rats, for unscheduled synthesis of DNA in human fibroblasts, and for heritable translocation in mice have given negative results.

E. Cytogenetic Effects

1. Metronidazole, in the dosage regimen used for trichomoniasis produced no meaningful increase in chromosomal abnormalities in the circulating lymphocytes of women patients.
2. Metronidazole and its two main oxidative metabolites had no genotoxic activity on cultures of human lymphocytes containing from 10 to 100 μg/ml of these substances.
3. Neither metronidazole nor its main human metabolites inhibited DNA synthesis in unstimulated peripheral lymphocytes and DNA repair synthesis was not evoked.
4. Although metronidazole increased the yield of chromosomal abnormalities in lymphocytes produced by irradiating anoxic blood such enhancement did not occur in fully oxygenated blood.

F. Carcinogenic Potential

Increased incidences of lung tumors in each of three mouse studies and of lymphoreticular neoplasms in one of those studies and a slight possible increased incidence of mammary tumors in one of two rat studies are probably secondary to the effects of metronidazole in prolonged high dosage on gut flora and nutritional status.

Animal studies have produced no evidence that metronidazole is a primary carcinogen. Studies in which the substance has been administered at therapeutic dosages showed no evidence of increased tumor incidence.

V. Metronidazole in the Treatment of Anaerobic Bacterial Infections

Although the marked antimicrobial activity of metronidazole against some species of anaerobic bacteria had been revealed by Davies *et al.* (1964) and by Freeman *et al.* (1968), and metronidazole had been shown to be highly effective in the treatment of acute ulcerative gingivitis by Shinn (1962), Davies *et al.* (1964), and Shinn *et al.* (1965), clinical studies to demonstrate the efficacy of the drug in preventing tetanus or gas gangrene could not be arranged and the credit for suggesting and investigating the use of metronidazole to treat *Bacteroides* infections must go to Tally *et al.* (1972).

Reports on the use of metronidazole to treat infections in which anaerobic bacteria were known or thought to be involved have mainly concerned open studies made on single cases or small groups of patients having similar infections or larger collections of miscellaneous infections. Reliable assessments of the chemotherapeutic role of metronidazole have sometimes been impaired by incomplete bacteriological assessments, by the administration of other antimicrobial agents having varying degrees of activity against anaerobes, and by the fully justifiable use of surgical procedures for aspiration and drainage of abscesses. Nevertheless, there is sound evidence of metronidazole's therapeutic value in the following sections.

A. Infections of the Head, Neck, and Oropharynx

1. *Brain Abscess*

George and Bint (1976) described the successful treatment of a 3-year-old girl with brain abscess caused by *B. fragilis*. The patient had Fallot's tetralogy and had been treated 5 months previously with penicillin, sulfadiazine, and chloramphenicol for meningitis. On readmission to the hospital she was found to have a left parietal abscess from which 60 ml pus was aspirated. *B. fragilis* was isolated from the pus and oral clindamycin was given for 1 week and then replaced by erythromycin because of severe diarrhea. There was little or no clinical response after three further aspirations and instillations of chloramphenicol. Metronidazole, 100 mg four times daily (8 mg/kg) was substituted and microbiological assay of pus aspirated 7 days later showed a concentration of 42 mg/liter (42 μg/ml). The abscess was aspirated once more and the child recovered and was discharged 7 weeks after metronidazole therapy was started; the drug was given for 10 weeks.

Ingham *et al.* (1977b) described a comprehensive study of nine consecutive patients with otogenic cerebral abscesses who were treated by surgical aspiration of the abscess contents and, in severe cases, by the instillation of lincomycin (one case), chloramphenicol (six cases), penicillin (five cases), and streptomycin (two cases) into the abscess cavity. Systemic chemotherapy comprised metronidazole, 400–600 mg 8-hourly orally (for 3 to 5 weeks in four patients) or intravenously (for 1 to 14 days in five patients) and then orally (for 4 weeks in three patients), together with gentamicin (three patients), penicillin (two patients), ampicillin (three patients), or chloramphenicol (one patient). Mixed growths of aerobic and obligately anaerobic bacteria were isolated from the pus in five patients and obligate anaerobes only were isolated from the other four; *Bacteroides fragilis* was present in eight and an unidentifiable *Bacteroides* in the ninth, invariably in much larger numbers than the other organisms.

Metronidazole concentrations measured polarographically in pus or ventricular fluid and concurrently in serum are given in Table I.

All patients subsequently had a mastoidectomy and in two patients the abscess capsule was later incised. One of these remained comatose for many weeks before recovering albeit with residual cerebellar ataxia. The

TABLE I

METRONIDAZOLE CONCENTRATIONS

	Pus (μg/ml)	Serum (μg/ml)
After 400 mg 8-hourly orally	35.0	11.5
After 400 mg 8-hourly orally	34.4	35.1
After 600 mg 8-hourly intravenously	45.0	12.5
	Ventricular fluid	
After 400 mg 8-hourly intravenously	20.7	

other patients, including three who were stuporose and one who was unconscious, recovered rapidly and aspirations of abscess contents repeated after 48 hours gave no bacterial growth.

The authors concluded that metronidazole was of prime importance in the chemotherapy of the anaerobic component of otogenic cerebral abscesses, particularly *B. fragilis*. They also suggested that with metronidazole shorter treatments might be sufficient. The availability of "Flagyl" injection for intravenous infusion appears to have been of crucial importance in the treatment of patients who were stuporose or unconscious.

Ingham *et al.* (1978b) reported that the bacterial species found in pus aspirated from frontal lobe brain abscesses in two patients were typical of those found in dental sepsis; apical root abscesses were later found in the upper jaws of both patients. The addition of intravenous metronidazole (400 mg 8-hourly) to intravenous ampicillin and gentamicin after aspiration of the abscess contents sterilized the abscesses, the capsules of which were later incised. Both patients were discharged symptom-free.

2. *Meningitis*

W. Roberts (personal communication) reported the successful use of oral metronidazole in a 4-year-old boy with *Bacteroides* meningitis.

Feldman (1976) described two cases of *Bacteroides fragilis* ventriculitis and meningitis which responded to metronidazole after the failure of ampicillin, chloramphenicol, and clindamycin.

O'Grady and Ralph (1976) discussed the cases of a $4\frac{1}{4}$-year-old girl and a 16-year-old boy who developed a *Fusobacterium* meningitis after upper respiratory tract infection and responded to metronidazole. However, the role of this agent was obscured by previous chemotherapy which included chloramphenicol.

Such efficacy was demonstrated by Chattopadhyay (1977) who described the case of an 83-year-old man with a long-standing history of chronic otitis media who was admitted to the hospital with meningitis due to *Bacteroides fragilis*. The patient was treated with metronidazole and recovered uneventfully. This case prompted the author to insist on the need for routine anaerobic culture of CSF specimens from patients having signs and symptoms of pyogenic meningitis.

Bryan *et al.* (1979) described two adult patients with *Bacteroides fragilis* meningitis in whom treatment that included intravenous metronidazole was curative after treatment with chloramphenicol alone or in combination with nafcillin proved ineffective.

Christensson *et al.* (1979) cured a 6-month-old girl, who had mixed anaerobic aerobic bacterial meningitis, with metronidazole and lincomycin; however, the use of the latter might have obscured the role of metronidazole.

3. *Orbital Cellulitis*

Eykyn (1979) described the successful treatment with metronidazole, amoxycillin, and surgical drainage of three patients with severe orbital cellulitis from acute sinusitis.

4. *Thrombophlebitis of the Internal Jugular Vein*

One of the earliest reports of successful treatment with metronidazole by Mitre and Rotheram (1974) concerned a patient with anaerobic septicemia associated with thrombophlebitis of the internal jugular vein which had failed to respond to gentamicin, tetracycline, chloramphenicol, clindamycin, and penicillin.

5. *Anginose Infectious Mononucleosis*

Heldstrom *et al.* (1978) studied 29 consecutive patients, 15 boys and 14 girls, aged 10–20 years. Eighteen had received antibiotic therapy before admission to the hospital, phenoxymethyl penicillin in sixteen and erythromycin in two. In 10 of the 16 patients who received metronidazole, 600–1200 mg orally per day for 5 to 7 days, temperature became normal and there was no sign of tonsillitis after 3 days. The remaining six patients had completely recovered by the fifth day. In 10 unmedicated patients, tonsillitis was present for 4 to 7 days after admission and elevated temperatures were noted for 5 to 10 days.

6. *Acute Dental Infections*

Metronidazole has been shown to be as effective as penicillin in treatment of pericoronitis and acute apical infection (Ingham *et al.*, 1977a; McGowan *et al.*, 1977; Hood, 1978); but the more consistent bactericidal activity of the former against strains of *Bacteroides melaninogenicus* and *B. oralis* has been particularly evident in cases of osteomyelitis of the mandible which responded to metronidazole after penicillin, ampicillin, and gentamicin had failed (Bradnum and Hood, 1977; Webb, 1977).

B. Pleuropulmonary Infections

Although metronidazole alone has often proved to be adequate antimicrobial therapy for mixed anaerobic aerobic sepsis involving the microflora of the gastrointestinal and female genital tracts (Study Group, 1975; Willis *et al.*, 1976, 1977; Eykyn and Phillips, 1976), its performance in analogous pleuropulmonary infections has not been so consistently good (Sanders *et al.*, 1979).

However, many cases of necrotizing pneumonia, pulmonary abscess, aspiration pneumonitis, and empyema from which anaerobes only were isolated have responded well provided that adequate drainage or aspiration had been carried out (Tally *et al.*, 1975; Giamarellou *et al.*, 1977; Eykyn, 1979). Eykyn (1979) pointed out that anaerobic empyema is often encountered as a postoperative complication of thoracic surgery, particularly esophagectomy.

Cameron (1978) made a clinical study of 230 patients admitted to the hospital with chronic destructive pneumonia and found that the addition of penicillin G or V and metronidazole to cephalosporin medication reduced mortality and the incidence of postoperative infection.

C. Cardiovascular Infections

Metronidazole has been used successfully in the management of endocarditis and *Fusobacterium* bacteremia (Seggie, 1978), *Bacteroides fragilis* bacteremia and endocarditis (Galgiani *et al.*, 1978), and four other cases of endocarditis (Hunt *et al.*, 1978).

D. Infections of the Gastrointestinal Tract

1. *Infections Developing after Surgery or Evident at Laparotomy in Unprotected or Inadequately Protected Patients*

Willis *et al.* (1976) used rectal metronidazole alone with rapid success in the management of five unmedicated control appendectomy patients who developed deep-seated anaerobic infections. In a similar fashion Willis *et al.* (1977) successfully treated severe anaerobic sepsis in 11 of 19 unmedicated control patients in a double-blind randomized chemoprophylactic trial in elective colorectal surgery.

Fiddian (1978) elaborated on the findings in patients who received metronidazole prophylactically during or after the trial by Willis *et al.* (1977). Thus of 18 patients who survived operation without serious infection, 13 had fecal peritonitis resulting from carcinoma of the colon (6) and other pathological conditions such as volvulus, diverticular disease, and rectal injury (7); two had purulent peritonitis associated with colonic carcinoma and two with malignant large bowel obstruction at emergency operation in which the proximal distended loop was ruptured causing fecal flooding of the abdominal cavity; one young man with Crohn's disease and peritonitis who was submitted to appendectomy suffered no fistula formation or deep infection. A patient with perforated diverticular disease and subphrenic gas on erect films who received metronidazole in preparation for surgery, made a rapid and uneventful recovery without operation.

Giamarellou *et al.* (1977) used metronidazole orally or rectally in the treatment of 48 patients with serious anaerobic infections. Thirty-seven of these were said to be postoperative infections and included 11 which were clearly identified as such: generalized peritonitis (3), subdiaphragmatic abscess (5), and abdominal wound infections (3); there were also six patients with perforated and gangrenous appendicitis and local peritonitis found at operation. All except two responded to metronidazole therapy: one of generalized peritonitis and one an abdominal wound infection.

Baron *et al.* (1977) described severe *Bacteroides fragilis* infections with septicemia in five patients who had undergone gastrointestinal surgery (three appendectomies, one gastroduodenectomy, and one pancreatectomy) and in one patient with a gun-shot wound in the left iliac fossa. All responded satisfactorily to orally administered metronidazole (usually 50 mg/kg/day), in some instances after failure to respond to other antimicrobial agents including lincomycin (2), tetracycline (1), and chloramphenicol (1).

Coulbois *et al.* (1977) reported the successful use of metronidazole given orally in three patients: one had a *Bacteroides fragilis* septicemia, one had a subhepatic appendicitis (*B. fragilis* isolated), and the other had cellulitis of the abdominal wall (mixed anaerobic flora).

Tennican *et al.* (1978) included 26 intraabdominal infections (12 abscess, 10 peritonitis, 2 liver, and 2 biliary) among 50 patients with serious anaerobic infections from all except one of which anaerobic infection was eliminated by means of intravenous infusion of metronidazole.

Eykyn and Phillips (1978) reviewed 30 patients, aged 6 to 80 years, with anaerobic sepsis who had been treated with metronidazole alone, intravenously in 4, orally in 10, and intravenously and orally in 16. Twenty of these involved the gastrointestinal tract, viz. sepsis after colonic surgery (9), perforated gangrenous appendix (8), diverticulosis with abscess (2), and sepsis after laparotomy for adhesions (1). There were good responses in fifteen, initial improvements in four, and one failure.

Only three of these infections were wholly anaerobic and, as expected, all responded well to specific anaerobicidal therapy. However, 11 mixed anaerobic/aerobic infections responded equally well—for although cultures during treatment yielded aerobes only, these eventually disappeared as the sepsis resolved and no specific chemotherapy was required.

These and similar findings in 10 nonintestinal infections described in this article led the authors to suggest that it was likely that for sepsis associated with intestinal surgery and perhaps in other sites, metronidazole could reasonably be used alone in mixed infections with impressive results.

2. *Other Infections Involving the Gastrointestinal Tract*

Perera *et al.* (1980) reviewed their experience in treating 90 patients of whom 42 had bacteriologically confirmed anaerobic sepsis (33 associated with gastrointestinal pathology) and 47 had presumed anaerobic sepsis. Patients in the first category received metronidazole only (13 courses), metronidazole + gentamicin (24 courses), metronidazole + ampicillin (3 courses), metronidazole + co-trimoxazole (2 courses), flucloxacillin (4 courses), and penicillin (2 courses). Complete bacteriological and clinical cure was achieved in 33 courses of treatment (76%). Patients with presumed anaerobic sepsis who received metronidazole alone responded similarly with only 25% responding poorly.

Goodwin (1979) studied the use of intravenous metronidazole as an adjunct to the treatment of severely shocked patients with abdominal infections in an intensive care unit in Durban, South Africa. The use of this adjunct was associated with an improvement of survival rate in general surgical cases from 14.8 to 38.5%. Of particular interest was the survival of three out of five cases of fulminating amebic dysentery, with perforation and massive peritoneal contamination, that underwent colectomy. Previously no such patient had survived.

3. *Liver Abscess*

The remarkable chemotherapeutic efficacy of metronidazole in the treatment of amebic liver abscess (Powell, 1972) appears to extend to liver abscesses which have been shown to be either pure or mixed anaerobic bacterial infections.

Thus good responses to metronidazole therapy have been reported by Giamarellou *et al.* (1977), Back *et al.* (1978), and Rissing *et al.* (1978).

4. *Jejunoileal Bypass Enteropathy*

The value of metronidazole therapy in controlling the postoperative abdominal distension, persisting diarrhea, foul-smelling flatulence, and abdominal pain of the intestinal bypass operation for obesity has been established by Solhaug (1977), Barry *et al.* (1977), Corrodi *et al.* (1978), Wandtke *et al.* (1977), and Knipp *et al.* (1978).

5. *Acute Diverticular Disease*

Pashby (1979) reviewed patients with acute diverticular disease admitted to the same hospital during the periods 1969–1972 (42 patients who received no metronidazole and all needed emergency surgery) and 1975–1978 (51 patients who received metronidazole and of whom 26 needed surgery and 25 who were treated conservatively and required no surgery). Thus, there was a significant reduction in the proportion of patients needing surgery and among those who did there was a lower mortality rate, fewer wound infections, and no fecal fistulas or pelvic abscesses.

6. *Neonatal Necrotizing Enterocolitis* (*NNEC*)

Khan and Nixon (1978a) in the Hospital for Sick Children, London, compared the results of the conservative treatment of 10 consecutive cases of neonatal necrotizing enterocolitis by means of intravenous cloxacillin and gentamicin with those of a subsequent series of 10 consecutive cases who received similar chemotherapy plus intravenous metronidazole. All patients in both series had abdominal distension, blood in the stools, and pneumatosis intestinalis, most had bile-stained vomit, and some had peritonitis or septicemia. Surgery was performed when indicated. The difference in the number of uneventful recoveries (seven in the metronidazole group and three in the control group) was not statistically significant, but the authors also noted that whereas three deaths in the control group were due to NNEC, there was no postmortem evidence of this in the two metronidazole-treated patients who died from other causes. In addition, it was noted that recovery took place more quickly in the metronidazole series (third day versus seventh day); there were fewer bowel perforations (one versus four); and there was no damage to the bowel wall in the metronidazole-treated patients whereas two babies in the control series had strictures and two others developed disaccharide intolerance. Finally, the addition of metronidazole to the intravenous antimicrobial therapy appeared to be useful in preventing infection after bowel surgery.

7. *Pseudomembranous Colitis* (*PMC*)

Trinh Dinh *et al.* (1978) described a 27-year-old woman who developed pseudomembranous colitis 3 days after completing a 7-day course of ampicillin (2 gm/day) for bronchitis; she responded promptly to oral metronidazole, 1.5 gm/day for 7 days.

Malcolm (1978) described a case of PMC causing colostomy dysfunction in a 69-year-old woman with a history of Crohn's disease who had not received antibiotics in the preceding 2 years. Cultures of feces failed to grow *Clostridium sordellii* or *Cl. difficile.* Treatment with metronidazole (1.5 gm/day orally) was followed by disappearance of plaques and improvement of symptoms within 7 days and the patient was discharged without requiring surgery.

Matuchansky *et al.* (1978) reported the successful treatment, with oral metronidazole, 1.5 gm/day for 15 days, of three patients with antibiotic-induced colitis; one had received lincomycin and two had received ampicillin. All patients had persistent diarrhea (8–18 watery stools per day), despite stopping the incriminated antibiotic, for 5 days to 4 weeks. The diagnoses were confirmed by proctosigmoidoscopy and histology of biopsy specimens. The patients showed a dramatic clinical response to metronidazole therapy; diarrhea stopped within 24 to 48 hours and the rectal mucosa was endoscopically normal within 2, 4, and 6 days, respectively. Two weeks after treatment had been stopped there was no evidence of relapse, clinically, proctoscopically, or radiographically.

Metronidazole was used successfully in the treatment of *Clostridium difficile* colitis in two patients who had been treated with clindamycin (Pashby *et al.*, 1979) and in one patient who had received neomycin (Bolton, 1979).

8. *Primary Pneumatosis Coli*

Ellis (1980) reported the successful use of metronidazole in two elderly women who had long histories of diarrhea with excessive flatus and mucus and vague lower abdominal pain. Oxygen treatment gave temporary relief in one case but oral metronidazole controlled intestinal symptoms in both patients.

9. *Crohn's Disease*

In open studies (Ursing and Kamme, 1975; Montgomery, 1975; Holdstock, 1975; Ursing, 1977), metronidazole was considered to have produced improvement based on clinical, radiographic, and laboratory findings and attributed by the last-named investigator to an antimicrobial effect on the gut microflora and on infected lesions in the gut wall.

Controlled studies (Allan and Cooke, 1977; Blichfeldt *et al.*, 1978) failed to demonstrate any significant beneficial effect on the general clinical condition of patients with active Crohn's disease. Nevertheless, these investigators and Bardet *et al.* (1977) reported improvement in some features of colonic and perianal involvement such as diarrhea and ulceration.

Of possible relevance are the findings of Krook *et al.* (1979) who studied changes in the fecal flora of six patients with Crohn's disease during treatment with metronidazole. The anaerobic bacterial counts were greatly reduced in the three patients who responded well to treatment and of whom two had the most extensive colonic damage. Of two nonresponding patients, one showed no reduction in the anaerobic counts and the other gave reduced total counts but persistence of metronidazole-resistant Gram-negative rods. One patient who had only moderate benefit also showed some reduction in total anaerobe count.

LaMont and Trnka (1980) found *Clostridium difficile* toxin in the ileostomy fluid of a patient with Crohn's disease during an episode of duodenal ulceration but not after clinical improvement. The same toxin was also found in the stools of two patients with proctitis and three with ulcerative colitis during a period of relapse.

Bolton *et al.* (1980) in screening 56 patients with diarrhea for *Clostridium difficile* toxin in stools found that, of the nine patients with organism and toxin in the stools, five had severe inflammatory bowel disease (one with Crohn's disease and four with ulcerative colitis) and were receiving systemic steroids. Four of these five patients were subsequently treated with vancomycin or metronidazole and all improved clinically with disappearance of toxin from the stools. The patient with Crohn's disease improved so much that steroids and azathioprine could be withdrawn.

Most of the reported cases of peripheral sensory neuropathy have occurred in patients with Crohn's disease who received oral metronidazole in moderately high dosage for several months and this should be borne in mind if metronidazole therapy is specifically indicated.

Although this anaerobicide is not generally indicated for the medical management of Crohn's disease, its value for the prevention or early treatment of postoperative anaerobic sepsis in such patients appears to be widely appreciated.

E. Infections of the Female Genital Tract

1. *Systemic Infections*

Baron *et al.* (1977) describe three cases of local and systemic infection due to *Bacteroides fragilis* with septicemia and metastatic lung infection. One patient had had surgery for cancer of the cervix and the other two had needed surgery for retained placenta. Antibiotic therapy had proved ineffective, tetracycline in the first patient and cephalothin and gentamicin in the parturient patients. Metronidazole, 25 mg/kg/day orally for 23 days in the first patient, 70 mg/kg/day orally for 21 days in the second patient, and 50 mg/kg/day for 30 days in the third patient, was completely effective in all these cases.

Sharp *et al.* (1977) described a patient who produced a copious foul-smelling vaginal discharge and bacteremia after vaginal hysterectomy and anterior repair. *Bacteroides fragilis* was isolated in pure culture from the discharge and blood before and after five days therapy with clindamycin, 400 mg q.d.s. orally, despite the fact that the organism remained sensitive *in vitro* to that antibiotic. A change of therapy to metronidazole, 400 mg q.d.s. orally, produced clinical and bacteriological cure.

Goodwin (1979) compared the survival rates of women admitted to an intensive care unit with septic abortions with pelvic infections and multiple organ failure before and after the addition of intravenous metronidazole to the many other measures taken for moribund patients. Before the use of metronidazole 10 out of 18 patients survived and with metronidazole 6 out of 9 patients survived.

2. *Postoperative Infections*

a. After Hysterectomy. Anaerobic infections after abdominal or vaginal hysterectomy have been effectively treated with metronidazole. These comprise wound infection or abscess, pelvic abscess, or cellulitis (Study Group, 1975; Eykyn and Phillips, 1976; Giamarellou *et al.*, 1977; Appelbaum *et al.*, 1978).

b. After Cesarean Section. Metronidazole therapy has been successful in generalized peritonitis, pelvic abscess (Study Group, 1974; Eykyn and Phillips, 1976; Giamarellou *et al.*, 1978), and endometritis (Christensson *et al.*, 1979).

3. *Postpartum Infections*

Good responses have been recorded in (a) endomyometritis (Study Group, 1974; Ledger *et al.*, 1976; Giamarellou *et al.*, 1977) and (b) necrotizing fasciitis (Golde and Ledger, 1977; Ledger *et al.*, 1977).

4. *Other Gynecological Infections*

Metronidazole has been found effective in (a) septic abortion (Study Group, 1974; Christensson *et al.*, 1979); (b) salpingitis (Eykyn and Phillips, 1976; Christensson *et al.*, 1979); (c) adnexal abscesses (Eykyn and Phillips, 1976; Giamarellou *et al.*, 1977); and (d) nonspecific vaginitis.

Although *Haemophilus vaginalis* is a facultative anaerobe showing variable *in vitro* susceptibility to metronidazole there is increasing evidence that the antimicrobial agent is effective in the treatment of cases of nonspecific vaginitis from which the organism has been isolated (Pheifer *et al.*, 1978; Durfee *et al.*, 1979, Balsdon *et al.*, 1980).

F. Other Anaerobic Infections

Metronidazole has been found effective in:

1. Osteomyelitis (Tally *et al.*, 1975; Eykyn and Phillips, 1976; Warner and Prior, 1977; Raff *et al.*, 1978; Tennican *et al.*, 1978; Giamarellou *et al.*,

1978; Galgiani *et al.*, 1978; Hunt *et al.*, 1978; Rissing *et al.*, 1978; Eykyn, 1979; Zimmerman *et al.*, 1980).

2. Septic arthritis (Hunt *et al.*, 1978; Eykyn, 1979).
3. Breast abscess in nonpuerperal women (Hale *et al.*, 1976; Leach *et al.*, 1979; Ingham *et al.*, 1979).
4. Hidradenitis suppuritiva (Leach *et al.*, 1979).
5. Scrotal abscess (Eykyn, 1979).
6. Soft tissue abscess (Hanna *et al.*, 1976; Eykyn and Phillips, 1976; Giamarellou *et al.*, 1978).
7. Pressure sores (Jones *et al.*, 1978; Galgiani *et al.*, 1978; Rissing *et al.*, 1978).
8. Leg ulcers (Khanna *et al.*, 1979).
9. Synergistic gangrene (Eykyn, 1979).
10. Gas gangrene (Eykyn, 1979).
11. Diabetic gangrene (Giamarellou *et al.*, 1977).
12. Clostridial septicemia (Pieron *et al.*, 1977).
13. Neonatal anaerobic sepsis (Rom *et al.*, 1977).
14. Necrotizing snake bite wounds (Russell, 1966).
15. Rosacea (Pye and Burton, 1976; Guilhou *et al.*, 1979).
16. Urinary tract infections (Ingham *et al.*, 1975; Eykyn and Phillips, 1976; Giamarellou *et al.*, 1977; Warner and Prior, 1977).
17. Foul odors in patients with cancer and mouth infection (Ohkawa *et al.*, 1969; Sparrow *et al.*, 1980).

VI. Metronidazole in the Prevention of Anaerobic Bacterial Infections

Chemoprophylaxis for surgery is a controversial subject on which many widely different but strongly held opinions have been and continue to be stated.

There are numerous causes for this situation which is gradually becoming somewhat less confused as investigators turn to the use of specific antimicrobial agents for anaerobes, with or without antiaerobic agents. The commonest are failures by many investigators to define accurately the therapeutic objective in terms of:

1. The Nature and Incidence of the Postoperative Infections Known to Occur or Which Might Be Expected

Failure to make this definition is exemplified by inability or unwillingness to separate exogenous from endogenous infections; thus, preoccupation with wound infections has led some workers to overlook the more serious septic complications such as subphrenic abscess, pelvic abscess, peritonitis, thrombophlebitis, and septicemia leading to metastatic abscess formation.

The main cause of confusion has been the failure by many surgeons and microbiologists to recognize nonsporing anaerobic bacteria as the major pathogens in sepsis occurring after surgery involving the gastrointestinal, female genital, and upper respiratory tracts. Such recognition was prevented for many years by the lack of facilities for reliable anaerobic bacteriological culture, isolation, and identification.

2. The Required Properties of the Most Suitable Antimicrobial Agents

The use of many different antimicrobial agents, often in association, which for many years were intended to combat aerobic bacteria, but which also had variable and, in some cases, gradually diminishing activity against nonsporing anaerobes, tended to obscure the involvement of anaerobes and to overemphasize the importance of aerobes and facultative anaerobes in postoperative sepsis.

3. The Route and Timing of Administration of the Antimicrobial Agent(s)

Some investigators have insufflated antiseptic or antibiotic powders into the peritoneal cavity and/or into the wound before closure. Others have instilled solutions of antibiotics into the peritoneal cavity before closure and gynecologists have quite rationally sought to diminish or eliminate the vaginal and cervical microflora with topically applied antibacterial agents before surgery.

The oldest example of preoperative chemotherapy was the use of nonabsorbed sulfonamides and/or nonabsorbed antibiotics given orally for several days in an attempt to reduce the numbers of potential pathogens in the bowel lumen before surgery. Such procedures were of dubious efficacy until antibiotics such as lincomycin or clindamycin, with significant activity against anaerobic bacteria, were used; but the risks of inducing pseudomembranous colitis or of encouraging the emergence of antibiotic-resistant strains of gut-dwelling aerobes or facultative anaerobes have been such as to cause many workers to eschew such preoperative antibiotic therapy for bowel surgery.

In the face of the plethora of chemoprophylactic agents and regimens and other procedures which have been advocated during the past 30 years, it seems reasonable to conclude that none of them was entirely satisfactory for the prevention of endogenous postoperative sepsis until a specific anaerobicidal agent—metronidazole—was used systemically with dramatic success by workers in the Luton and Dunstable Hospital for patients undergoing major gynecological surgery (Study Group, 1975), appendectomy (Willis *et al*., 1976), and colon surgery (Willis *et al*., 1977).

These workers observed the principles already enunciated and, because they used a specifically anaerobicidal agent, they were able to demonstrate that in the endogenous bacterial infections which frequently complicate the types of surgery that they selected for study, obligately anaerobic bacteria were the main causes of severe postoperative sepsis. With the elimination of such pathogens, aerobic and facultatively anaerobic bacteria from the microflora of the gut and the female genital tract appear to have lost much of their pathogenic propensities.

During the past 4 years, metronidazole has been employed by many investigators who were reluctant to make radical changes in the chemoprophylactic procedures which they believed to be effective. Consequently, most of the published reports on prophylactic studies which are summarized in this section show major differences in concept, execution, and interpretation, although the results have been consistently good.

A. Chemoprophylaxis for Gynecological Surgery and Cesarean Section

The potentialities of metronidazole given orally for this purpose were first appreciated by Willis and his colleagues in the Luton and Dunstable Hospital whose preliminary communication appeared in December 1974 (Study Group, 1974).

These workers subsequently provided a full account (Study Group, 1975) of their completed trial of prophylactic metronidazole in 202 patients who had elective gynecological surgery. One hundred patients received metronidazole medication according to one or two schedules: those admitted 24 hours before operation were given 2 gm on admission and those admitted 48 hours before operation were given 2 gm on admission and 200 mg three times on the day before operation. All patients in this group received 200 mg three times daily after operation to the end of the seventh postoperative day. One hundred and two patients received no metronidazole during the pre- and postoperative periods.

During their stay in the hospital and later in a convalescent home (average 14 days), none of the medicated patients developed an anerobic infection but one patient did develop an anaerobic pelvic infection 28 days after operation (14 days after discharge from the hospital). She was readmitted with a pelvic abscess which on drainage yielded a heavy growth of *Bacteroides fragilis* and an anaerobic streptococcus.

In contrast, bacteriologically confirmed clinical anaerobic infections developed in 19 of the unmedicated patients (18 hysterectomies and 1 vaginal repair).

Within each group of patients, some infections developed due exclusively to facultative bacteria: two urinary tract infections among medicated patients and three among the unmedicated; two wound infections among medicated patients and three among the unmedicated.

The clinical infections developed between the second and seventh days after operation and were manifested by local inflammation, pus and abscess formation, and pyrexia. In 12, nonsporing anaerobes were the only pathogens isolated; in the remaining 7 patients, facultatively anaerobic pathogens such as *E. coli* and *Proteus* species were isolated in addition to obligate anaerobic bacteria, but were present in insignificant numbers. Frequently, organisms such as *Staphylococcus epidermidis*, diphtheroids, and lactobacilli were present in small numbers in the pathological material but these were disregarded.

These workers calculated that the prophylactic use of metronidazole in the medicated patients saved bed-days to the value of almost £2000 or enabled their gynecological ward to handle 26 additional major surgical cases each year.

Preoperative vaginal anaerobe carriage rates in the two groups of patients were similar, 45 to 50%. Postoperatively the rate for patients in the medicated group fell to 6% whereas that for the unmedicated patients increased to 65%.

Serum concentrations of metronidazole in samples taken at operation showed that an effective tissue barrier to anaerobic infection had been provided by the preoperative oral medication.

The investigators terminated the controlled study as soon as the findings led them to believe that it was improper to withhold metronidazole prophylaxis from patients undergoing hysterectomy.

Since this trial was completed, A. T. Willis (personal communication) has observed that none of 618 hysterectomy patients who received metronidazole prophylaxis experienced postoperative anaerobic sepsis.

Seligman (1978), in seeking the optimal prophylactic metronidazole regimen for women undergoing hysterectomy, compared three regimens with that used by the Study Group (1975). All of these procedures were completely effective in preventing bacteriologically diagnosible sepsis and it was therefore necessary to measure the incidence and duration of postoperative pyrexia (over 37.2°C). The best regimen comprised a single preoperative oral dose of 2 gm (later reduced to 1.2 gm) followed by 1 gm rectal suppository with the anesthetic premedication and repeated 8-hourly for 48 hours.

In Auckland, New Zealand, Jackson *et al*. (1979), who sought to administer a single dose of metronidazole preoperatively at such a time as would ensure bactericidal tissue concentrations during gynecological surgery, measured serum concentrations during a 24-hour period in six patients who were given two 1 gm metronidazole rectal suppositories just before they underwent abdominal hysterectomy. Bactericidal serum levels (> 2.7 μg/ml) were present within 2 hours and maintained for at least 24 hours.

These workers then proceeded to make a double-blind study of 200 patients undergoing abdominal hysterectomies, vaginal hysterectomies, and vaginal repairs. Their observations show that a single rectal dose of 2 gm metronidazole was associated with a significant reduction in the extent and duration of postoperative pyrexia and a dramatic reduction from 18 to 1% of major postoperative wound and pelvic infections. *Bacteroides spp.* were isolated from 4 of the 18 infections in the placebo group.

Appelbaum *et al.* (1978), in the University of Natal, studied the influence of prophylactic metronidazole on the vaginal carrier rates of anaerobes and on the development of postoperative anaerobic infection in 104 women who underwent abdominal hysterectomy. Their results confirmed the efficacy of metronidazole in the prophylaxis of anaerobic sepsis associated with this surgical procedure. It was observed that, in the light of these findings and those of the Study Group (1975), the withholding of metronidazole prophylaxis from patients undergoing gynecological surgery seemed questionable.

In New Zealand, Heginbotham and Rutherford (1979) compared oral metronidazole given pre- and postoperatively, with placebo in the prophylaxis of 100 patients undergoing abdominal hysterectomy, vaginal hysterectomy with or without vaginal repair, or vaginal repair alone.

Four patients in the placebo group had anaerobic postoperative wound infections and five had aerobic infections, whereas among the medicated patients there were no anaerobic infections and four instances of aerobic wound infection. Medicated patients had less postoperative pyrexia and spent less time in the hospital than the patients in the placebo group.

Chowdhury *et al.* (1978), working in Calcutta, studied the prophylactic and therapeutic activity of metronidazole in 1029 patients who underwent medical termination of pregnancy (MTP) and insertion of an intrauterine contraceptive device (IUCD).

Among 486 patients who received metronidazole orally, 1 gm on admission followed, on the day after operation, by 200 mg three times a day for 7 days, there was no postoperative infection.

Of 543 patients who received benzathine penicillin according to a similar schedule, 88 developed postoperative infections. Anaerobic cultures of high vaginal swabs from 40 infected patients, who had been selected at random, grew anaerobic cocci (34 cases) and anaerobic Gram-negative rods (20 cases).

The 88 patients who developed postoperative infections in spite of benzathine penicillin therapy were treated with metronidazole orally, 1 gm statim followed by 200 to 400 mg three times daily for 5 to 10 days. Excellent or good responses occurred in 72 patients. It was therefore concluded that about 16% of patients had experienced anaerobic infections after MTP with IUCD and that such infections had been prevented in patients medicated with metronidazole.

Hughes *et al*. (1979) made a controlled study on 120 patients undergoing elective hysterectomy, abdominal or vaginal, or repair of uterovaginal prolapse. Forty-one patients received metronidazole 500 mg by intravenous infusion at the start of the operation and a similar administration 12 hours later; 39 patients received only the initial intravenous dose of metronidazole at the start of the operation and a placebo infusion 12 hours later. Forty patients received placebo infusion during and 12 hours after the operation. The incidence of postoperative sepsis was reduced from 25% in the placebo group to 10.3% in the group receiving only one medication and to 2.4% in those receiving two intravenous doses.

Vaughan (1979) in Pietermaritzburg, South Africa, studied 200 women undergoing emergency cesarean section. Of 40 patients who received metronidazole 500 mg iv preoperatively and three similar doses postoperatively at 8-hourly intervals, two showed clinically significant wound sepsis. Eleven of 42 patients who received placebo infusions had such sepsis. Of 78 patients who received cephradine 1 gm iv as a preoperative dose and a similar dose 4 hours later, six developed wound sepsis. Of 40 patients who received both metronidazole and cephradine, two had significant wound sepsis and the author concluded that the addition of cephradine to metronidazole conferred no advantage.

Recommended Regimens

It would appear that effective and well-tolerated systemic prophylaxis with metronidazole for gynecological surgery and cesarean section should provide serum concentrations of 6 to 10 μg/ml at the start of an operation and for the following 2 or 3 days.

The simplest means of achieving such an effective tissue barrier to anaerobic infection are by administering either (1) *rectal suppositories* (1 gm at least 4 hours before operation and repeated 8-hourly during the next 24 or 48 hours); (2) *intravenous infusions* (500 mg immediately before operation and repeated 8-hourly during the next 24 or 48 hours).

In circumstances where only oral medication is possible, a logical regimen would comprise 400 mg 8-hourly on day −1 to be continued postoperatively, as soon as the patient can ingest food, for 2 to 3 days.

B. Chemoprophylaxis for Appendectomy

1. *Clinical Trials*

Willis *et al.* (1976) were members of a second Study Group formed at the Luton and Dunstable Hospital to assess, by means of a double-blind trial, the efficacy of metronidazole in the prophylaxis of sepsis after appendectomy. These workers had noted the recovery by Leigh *et al.* (1974) of *Bacteroides fragilis* from 90% of wound infections after appendectomy and had been impressed by the performance of orally administered metronidazole in preventing anaerobic sepsis in patients undergoing gynecological surgery (Study Group, 1975).

Preoperative oral medication with metronidazole was not possible in patients undergoing emergency appendectomies and the investigators considered intravenous medication to be inappropriate. They had already shown (Study Group, 1975) that metronidazole, given in the form of rectal suppositories, provided anaerobicidal serum concentrations of metronidazole within 1 hour of administration and peak levels after 4 hours. They therefore selected a prophylactic regimen that involved the administration of a rectal suppository containing 1 gm metronidazole (0.5 gm for children under 12 years) with the anesthetic premedication and repeated every 8 hours until oral medication with 200 mg three times daily became possible. This was continued until the end of the seventh day.

In the medicated group of 49 patients, of whom 33 had acute appendicitis and 13 had gangrenous appendices, there was no anaerobic postoperative infection but 5 had mild superificial aerobic infections. In the placebo group of 46 patients, of whom 24 had acute appendicitis and 7 had gangrenous appendices, there were 9 anaerobic infections, 5 of which required treatment with metronidazole; there were also 2 mild superficial and 1 urinary tract aerobic infections.

Pashby and Mee (1978) reviewed 302 consecutive appendectomies carried out in the Luton and Dunstable Hospital and found that there had been no anaerobic infection and four aerobic infections in 241 patients who had received metronidazole prophylaxis; among 14 antibiotic-treated patients there had been six anaerobic infections and one aerobic infection; in 47 unmedicated patients there had been 15 anaerobic and 1 aerobic infection.

These authors therefore studied 99 patients who received 1 gm metronidazole rectally with their anesthetic premedication followed by the same dose 8-hourly for at least 3 days. No other antibacterial agent, systemic or local, was used, peritoneal toilet was by suction and swabbing, drains were not used, and primary wound closure was carried out.

Careful follow-up examinations showed that after 10 days, 64 wounds were in excellent condition, 26 were assessed as average, and 9 were infected with aerobes only. Five of these wound infections were in patients whose appendix had been gangrenous or perforated, three were in patients with an acutely inflamed appendix, and one was in a patient with a normal appendix. The last four infections were superficial, required no chemotherapy, and did not delay the patients' discharges from the hospital.

The authors speculated that aerobic wound infections in patients found to have a gangrenous or ruptured appendix might be prevented by starting gentamicin therapy preoperatively. In the other 84 patients, metronidazole alone reduced serious sepsis to nil and trivial sepsis to about 5%. Before metronidazole was used, the average stay in the hospital was about 10 days. With metronidazole prophylaxis, it had been reduced to 5 days.

Rodgers *et al.* (1979) made a controlled trial of rectal metronidazole which closely resembled that of Willis *et al.* (1976); the main difference was that medication was solely by suppositories given at diagnosis and continued for only 2 days.

Their observations confirmed the findings of the Luton and Dunstable Hospital workers that postoperative anaerobic sepsis did not occur in patients protected with systemic metronidazole.

McMahon *et al.* (1979) made a controlled trial in which medication was limited to a single dose of 500 mg of metronidazole infused intravenously at the start of the operation. They found that postoperative anaerobic infection was completely prevented by preoperative systemic metronidazole.

In Denmark, Finn Gottrup (1978) made a controlled trial in 406 patients of a single intravenous dose of 500 mg metronidazole given preoperatively. This was the only medication given to those patients whose appendices were seen to be nonperforated at operation; patients with perforated appendices were also given metronidazole suppositories postoperatively. The postoperative infection rates in patients with nonperforated appendices were 1% in the metronidazole group and 8% in the control group. The corresponding rates for the patients with perforated appendices were 0 and 45%, respectively. *Bacteroides fragilis* and *E. coli* were isolated from most of the wound infections.

Foster *et al.* (1979) compared rectal metronidazole, 1 gm given only 40 minutes before operation and continued 8-hourly for 3 days, povidone iodine dry powder sprayed on the wound, and no medication in a series of 200 patients, the main aim being to evaluate quantitatively the economic consequences of wound infection both to the patient and to the National Health Service of the United Kingdom. The incidences of postoperative wound sepsis were 30% in both the control and povidone iodine groups and 12% in the metronidazole group; no *Bacteroides* species was isolated from the latter but such organisms were found in 12 wound infections in the control and povidone iodine group. These differences were paralleled by shorter stays in the hospital and periods of incapacity and by fewer District Nurse visits which resulted in a saving of at least £120 per patient. It was calculated that the use of short-term metronidazole prophylaxis in all of the appendectomies carried out in England and Wales on patients between the ages of 16 and 65 (54,150 in 1973) might save the National Health Service over £6 million per year.

Corbett *et al.* (1979), who started rectal metronidazole (1 gm for adults and 500 mg for children under 14 years) 1 hour before operation and continued it 8-hourly for 3 days, found anaerobes in two out of four deep wound infections in a group of 52 metronidazole-medicated patients. Nine out of 53 unmedicated patients had deep wound infections; all of the five which were examined bacteriologically had anaerobes.

Such failure of metronidazole to prevent completely postoperative infections from which anaerobes could be isolated was also reported by Pinto and Sanderson (1979), who also gave a single rectal dose of 1 gm (500 mg for children under 12 years) when it was decided to operate. At operation they classified appendices as normal or inflamed and "gangrenous or perforated."

Patients in the former group received two more rectal doses at 8-hourly intervals whereas patients in the latter group continued to receive rectal doses 8-hourly for 5 days or until oral medication became possible.

Salem (1979) compared rectal metronidazole (1 gm 1 to 2 hours before operation and 8-hourly thereafter for 3 days) with povidone iodine powder (sprayed into the wound after closure of the peritoneum and again after skin closure). Four out of 65 patients in the metronidazole group developed wound infections of which two were superficial. Sixteen out of 60 patients in the povidone iodine group developed wound infections of which six were superficial and seven of the more severe infections yielded *Bacteroides*. Three of these presented after the patients left the hospital and necessitated readmission to the hospital.

Morris *et al.* (1979) compared rectal metronidazole, 1 gm 8-hourly on four occasions, starting 15 minutes to 2 hours before operation, parenteral cephazolin, 0.5 gm 8-hourly on four occasions, rectal metronidazole and parenteral cephazolin in the same regimens with double placebos. Wound sepsis in the hospital occurred in 2/67, 7/71, 1/67, and 11/66 in the respective groups but sepsis after discharge from the hospital occurred in 12/67, 7/71, 1/67, and 9/66, respectively. No bacteriological assessment of such wound sepsis was reported.

2. *Commentary*

a. Metronidazole Alone vs Metronidazole and an Antiaerobic Agent. In 5 of the 10 studies under review, the authors appeared to have been satisfied that metronidazole alone reduced the incidence of postoperative sepsis to acceptable levels.

In the remaining 6 studies, however, the authors considered that a supplementary systemic antiaerobic agent should be used, especially for patients with gangrenous or perforated appendices or peritonitis.

Corbett *et al.* (1979) favored an aminoglycoside. Pashby and Mee (1978) suggested the addition of gentamicin for patients found to have gangrenous or perforated appendices. Pinto and Sanderson (1979) considered that metronidazole should be one in a combination of drugs needed for the management of patients found to have gangrenous or perforated appendices; they did not specify the other agent(s).

Morris *et al.* (1979) claimed that metronidazole and cephazolin was more effective than metronidazole alone in preventing aerobic infections.

Salem (1979) stated that additional antimicrobial agents should be considered in cases of gangrenous or perforated appendicitis.

b. Recommended Regimens. Since it is impossible to differentiate accurately normal or inflamed appendices from gangrenous or perforated appendices until the abdomen is opened, and because some anaerobic infections do occur after the removal of the former, there is everything to be gained and nothing to be lost by adhering to the principle of preoperative metronidazole medication for all patients to ensure that anaerobicidal tissue concentrations are present at operation. These can be achieved by the following.

i. Preoperative medication. Rectal suppositories: 1 gm for patients of ≥12 years and 500 mg for patients of <12 years to be administered at the earliest possible time once it is decided to operate; ideally this should be at least 4 hours before the operation. Intravenous infusion: 500 mg for patients of ≥12 years and 7.5 mg/kg bodyweight for patients of <12 years to be administered immediately before the operation.

ii. Postoperative medication. After preoperative rectal dose: the preoperative dose should be repeated 8-hourly for 2 to 3 days. After preoperative intravenous dose: for patients with gangrenous or perforated appendices or peritonitis, metronidazole medication should be continued for 3 days, either by repeating the preoperative intravenous dose 8-hourly or by changing to the corresponding rectal dose (1 gm or 500 mg) also given 8-hourly.

For patients with normal or inflamed appendices, the surgeon may choose one of three courses of action: (1) to continue medication for 3 days as for patients with gangrenous or perforated appendices; (2) to continue such medication for a shorter period; (3) to give no postoperative metronidazole.

C. Chemoprophylaxis for Colorectal Surgery

1. *Metronidazole in Preoperative Bowel Preparation*

Metronidazole given orally has been added to nonabsorbed antimicrobial agents in order to diminish the aerobic and anaerobic microflora of the colon before surgery.

Thus, Gillespie and McNaught (1978) gave metronidazole 200 mg and kanamycin 1 gm, both 6-hourly for 3 days, and eliminated postoperative anaerobic sepsis and reduced the incidence of aerobic infections.

Taylor *et al*. (1979) gave metronidazole, 400 mg three times daily and phthalylsulfathiazole, 2.5 gm four times daily, both for 4 days and obtained results similar to those of Gillespie and McNaught.

Almost identical results were obtained by Matheson *et al.* (1978) who gave metronidazole 200 mg and neomycin 1 gm both 8-hourly on days −2 and −1.

Brass *et al.* (1978) compared the addition of metronidazole, 750 mg three times daily on days −2 and −1, with that of erythromycin, 1 gm three times on day −1, to neomycin, 1 gm three times on day −1. Both groups of patients were also given cephalothin intravenously 1 hour before operation and at 5 and 12 hours afterward. In the metronidazole group endogenous wound infections were completely suppressed whereas in the erythromycin group, 25% of patients had infections associated with gut-derived coliforms, enterococci, and *Bacteroides*.

Proud *et al.* (1978) compared three groups of patients. One group received only metronidazole, 400 mg 6-hourly for 3 days; the second group received metronidazole by the same regimen and kanamycin, 1 gm 6-hourly for 3 days; the third group had placebos only. There was no anaerobic sepsis in any patient who received metronidazole with kanamycin or metronidazole alone.

Vallance *et al.* (1979) also compared prophylactic efficacies of metronidazole, 200 mg 8-hourly for 48 hours before operation and of metronidazole in the same dosage with neomycin, 1 gm 8-hourly for the same period. They found that metronidazole alone was significantly less effective than metronidazole with neomycin in reducing the incidence of infections associated with *Bacteroides* spp. This study included more patients than that of Proud *et al.* but the latter used larger doses of metronidazole which could have provided anaerobicidal serum concentrations during surgery.

2. *Medication for Postoperative Systemic Protection*

Willis *et al.* (1977) gave metronidazole orally 1 gm statim and 200 mg 8-hourly on day −1, 1 gm rectal suppository with anesthetic premedication and repeated 8-hourly until oral medication with 200 mg 8-hourly could be substituted and continued until the end of day +7. A single intramuscular injection of 80 mg gentamicin was also given with the preoperative medication. Anaerobic sepsis was eliminated in all of 27 patients in the controlled trial and in 200 patients operated on subsequently (Willis and Jones, 1979).

Feathers *et al.* (1977) compared patients who had only mechanical bowel preparation with others who were similarly prepared and also given gentamicin, 1.6 mg/kg im or iv with anesthetic premedication and 8-hourly until monitored dosage became possible for 5 days, and metronidazole, 1 gm suppository with anesthetic premedication and 8-hourly for 5 days (11 patients). Three patients who needed low anterior resections received metronidazole 500 mg intravenously at 8-hourly intervals for 5 days. Only one of these fourteen patients had a postoperative infection; this was superficial and grew *E. coli*.

Bjerkeset and Digranes (1978) obtained a similar result with 25 patients whose systemic metronidazole protection was provided by a single oral dose of 2 gm on day −1 and by oral doses of 400 mg 8-hourly on days +1 to +5.

Watt-Boolsen *et al.* (1979) gave metronidazole orally 1 gm three times on day −1 and intravenously 500 mg three times daily on days 0, +1, +2, +3, and +4. Anaerobes were isolated from one of four abdominal wound infections in the metronidazole group and from two of four such infections in the tetracycline group.

Eykyn *et al.* (1979) gave only metronidazole, 500 mg by intravenous infusion before operation and repeated at 8 and 16 hours later and compared the regimen with placebo medication. Anaerobes were isolated from six deep infections (five associated with anastomotic leak) in metronidazole-medicated patients and from 16 of 20 deep infections (10 associated with anastomotic leak) in the unmedicated patients. These authors commented on the dramatic reduction in postoperative infection provided by three intravenous infusions of metronidazole, despite an abnormally high incidence of leaking anastomoses; this suggested that lengthy chemoprophylaxis with metronidazole might be unnecessary and that a supplementary agent active against colonic aerobes might not be needed.

3. *Comparison of Preoperative Oral Medication with Perioperative Parenteral Medication*

Richards *et al*. (1979) compared patients who received oral neomycin (1 gm three times on day −1) and oral metronidazole (750 mg three times on days −2 and −1) with patients similarly medicated with neomycin but given metronidazole intravenously (1 gm 1 hour before surgery and 500 mg 8 hours and 16 hours later). Among the 78 patients in the trial there was no anaerobic wound infection and only four aerobic infections (one in the oral group and three in the intravenous group). The only unexpected finding was that the intralumenal colon contents of metronidazole were of the same order in both groups, and were associated with similar marked reductions in the *Bacteroides* content of the colon.

Burdon and Keighley (1979) and Aeberhard *et al.* (1979) used a common protocol for trials in Birmingham and Berne in which preoperative oral medication (metronidazole 1.2 gm daily on days −3 and −2 and kanamycin 3 gm daily on days −3, −2, and −1) was compared with parenteral medication (metronidazole 500 mg iv and kanamycin 1 gm iv or im immediately before operation and repeated in the evening after the operation and again on the following morning.

The Swiss workers found no significant difference in the rates of postoperative infection, anastomotic dehiscence, wound dehiscence, and the need for reoperation.

In Birmingham, however, postoperative sepsis occurred in 17 patients in the oral group and in only three patients in the parenteral group; *Bacteroides fragilis* was isolated from only one patient in the oral group and from two patients in the parenteral group. Thus most of the sepsis in the oral group was due to aerobes and facultative organisms many of which, especially *E. coli* and *Staphylococcus aureus,* were kanamycin-resistant.

The foregoing comparisons of preoperative oral medication using metronidazole and antiaerobic agents, with perioperative parenteral medication show that they are equally effective in preventing postoperative anaerobic infection. However their efficacies in preventing aerobic sepsis vary according to the antiaerobic agents used and the sensitivities to them of the aerobes and facultative organisms in the colonic microflora. The so-called preoperative bowel sterilization procedure has the following disadvantages:

a. Tendency to cause pseudomembranous colitis which, however, was reported only by the Birmingham workers and has not so far been reported even by them in patients who received metronidazole alone.

b. Nonabsorbed sulfonamides and aminoglycosides are not effective against all of the facultative and aerobic organisms in the colonic microflora: consequently resistant strains of these bacteria may give rise to postoperative sepsis.

c. Failure to prevent delayed postoperative anaerobic infection caused by anastomotic leakage or dehiscence.

d. They are unsuitable for emergency surgery.

4. *Combined Preoperative Antimicrobial Bowel Preparation and Postoperative Systemic Metronidazole Medication*

For children undergoing elective large bowel surgery, Khan and Nixon (1978a,b) successfully employed oral neomycin and metronidazole before surgery and metronidazole suppositories (125 mg for children of less than 1 year, 250 mg, 1 to 5 years, or 500 mg, more than 5 years) given per rectum or via a colostomy after the operation and repeated 8-hourly for 48 hours.

5. *Recommended Procedures*

The most effective and convenient procedure with the least disadvantages is one which provides bactericidal tissue concentrations during and after colorectal surgery. There is substantial evidence that metronidazole alone is adequate for this purpose when administered systemically before and after surgery. For those who still wish to provide chemoprophylaxis against endogenous infection by facultative and aerobic bacteria the choice is at present limited to gentamicin or one of the recently introduced aminoglycosides; but these are not as uniformly and incisively effective against their target organisms as metronidazole is against obligately anaerobic bacteria. Moreover, because of their dosage related toxicity, they are not as suitable as metronidazole for multiple dose postoperative medication.

For metronidazole, used alone or in association with an antiaerobic agent, the choice lies between rectal and intravenous administration.

a. Rectal Administration. Adults and children over 12 years: 1 gm suppository given at least 4 hours before operation and repeated 8-hourly for 2 or 3 days. Children (5 to 12 years): 500 mg suppository in the same regimen.

b. Intravenous Administration. Adults and children over 12 years: 500 mg infused immediately before operation and repeated 8-hourly for 2 to 3 days. Children under 12 years: As for adults but the single intravenous dose is based on 7.5 mg metronidazole per kg bodyweight.

D. Chemoprophylaxis against Systemic Infection after Transrectal Biopsy for Suspected Prostatic Carcinoma

Ashby *et al.* (1978) gave oral doses of ampicillin 500 mg and of metronidazole 400 mg at 8-hourly intervals for 48 hours to 21 patients who had undergone transrectal prostatic biopsy. Blood for culture was withdrawn 5 minutes after the biopsy procedure and medication was then started. Sixteen blood samples were positive on culture yielding 10 aerobes comprising nonhemolytic streptococci (2), *E. coli* (6), and enterococci (2); all were sensitive to ampicillin except two coliforms. Fourteen anaerobes were isolated, comprising *Bacteroides* spp. (110) and nonhemolytic streptococci (3); all were sensitive to metronidazole. Blood samples taken 3 to 4 days after the biopsy were negative on culture in every case and only four patients had rigors, malaise, and flushes which resolved in 1 to 5 days.

E. Chemoprophylaxis for Ear, Nose, and Throat Surgery and Thoracic Surgery

This article on the widespread use of a specific anaerobicide, metronidazole, to prevent endogenous postoperative infection after surgery involving those parts of the body where anaerobic bacteria abound, viz. the female genital and intestinal tracts, is remarkable for the absence of published reports on chemoprophylaxis for surgery involving the oropharynx where anaerobic bacteria also predominate. From Section V, it is evident that many ENT infections involving anaerobes have been successfully treated with metronidazole and it would appear logical to use this agent prophylactically for many operative procedures in which there is a substantial risk of endogenous anaerobic infection.

An analogous situation obtained with some forms of thoracic surgery, e.g., esophagectomy and intervention in the presence of suppurative pleuropulmonary infections.

VII. Concluding Observations

There are few if any other antimicrobial agents that, like metronidazole, have been considered worthy of three inclusions in *Advances in Chemotherapy* or *Advances in Pharmacology and Chemotherapy* during a 20-year life.

The product's introduction as the first systemically effective chemotherapeutic agent for urogenital trichomoniasis in 1960 provided an undoubted advance in therapy in terms of efficacy, convenience, and brevity. It is still used with undiminished efficacy throughout the world and many venereologists prefer to administer it as a single dose—a veritable "magic bullet" as envisaged by Ehrlich.

Six years elapsed before the late Professor John Powell and his colleagues in Durban were able to demonstrate metronidazole's remarkable efficacy as a systemic amebicide (Powell *et al.*, 1966) and it was largely due to his further efforts up to his untimely death in 1973 that metronidazole became and still is the product of choice for the effective treatment of amebic dysentery and amebic liver abscess.

The third and, we believe, the most important use of metronidazole as an anaerobicide for the treatment and prevention of infections involving anaerobic bacteria had to await the anaerobic renaissance which started in the United States in the late 1960s with the technological advances of the Virginia Polytechnic Institute in the culture, isolation, and identification of nonsporing anaerobes by the use of prereduced anaerobically sterile media.

The initiative in demonstrating that metronidazole was active *in vitro* and clinically against *Bacteroides fragilis* was taken in Finegold's laboratory in Los Angeles (Tally *et al.*, 1972), but it soon passed to Britain where the product's potentialities for the prevention and treatment of infections involving nonsporing anaerobes were quickly recognized and investigated from 1974 onward.

The worldwide recognition of the importance of anaerobic bacteria in the pathogenesis of many forms of serious sepsis has been helped by the fact that metronidazole's direct bactericidal activity is specific for anaerobes, but the demonstration of the outstanding value of the product as a chemotherapeutic agent has mainly resulted from the pioneering work of microbiologists and their surgeon colleagues in British hospitals.

Outstanding among these are Willis *et al.*, Luton and Dunstable Hospital; Selkon, Ingham *et al.*, General Hospital, Newcastle-upon-Tyne; Phillips, Eykyn *et al.*, St. Thomas's Hospital, London; and McNaught *et al.*, Victoria Infirmary, Glasgow.

This substance's potentialities in treatment and in chemoprophylaxis for surgery have still to be fully realized.

References

Aeberhard, P., Berger, J., and Casey, P. (1979). *In* "Metronidazole Proc. Geneva Conf." (I. Phillips and J. Collier, eds.), pp 173–177. Royal Soc. Med. Int. Ser. No. 18. Academic Press, New York.

Ahart, J., Landrigan, J., Jacobus, N. V., Gorbach, S. L., and Tally, F. P. (1979). *Int. Congr. Chemother, 11th, Boston* 960.

Allan, R., and Cooke, W. T. (1977). *Gut* **18,** 422.

Appelbaum, P. C., and Chatterton, S. A. (1978). *Antimicrob. Ag. Chemother.* **14,** 371.

Appelbaum, P. C., Moodley, J., Chatterton, S. A., Cowan, D. B., and Africa, C. W. (1978). *S. Afr. Med. J.* **54,** 703.

Arabi, Y., Dimock, F., Burdon, D. W., Alexander-Williams, J., and Keighley, M. R. B. (1977). *Gut* **18,** A969.

Ashby, E. C., Rees, M., and Dowding, C. H. (1978). *Br. Med. J.* **2,** 1263.

Back, E. Hermanson, J., and Wickman, M. (1978). *Scand. J. Infect. Dis.* **10,** 152.

Baines, E. J. (1977). *In* "Proc. Int. Metronidazole Conf. Montreal, 1976" (S. M. Finegold, J. A. McFadzean, and F. J. C. Roe, eds.), pp. 61–71. Elsevier, Amsterdam.

Baines, E. J. (1978). *J. Antimicrob. Chemother.* **4**(Suppl.C), 97.

Balsdon, M. J., Taylor, G. E., Pead, L., and Maskel, R. (1980). *Lancet* **1,** 501.

Banerjee, A. K. (1978). *Drugs Exp. Clin. Res.* **4,** 39.

Bardet, J.-C., Besançon, F., Bourdais, J.-P., Delavierre, P., Guerre, J., Laverdant, C., Leblanc, L., Roy, J-L., Teyssou, R., and Verduron, J. (1977). *Nouv. Presse Med.* **6,** 2077.

Baron, D., Drugeon, H., Nicolas, F., and Courtieu, A. (1977). *Med. Malad. Infect.* **7,** 158.

Barry, R. E., Chow, A. W., and Billesdon, J. (1977). *Gut* **18,** 356.

Bartlett, J. G. (1978). *J. Antimicrob. Chemother.* **4,** 392.

Bjerkeset, T., and Digranes, A. (1978). *World Congr.* Gastroenterol., *6th, Madrid, June* Communication

Blichfeldt, P., Blomhoff, J. P., Myre, E., and Gjone, E. (1978). *Scand. J. Gastroenterol.* **13,** 123.

Bolton, R. P. (1979). *Br. Med. J.* **2,** 1479.

Bolton, R. P., Sherriff, R. J., and Read, A. E. (1980). *Lancet* **1,** 383.

Bradnum, P., and Hood, F. J. C. (1977). *Br. Dent. J.* **142,** 313.

Brass, C., Richards, G. K., Ruedy, J., Prentis, J., and Hinchey, E. J. (1978). *Am. J. Surg.* **135,** 91.

Britz, M. L., and Wilkinson, R. G. (1979). *Antimicrob. Ag. Chemother.* **16,** 19.

Bryan, C. S., Huffman, L. J., Del Bene, V. E., Sanders, C. V., and Scalcini, M. C. (1979). *South. Med. J.* **72,** 494.

Burdon, D. W., and Keighley, M. R. B. (1979). *In* "Metronidazole Proc. Geneva Conf." (I. Phillips and J. Collier, eds.), Royal Soc. Med. Int. Ser. No. 18, pp. 179–183. Academic Press, New York.

Burke, M. F. (1979). *In* "Metronidazole Proc. Geneva Conf." (I. Phillips and J. Collier, eds.), Royal Soc. Med. Int. Ser. No. 18, pp. 211–214. Academic Press, New York.

Cameron, E. W. J. (1978). *S. Afr. Med. J.* **54,** 57.

Chattopadhyay, B. (1977). *Lancet* **1,** 1371.

Chow, A. W., Bednorz, D., and Guze, L. B. (1977). *In* "Proc. Int. Metronidazole Conf. Montreal, 1976" (S. M. Finegold, J. A. McFadzean, and F. J. C. Roe, eds.), pp. 286–292. Elsevier, Amsterdam.

Chow, A. W., Patten, V., and Bednorz, D. (1978). *Antimicrob. Ag. Chemother.* **13,** 416.

Chowdhury, N., Basak, A., and Sanyal, S. (1978). *Indian Pract.* **31,** 437.

Christensson, B., Hedstrom, S. A., and Ursing, Bo. (1979). *Scand. J. Infect. Dis.* **11,** 69.

Churcher, G. M., and Human, R. P. (1977). *J. Antimicrob. Chemother.* **3,** 363.

Connor, T. H., Stoeckel, M., Evrard, J., and Legator, M. S. (1977). *Cancer Res.* **37,** 629.

Coombs, G. H. (1976). *In* "Biochemistry of Parasites and Host-Parasite Relationships" (H. Vanden Bosch, ed.), pp. 545–552. Biomedical Press, Amsterdam.

Corbett, R., Prout, W. G., Hewitt, C. W., Tuke, W., and Okubadejo, O. A. (1979). *In*

"Metronidazole Proc. Geneva Conf." (I. Phillips and J. Collier, eds.), pp. 111–113. Royal Soc. Med. Int. Ser. No. 18. Academic Press, New York.

Corrodi, P., Wideman, P. A., Sutter, V. L., Drenick, E. J., Passaro, E., Jr., and Finegold, S. M. (1978). *J. Infect. Dis.* **137,** 1.

Coulbois, B., Legall, N., Blondel, P., Riche, D., Curtet, N., Guesnon, P., and Guéry, J. (1977). *Anaesthesiol. Analges. Reanim.* **34,** 367.

Davies, A. H., McFadzean, J. A., and Squires, S. (1964). *Br. Med. J.* **1,** 1149.

Davies, P. S., Rhodes, J., Heatley, R. V., and Owen, E. (1977). *In* "Proc. Int. Metrondazole Conf. Montreal, 1976" (S. M. Finegold, J. A. McFadzean, and F. J. C. Roe, eds.), pp. 422–425. Elsevier, Amsterdam.

Dublanchet, A., Durieux, R., and Fevre, D. (1977). *Med. Malad. Infect.* **7,** 317.

Durfee, M. A., Forsyth, P. S., Hale, J. A., and Holmes, K. K. (1979). *Antimicrob. Ag. Chemother.* **16,** 635.

Ellis, B. W. (1980). *Br. Med. J.* **280,** 763.

Eykyn, S. J. (1979). *In* "Metronidazole Proc. Geneva Conf." (I. Phillips and J. Collier, eds.), pp. 75–81. Royal Soc. Med. Int. Ser. No. 18. Academic Press, New York.

Eykyn, S. J., and Phillips, I. (1976). *Br. Med. J.* **2,** 1418.

Eykyn, S. J., and Phillips, I. (1978). *J. Antimicrob. Chemother.* **4,** (Suppl. C), 75.

Eykyn, S. J., Jackson, B. T., Lockhart-Mummery, H. E., and Phillips, I. (1979). *In* "Metronidazole Proc. Geneva Conf." (I. Phillips and J. Collier, eds.), pp. 167–171. Royal Soc. Med. Int. Ser. No. 18. Academic Press, New York.

Feathers, R. S., Lewis, A. A. M., Sagor, G. R., Amirak, I. D., and Noone, P. (1977). *Lancet* **2,** 4.

Feldman, W. E. (1976). *Am. J. Dis. Child.* **130,** 880.

Fiddian, R. V. (1978). *J. Antimicrob. Chemother.* **4,** Suppl C, 39.

Finn Gottrup, F. (1978). *Medit. Soc. Chemother., Madrid, Sept.* Communication.

Foster, G. E., Bourke, J. B., Holliday, A., Doran, J., Balfour, T. W., Hardcastle, J. D., and Marshall, D. J. (1979). *In* "Metronidazole Proc. Geneva Conf." (I. Phillips and J. Collier, eds.), pp. 105–110. Royal Soc. Med. Int. Ser. No. 18. Academic Press, New York.

Foster, J. L., and Willson, R. L. (1976). *In* "Chemotherapy," Vol. 7, pp. 215–222. Plenum, New York.

Freeman, W. H., McFadzean, J. A., and Whelan, J. P. F. (1968). *J. Appl. Bacteriol.* **31,** 443.

Füzi, M., and Csukás, Z. (1970). *Zentralbl. Bakteriol. Parasitenkd. Infectionskr. Hyg.* **213,** 258.

Gabriel, R., Page, C. M., Weller, I. V. D., Collier, J., Houghton, G. W., Templeton, R., and Thorne, P. S. (1979). *In* "Metronidazole Proc. Geneva Conf." (I. Phillips and J. Collier, eds.), pp. 49–54. Royal Soc. Med. Int. Ser. No. 18. Academic Press, New York.

Galgiani, J. N., Busch, D. F., Brass, C., Rumans, L. W., Mangels, J. I., and Stevens D. A. (1978). *Am. J. Med.* **65,** 284.

Garcia Rodriguez, J. A., Garcia Sanchez, J. E., Saenz Gonzalez, M. C., and Prieto Prieto, J. (1977). *Pharmatherapeutica* **1,** 573.

Garcia Sanchez, J. E., Gomez Garcia, A. C., Prieto Prieto, J., and Saenz Gonzalez, M. C. (1978). *Curr. Chemother.* **1,** 289.

George, R. H., and Bint, A. J. (1976). *J. Antimicrob. Chemother.* **2,** 101.

Giamarellou, H., Kanellakopoulou, K., Pragastis, D., Tagaris, N., and Daikos, G. K. (1977). *J. Antimicrob. Chemother.* **3,** 347.

Giamarellou, H., Tagaris, N., Kanellakopoulou, K., Avlami, A., Pragastis, D., and Daikos, G. K. (1978). *Medit. Soc. Chemother. Madrid, Sept.* Communication

Gillespie, G., and McNaught, W. (1978). *J. Antimicrob. Chemother.* **4**(Suppl.C), 29.

Gnarpe, H., and Lundback, A. (1978). *Curr. Chemother.* **1,** 718.

Golde, S., and Ledger, W. J. (1977). *Obstet. Gynecol.* **50,** 670.
Goldring, J., Scott, A., McNaught, W., and Gillespie, G. (1975). *Lancet* **2,** 997.
Goodwin, N. M. (1979). *In* "Metronidazole Proc. Geneva Conf." (I. Phillips and J. Collier, eds.), pp. 59–62. Royal Soc. Med. Int. Ser. No. 18. Academic Press, New York.
Grove, D. I., Mahmoud, A. A. F., and Warren K. S. (1977). *Int. Arch. Allergy. Appl. Immunol.* **54,** 422.
Guilhou, J.-J., Guilhou, E., Malbos, S., and Meynadier, J. (1979). *Ann. Dermatol. Venereol. (Paris)* **106,** 127.
Gustafsson, B. E., Gustafsson, J. A., and Carlstedt, D. B. (1977). *Acta Med. Scand.* **201,** 155.
Hale, J. E., Perinpanayagam, R. M., and Smith, G. (1976). *Lancet* **2,** 70.
Hanna, B. J., Sanders, C. V., Lewis, A. C., Williams, W. L., and Sands, M. L. (1976). *Intersci. Conf. Antimicrob. Ag. Chemother., 16th, Chicago* 458.
Heginbotham, D., and Rutherford, A. M. (1979). *N. Z. Med. J.* **89,** 246.
Heldström, S. A., Mardh, P.-A., and Ripa, J. (1978). *Scand. J. Infect. Dis.* **10,** 7.
Holdstock, D. J. (1975). *Lancet* **2,** 1260.
Hood, F. J. C. (1978). *J. Antimicrob. Chemother.* **4** (Suppl.C), 71.
Houghton, G. W., Thorne, P. S., Smith, J., Templeton, R., and Collier, J. (1979). *Br. J. Clin. Pharmacol.* **8,** 337.
Hughes, T. B. J., Frampton, J., Begg, H. B., and Khan, M. S. (1979). *In* "Metronidazole Proc. Geneva Conf." (I. Phillips and J. Collier, eds.), pp. 207–210. Royal Soc. Med. Int. Ser. No. 18. Academic Press, New York.
Hunt, W. L., Agre, K., Oppermann, J., and Nissen, C. H. (1978). *Annu. Meet. Am. Soc. Microbiol.* **A66,** p. 12.
Hutchinson, M., Lambert, H. P., Loughman, D., and Morgan, M. W. E. (1977). *In* "Proc. Int. Metronidazole Conf. Montreal, 1976" (S. M. Finegold, J. A. McFadzean, and F. J. C. Roe, eds.), pp. 320–328. Elsevier, Amsterdam.
Ingham, H. R., Rich, G. E., Selkon, J. B., Hale, J. H., Roxby, C. M., Betty, M. J., Johnson, R. W. G., and Uldall, P. R. (1975). *J. Antimicrob. Chemother.* **1,** 235.
Ingham, H. R., Hood, F. J. C., Bradnum, P., Tharagonnet, D., and Selkon, J. B. (1977a). *Br. J. Oral Surg.* **14,** 264.
Ingham, H. R., Selkon, J. B., and Roxby, C. M. (1977b). *Br. Med. J.* **2,** 991.
Ingham, H. R., Eaton, S., Venables, C. W., and Adams, P. C. (1978a). *Lancet* **1,** 214.
Ingham, H. R., High, A. S., Kalbag, R. M., Sengupta, R. P., Tharagonnet, D., and Selkon, J. B. (1978b). *Lancet* **2,** 497.
Ingham, H. R., Hall, C. J., Sisson, P. R., Tharagonnet, D., and Selkon, J. B. (1979). *J. Antimicrob. Chemother.* **5,** 734.
Ingham, H. R., Selkon, J. B., Sisson, P. R., and Middleton, R. L. (1980). *Lancet* **1,** 659.
Ings, R. M. J. (1973). Ph.D. Thesis. Council for National Academic Awards. London, England.
Ings, R. M. J., Law, G. L., and Parnell, E. W. (1966). *Biochem. Pharmacol.* **15,** 515.
Ings, R. M. J., McFadzean, J. A., and Ormerod, W. E. (1974). *Biochem. Pharmacol.* **23,** 1421.
Jackson, B., and Dessau, F. I. (1961). *Lab. Invest.* 909.
Jackson, P., Ridley, W. J., and Pattison, H. S. (1979). *N. Z. Med. J.* **89,** 243.
Jokipii, L., and Jokipii, A. M. M. (1977). *J. Antimicrob. Chemother.* **3,** 571.
Jones, P. H., Willis, A. T., and Ferguson, I. R. (1978). *Lancet* **1,** 214.
Khan, O., and Nixon, H. H. (1978a). *Br. J. Surg.* **65,** 804.
Khan, O., and Nixon, H. H. (1978b). *Z. Kind. Chir.* **25,** 196.
Khanna, N. N., Sen, P. K., Ahmed, K., and Agarwal, R. K. (1979). *In* "Metronidazole Proc.

Geneva Conf." (I. Phillips and J. Collier, eds.), pp. 69–73. Royal Soc. Med. Int. Ser. No. 18. Academic Press, New York.

Knipp, J., Flood, S., and Faloon, W. W. (1978). *Gastroenterology* **74,** (5), 1128.

Koch, R. L., and Goldman, P. (1978). *J. Pharm. Exp. Ther.* **208,** 406.

Koch, R. L., Chrystal, E. J. T., Beaulieu, B. B., Jr., and Goldman, P. (1979). *Biochem. Pharmacol.* **28,** 3611.

Kostakis, A., and Calne, R. Y. (1977). *IRCS Med. Sci. Cardiovasc. System Immunol. Allergy Pharmacol. Surg. Transplant.* **5,** 142.

Krook, A., Danielsson, D., Kjellander, J., and Järnerot, G. (1979). *Scand. J. Gastroenterol.* **14,** 705.

LaMont, J. T., and Trnka, Y. M. (1980). *Lancet* **1,** 381.

Laufer, J., Mignon, H., and Videau, D. (1973). *Rev. Stomatol. Chir. Maxillo Fac.* **74,** 387.

Leach, R. D., Eykyn, S. J., Phillips, I., and Corrin, B. (1979). *Lancet* **1,** 35.

Ledger, W. J., Gee, C. L., Pollin, P. A., Lewis, W. P., Sutter, V. L., and Finegold, S. M. (1976). *Am. J. Obstet. Gynecol.* **126,** 1.

Ledger, W. J., Lewis, W., Golde, S., and Gee, C. (1977). *In* "Proc. Int. Metronidazole Conf. Montreal, 1976" (S. M. Finegold, J. A. McFadzean, and F. J. C. Roe, eds.), pp. 353–358. Elsevier, Amsterdam.

Leigh, D. A., Simmons, K., and Norman, E. (1974). *J. Clin. Pathol.* **27,** 997.

Lewis, R. P., Wideman, P., Sutter, V. L., and Finegold, S. M. (1977). In "Proc. Int. Metronidazole Conf. Montreal, 1976" (S. M. Finegold, J. A. McFadzean, and F. J. C. Roe, eds.), pp. 307–319. Elsevier, Amsterdam.

Lindmark, D. G., and Müller, M. (1976). *Antimicrob. Ag. Chemother.* **10,** 476.

Low-Beer, T. S., and Nutter, S. (1978). *Lancet* **2,** 1063.

McFadzean, J. A., Pugh, I. M., Squires, S., and Whelan, J. P. F. (1969). *Br. J. Vener. Dis.* **45,** 161.

McGowan, D. A., Murphy, K. J., and Sheiham, A. (1977). *Br. Dent. J.* **142,** 221.

McMahon, M. J., Greenall, M. J., and Cooke, E. M. (1979). *In* "Metronidazole Proc. Geneva Conf." (I. Phillips and J. Collier, eds.), pp. 133–136. Royal Soc. Med. Int. Ser. No. 18. Academic Press, New York.

Malcolm, A. J. (1978). *Br. Med. J.* **2,** 479.

Matheson, D. M., Arabi, Y., Baxter-Smith, D., Alexander-Williams, J., and Keighley, M. R. B. (1978). *Br. J. Surg.* **65,** 597.

Matuchansky, C., Aries, J., and Maire, P. (1978). *Lancet* **2,** 580.

Michaels, R. M. (1968). *In* "Advances in Chemotherapy" (A. Goldin, F. Hawking, and R. J. Schnitzer, eds.), Vol. 3, pp. 39–108. Academic Press, New York.

Milne, S. E., Stokes, E. J., and Waterworth, P. M. (1978). *J. Clin. Pathol.* **31,** 933.

Mitre, R. J., and Rotheram, E. B., Jr. (1974). *J. Am. Med. Assoc.* **230,** 1168.

Montgomery, R. D. (1975). *Lancet* **2,** 1149.

Morris, W. T., Ellis-Pegler, R. B., and Innes, D. B. (1979). *In* "Metronidazole Proc. Geneva Conf." (I. Phillips and J. Collier, eds.), pp. 129–131. Royal Soc. Med. Int. Ser. No. 18. Academic Press, New York.

Müller, M. (1979). *In* "Metronidazole Proc. Geneva Conf." (I. Phillips and J. Collier, eds.), pp. 223–228. Royal Soc. Med. Int. Ser. No. 18. Academic Press, New York.

Nastro, L. J., and Finegold, S. M. (1972). *J. Infect. Dis.* **126,** 104.

Nicol, C. S., Evans, A. J., McFadzean, J. A., and Squires, S. (1966). *Lancet* **2,** 41.

O'Grady, L. R., and Ralph, E. D. (1976). *Am. J. Dis. Child.* **130,** 871.

Okawa, T., Kimura, K., Sato, S., Sakai, K., Gunji, I., Honma, Y., and Suzuki, Y. (1969). *Shindan Chiryo* **44,** (7), 1287.

Onderdonk, A. B., Hermos, J. A., Dzink, J. L., and Bartlett, J. G. (1978). *Gastroenterology* **74,** 521.

Pashby, N. L. (1979). *In* "Metronidazole Proc. Geneva Conf." (I. Phillips and J. Collier, eds.), pp. 63–68. Royal Soc. Med. Int. Ser. No. 18. Academic Press, New York.

Pashby, N., and Mee, W. M. (1978). *J. Antimicrob. Chemother.* **4**(Suppl.C), 25.

Pashby, N. L., Bolton, R. P., and Sherriff, R. J. (1979). *Br. Med. J.* **1,** 1605.

Perera, M., Chipping, P. M., and Noone, P. (1980). *J. Antimicrob. Chemother.* **6,** 105.

Pheifer, T. A., Forsyth, P. S., Durfee, M. A., Pollock, H. M., and Holmes K. K. (1978). *New Engl. J. Med.* **298,** 1429.

Pieron, R., Debure, A., Mafart, Y., Lesobre, B., Bryskièr, A., and Vergez, P. (1977). *Sem. Hôp. Paris* **53,** 1709.

Pinto, D. J., and Sanderson, P. J. (1979). *In* "Metronidazole Proc. Geneva Conf." (I. Phillips and J. Collier, eds.), pp. 119–123. Royal Soc. Med. Int. Ser. No. 18. Academic Press, New York.

Powell, S. J. (1972). *In* "Advances in Pharmacology and Chemotherapy" (R. J. Schnitzer and F. Hawking, eds.), Vol. 10, pp. 91–103. Academic Press, New York.

Powell, S. J., Mcleod, I., Wilmot, A. J., and Elsdon-Dew, R. (1966). *Lancet* **ii,** 1329.

Prince, H. N., Grunberg, E., Titsworth, E., and DeLorenzo, W. F. (1969). *Appl. Microbiol.* **18,** 728.

Proud, G., Chamberlain, J., Ingham, H., Petty, A. H., Selkon, J. B., Venables, C. W., and Wilson, C. R. (1978). *Br. J. Surg.* **65,** 824.

Pye, R. J., and Burton, J. L. (1976). *Lancet* **1,** 1211.

Raff, M. J., Melo, J. C., Chun, C. H., Varghese, R., and Summersgill, J. (1978). *Intersci. Conf. Antimicrob. Ag. Chemother., 18th, Atlanta* Abstr. 367.

Ralph, E. D., and Clarke, D. A. (1978). *Antimicrob. Ag. Chemother.* **14,** 377.

Ralph, E. D., and Kirby, W. M. M. (1975). *Antimicrob. Ag. Chemother.* **8,** 409.

Richards, G. K., Dion, Y. M., Wink, R. T., and Hinchey, E. J. (1979). *In* "Metronidazole Proc. Geneva Conf." (I. Phillips and J. Collier, eds.), pp. 161–165. Royal Soc. Med. Int. Ser. No. 18. Academic Press, New York.

Rissing, P., Newman, C., Buxton, T., Edmundson, T., and Moore, W. (1978). *Annu. Meet. Am. Soc. Microbiol.* Abstr. A65, p. 11.

Rodgers, J., Ross, D., McNaught, W., and Gillespie, G. (1979). *Br. J. Surg.* **66,** 425.

Roe, F. J. C. (1979). *In* "Metronidazole Proc. Geneva Conf." (I. Phillips and J. Collier, eds.), pp. 215–222. Royal Soc. Med. Int. Ser. No. 18. Academic Press, New York.

Rom, S., Flynn, D., and Noone, P. (1977). *Arch. Dis. Child.* **52,** 740.

Rotimi, V. O., Duerden, B. I., Ede, V., and MacKinnon, A. E. (1979). *Lancet* **1,** 833.

Russell, F. E. (1966). *Mem. Inst. Butantan (San Paulo)* **33,** 845.

Salem, A. R., Jackson, D. D., and McFadzean, J. A. (1975). *J. Antimicrob. Chemother.* **1,** 387.

Salem, R. (1979). *In* "Metronidazole Proc. Geneva Conf." (I. Phillips and J. Collier, eds.), pp. 115–117. Royal Soc. Med. Int. Ser. No. 18. Academic Press, New York.

Sanders, C. V., Hanna, B. J., Lewis, A. C., and Scalcini, M. (1979). *In* "Metronidazole Proc. Geneva Conf." (I. Phillips and J. Collier, eds.), pp. 83–89. Royal Soc. Med. Int. Ser. No. 18. Academic Press, New York.

Seggie, J. (1978). *Br. Med. J.* **1,** 960.

Seligman, S. A. (1978). *J. Antimicrob. Chemother.* **4**(Suppl.C), 51.

Sharp, D. J., Corringham, R. E. T., Nye, E. B., Sagor, G. R., and Noone, P. (1977). *J. Antimicrob. Chemother.* **3,** 233.

Shinn, D. L. S. (1962). *Lancet* **1,** 1191.

Shinn, D. L. S., Squires, S., and McFadzean, J. A. (1965). *Dent. Pract.* **15,** 275.

Sisson, P. R., Ingham, H. R., and Selkon, J. B. (1978). *J. Med. Microbiol.* **11,** 111.
Solhaug, J. H. (1977). *Scand. J. Gastroenterol.* **12**(Suppl. 45), 100.
Sparrow, G., Minton, M., Rubens, R. D., Simmons, N. A., and Aubrey, C. (1980). *Lancet* **1,** 1185.
Speck, W. T., Stein, A. B., and Kosenkranz, H. S. (1976). *J. Natl. Cancer Inst.* **56,** 283.
Stambaugh, J. E., Feo, L. G., and Manthei, R. W. (1968). *J. Pharmacol. Exp. Ther.* **161,** 373.
Study Group (1974). *Lancet* **2,** 1540.
Study Group (1975). *J. Antimicrob. Chemother.* **1,** 393.
Sutter, V. L., and Finegold, S. M. (1975). *J. Infect. Dis.* **131,** 417.
Sutter, V. L., and Finegold, S. M. (1977). *In* "Proc. Int. Metronidazole Conf. Montreal, 1976" (S. M. Finegold, J. A. McFadzean, and F. J. C. Roe, eds.), pp. 279–285. Elsevier, Amsterdam.
Takazoe, I., Okuda, K., Yamamoto, A., and Nakamara, T. (1973). *Bull. Tokyo Dent. Coll.* **14,** 1.
Tally, F. P., Sutter, V. L., and Finegold, S. M. (1972). *Calif. Med.* **117,** 22.
Tally, F. P., Sutter, V. L., and Finegold, S. M. (1975). *Antimicrob. Ag. Chemother.* **7,** 672.
Tally, F. P., Goldin, B. R., Sullivan, N., Johnson, J., and Gorbach, S. L. (1978). *Antimicrob. Ag. Chemother.* **13,** 460.
Taylor, S. A., and Cawdery, H. M. (1977). *Proc. R. Soc. Med.* **70,** 481.
Taylor, S. A., Cawdery, H. M., and Smith, J. (1979). *Br. J. Surg.* **66,** 191.
Tennican, P. O., Tennican, F. L., Fowler, R. A., Friedman, B. A., Palpant, S. D., and Weinburg, M. (1978). *Intersci. Conf. Antimicrob. Ag. Chemother., 18th, Atlanta* Abstr. 368.
Trinh Dinh, H., Kernbaum, S., and Frottier, J. (1978). *Lancet* **1,** 338.
"The Nitroimidazole Family of Drugs" (1978). Editorial. *Br. J. Vener. Dis.* **54,** 69.
Ueno, K., Ninomiya, K., and Suzuki, S. (1971a). *Chemotherapy* (*Jpn.*) **19,** 111.
Ueno, K. Ninomiya, K., Sakisaka, K., Kamiya, H., and Suzuki, S. (1971b). *Clin. Rep.* (*Jpn.*) **5,** (4) 737.
Ursing, B. (1977). *In* "Proc. Int. Metronidazole Conf. Montreal, 1976" (S. M. Finegold, J. A. McFadzean, and F. J. C. Roe, eds.), pp. 415–421. Elsevier, Amsterdam.
Ursing, B., and Kamme, C. (1975). *Lancet* **1,** 775.
Vallance, S., Jones, A. B., Arabi, Y., and Keighley, M. R. B. (1979). *In* "Metronidazole Proc. Geneva Conf." (I. Phillips and J. Collier, eds.), pp. 155–159. Royal Soc. Med. Int. Ser. No. 18. Academic Press, New York.
Vanhoof, R., Vanderlinden, M. P., Dierickx, R., Lauwers, S., Yourassowsky, E., and Butzler, J. P. (1978). *Antimicrob. Ag. Chemother.* **14,** 553.
Vaughan, J. E. (1979). *In* "Metronidazole Proc. Geneva Conf." (I. Phillips and J. Collier, eds.), pp. 203–205. Royal Soc. Med. Int. Ser. No. 18. Academic Press, New York.
Videau, D. (1971). *Pathol. Biol.* **19,** 661.
Videau, D. Blanchard, J.-C., and Sebald, M. (1973). *Ann. Inst. Pasteur,* **124B,** 505.
Wandtke, J., Skucas, J., Spataro, R., and Bruneau, R. J. (1977). *Am. J. Roentgenol.* **129,** 601.
Warner, J. F., and Prior, R. B. (1977). *In* "Proc. Int. Metronidazole Conf. Montreal, 1976" (S. M. Finegold, J. A. McFadzean, and J. F. C. Roe, eds.) pp. 359–367. Elsevier, Amsterdam.
Watt, B., and Jack, E. P. (1977). *J. Med. Microbiol.* **10,** 461.
Watt-Boolsen, S., Justesen, T., Blichert-Toft, M., and Hansen, J. B. (1979). *Acta Chir. Scand.* **145,** 263.
Webb, C. H. (1977). *Lancet* **2,** 511.

Welkos, S., Toskes, P., and Baer, H. (1977). *Clin. Res.* **25,** (3), 320A.
Whelan, J. P. F., and Hale, J. H. (1973). *J. Clin. Pathol.* **26,** 393.
Willis, A. T., and Jones, P. H. (1979). *J. Pharmacother.* **2,** 122, 128.
Willis, A. T., Ferguson, I. R., Jones, P. H., Tearle, P. V., Berry, R. B., Fiddian, R. V., Graham, D. F., Harland, D. H. C., Innes, D. B., Mee, W. M., Rothwell-Jackson, R. L., Sutch, I., Kilbey, C., and Edwards, D. (1976). *Br. Med. J.* **1,** 318.
Willis, A. T., Ferguson, I. R., Jones, P. H., Phillips, K. D., Tearle, P. V., Fiddian, R. V., Graham, D. F., Harland, D. H. C., Huges, D. E. R., Knight, D., Mee, W. M., Rothwell-Jackson, R. L., Sutch, I., Kilbey, C., and Edwards, D. (1977). *Br. Med. J.* **1,** 607.
Willis, A. T., Jones, P. H., Phillips, K. D., and Gottobed, G. (1978). *Lancet* **1,** 721.
Zimmerman, J., Silver, J., Shapiro, M., Freidman, G., and Melmed, R. N. (1980). *Scand. J. Infect. Dis.* **12,** 79.

ADVANCES IN PHARMACOLOGY AND CHEMOTHERAPY, VOL. 18

Chemotherapeutic Inhibitors of the Enzymes of the *de Novo* Pyrimidine Pathway

THOMAS W. KENSLER*,† AND DAVID A. COONEY*

** Laboratory of Medicinal Chemistry and Biology*
National Cancer Institute
National Institutes of Health
Bethesda, Maryland
and
† Division of Toxicology
Department of Environmental Health Sciences
Johns Hopkins University School of Hygiene
and Public Health
Baltimore, Maryland

ISBN 0-12-032918-2

I. Introduction

The requirement for pyrimidines is ubiquitously distributed throughout the spectrum of living organisms and can be fulfilled by two synthetic pathways: a *de novo* and a salvage pathway. Uridine-5′-monophosphate is the common product of these two pathways. The *de novo* pathway is generally considered to consist of six enzymes: carbamyl phosphate synthetase II (CPS II), L-aspartate transcarbamylase (ATCase), L-dihydroorotase (DHOase), L-dihydroorotate dehydrogenase (DHO de-Hase), orotate phosphoribosyl transferase (OPRTase), and orotidine-5′-monophosphate decarboxylase (OMP deCase). Several excellent reviews of this pathway appear in the recent literature (Shambaugh, 1979; Jones, 1980). Additionally, the properties of the two enzymes catalyzing modification of the pyrimidine ring, namely, thymidylate synthetase and cytidylate synthetase have also been reviewed in the recent biochemical literature (Buchanan, 1973; Weinfeld *et al.*, 1978; Dunlap, 1978). An abbreviated discussion of the *de novo* pathway is presented at the outset of this article, its orientation is primarily from a perspective that considers the role of substrates and endogenous metabolites as modulators of enzymic activities and consequent flux through the pathway. It is felt that this perspective is necessary for an enlightened development and deployment of antipyrimidine therapy.

It has been the quest of considerable investigation to develop specific inhibitors of *de novo* pyrimidine biosynthesis and a substantial number of compounds (~50) have been described that exert inhibitory activities against one or more of the pyrimidine biosynthetic enzymes *in vitro*. However, two subsequent requirements, efficacy *in vivo* and managable host toxicity, have precluded admission of all but a handful of these drugs to clinical utility. In this presentation the activity of these drugs against crude or purified bacterial and mammalian enzymes has been summarized as has their efficacy *in vivo*, where known. Additionally, the antineoplastic activity of these inhibitors, singly and in combination with other pyrimidine inhibitors is described. Finally, in the Appendix (Section VI), we have attempted to summarize strategies that are presently or, perhaps, will in the future be useful for the measurement of pyrimidine enzymes and substrate levels. For, as our bias is sure to suggest, the successful clinical interruption of pyrimidine biosynthesis will require a well-defined attack on the *de novo* pathway based on the knowledge of the dynamic states of this pathway in host as well as target tissues.

II. Pyrimidine Biosynthetic Enzymes

Figure 1 is a diagram of the pyrimidine biosynthetic pathway. From this figure it can be appreciated that the main components of the pyrimidine ring are derived from L-aspartic acid and L-glutamine, respectively, while the ribosyl and phosphoryl moieties are transferred *en bloc* from phosphoribosyl pyrophosphate. This "geneology" of the pyrimidine ring is, so far as is known, universal, and serves to underscore the intimate interrelationship of the dicarboxylic amino acids and their amides with nucleic acid biosynthesis (Jayaram and Cooney, 1979).

At this point, each of the steps of the pyrimidine pathway will be considered in turn, first from the standpoint of the chemistry of the reactions involved; this will entail the pH optimum of the relevant enzymes, their equilibria at physiologic pH, substrate affinities, and specific activities both at saturation and under physiologic conditions. Next, the subcellular localization of the enzymes participating in pyrimidine biosynthesis and the nature of what is known of the polyfunctional complexes involved in certain of the steps of the pathway will be discussed. Lastly, the presentation will focus on endogenous or physiologic regulators of the catalytic activity of the six pyrimidine biosynthetic steps by way of background information for the discussion of exogenous, chemotherapeutic inhibitors which follows.

A. Carbamyl Phosphate Synthetase II

Under ordinary circumstances, the carbamyl phosphate necessary for pyrimidine biosynthesis is derived largely from the operation of CPS II, a soluble amidotransferase present in most tissues at concentrations proportionate to their rate of growth or mitotic activity (Mori and Tatibana, 1978). Because of the instability and/or rapid utilization of its principal product, carbamyl phosphate, it is likely that the reaction catalyzed by this enzyme is nearly irreversible, *in vivo.* From Table I it can be appreciated that CPS II, in the cytoplasm of liver at least, encounters concentrations of its ordinary substrates and cofactors which are greater than their K_ms. This feature should permit the catalytic operation of the enzyme at $\frac{1}{2}$ V_{max}; an exception to this general statement is ATP, which is present at roughly $\frac{1}{2}$ K_m. On this basis, it is plausible to suggest that alterations in the concentration of ATP *in vivo* might well regulate the availability of carbamyl phosphate for pyrimidine biosynthesis.

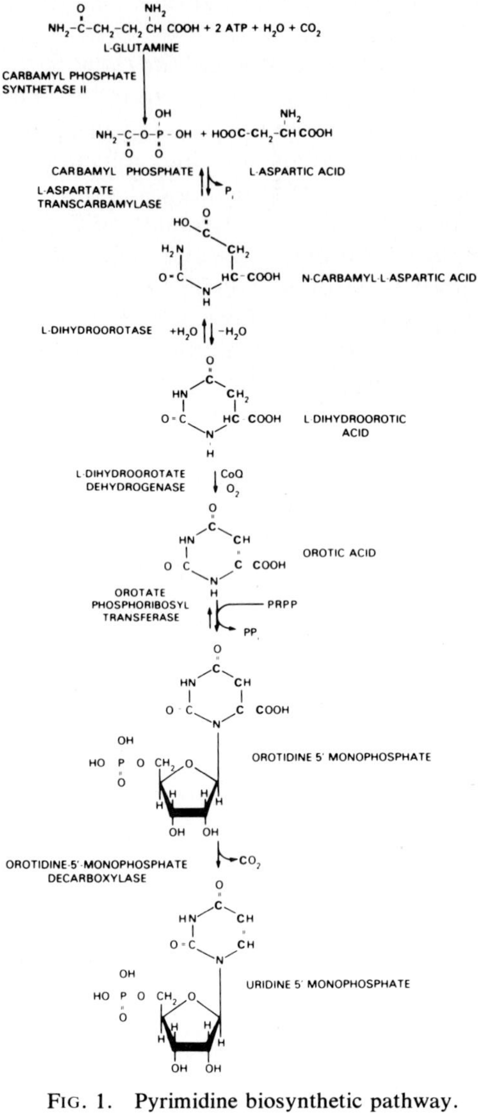

L-GLUTAMINE

CARBAMYL PHOSPHATE SYNTHETASE II

CARBAMYL PHOSPHATE

L-ASPARTIC ACID

L-ASPARTATE TRANSCARBAMYLASE

N-CARBAMYL-L-ASPARTIC ACID

L-DIHYDROOROTASE

L-DIHYDROOROTIC ACID

L-DIHYDROOROTATE DEHYDROGENASE

OROTIC ACID

OROTATE PHOSPHORIBOSYL TRANSFERASE

OROTIDINE 5' MONOPHOSPHATE

OROTIDINE-5'-MONOPHOSPHATE DECARBOXYLASE

URIDINE 5' MONOPHOSPHATE

FIG. 1. Pyrimidine biosynthetic pathway.

TABLE I

CARBAMYL PHOSPHATE SYNTHETASE II (CPS II)

$$HCO_3^- + 2\ ATP\text{-}Mg^{2+} + \text{L-glutamine (or Ammonia)} \rightleftharpoons \text{carbamyl phosphate} + 2\ ADP\text{-}Mg^{2+} + \text{L-glutamic acid (or } H_2O) + P_i$$

	References
a. Source: Ehrlich ascites tumor cells, rat hepatocytes, hepatoma cells, spleen, etc.	Mori and Tatibana (1978)
b. pH optima: 7.0 (L-glutamine as substrate) 7.8 (Ammonia as substrate)	Mori and Tatibana (1978)
c. Michaelis constants for substrates:	

Substrate	K_m (μM)	Concentration of substrate in the cell (μM)	References
HCO_3^-	1000–10,000	20,000	Mori and Tatibana (1978); Guyton (1971)
ATP	1700	1000	Jones (1980); Williamson and Brosnam (1974)
$MgCl_2$	2000–5000	25,000	Mori and Tatibana (1978); Guyton (1971)
K^+	18,000	140,000	Mori and Tatibana (1978); Guyton (1971)
L-Glutamine	21	500–5000	Jones (1980); Williamson and Brosnam (1974)
Ammonia	15,000	500	Jones (1980); Williamson and Brosnam (1974)

	References
d. Specific activity: 20 nmoles/mg protein/hour	Mori and Tatibana (1978)
e. Molecular weight (synthetase fragment, see text): 197,000	Shoaf and Jones (1973)
f. Equilibrium position: strongly in the biosynthetic direction	Shoaf and Jones (1973)
g. Substrate specificity: stringent, but ammonia can replace L-glutamine	Mori and Tatibana (1978)

The pH optimum is close to the pH of the cytoplasm, and not especially sharp, so that minor shifts in acid–base balance are unlikely to influence the activity of CPS II in normal tissues. However, in the more acidic microenvironment of certain tumor cells, it is possible that the velocity of the enzyme could be braked to an important degree.

In rat ascites hepatoma cells, the specific activity of crude CPS II approximates 20 nmoles per mg of protein per hour. However, as is discussed in the Appendix, this value is liable to underestimation on account of the inevitable dilution from $[^{12}C]CO_2$ in the atmosphere of the radioactive bicarbonate used to quantify it in tissues. Strategies for circumventing this problem are also suggested in the Appendix.

Although the molecular weight of CPS II is stated to be approximately 200,000 in the tabulation of the properties of the enzyme given in Table I, it is relevant at this point to note that the first three enzymes of pyrimidine biosynthesis all exist, in fact, as a multienzyme complex (*pyr* 1–3 in the nomenclature of Jones, 1980) whose molecular weight is close to 900,000. This aggregation of consecutive catalysts has obvious physiologic benefits—the principal of which is to channel products from the antecedent to the subsequent catalytic center without undue dilution or diffusion in the ambient cytoplasmic milieu.

Of the endogenous regulators of the activity of CPS II, phosphate esters are the most potent: thus, UMP,[1] UDP-glucose, CTP, dUTP, ADP, and, most effectively, UTP, all repress the catalytic activity of the enzyme by diminishing its affinity for ATP (Mori and Tatibana, 1978). Since, as was mentioned, ATP is unique among the substrates of CPS II in that its physiologic concentration is $<K_m$, such depressed affinity might assume exaggerated importance *in vivo* (Jones, 1980). The concentration of UTP required for 50% inhibition of CPS II is approximately 2 m*M* (Tatibana and Shigesada, 1972). Since the intracellular level of this nucleotide in liver is only 40 μM (Keppler *et al.*, 1974), at first glance it would appear unlikely that it could function as an inhibitory molecule *in vivo*. However, since many pyrimidine nucleotides repress the activity of CPS II, and since, in the aggregate, the net concentration of these nucleotides exceeds the median inhibitory concentration, it is likely that they do, in fact, modulate the function of the enzyme (Kensler *et al.*, 1981a; Jones, 1980).

Certain polyamines and amino acids also inhibit the activity of CPS II: thus glycine, L-alanine, spermine, spermidine, and putrescine all behave as retardants at concentrations between 1 and 4 m*M* (Mori and Tatibana,

[1] Jones (1980) reports that UMP is unique among the uridine nucleotides in not inhibiting CPS II. This difference between her results and those of Mori and Tatibana (1978) may arise from differences in the condition of analysis used.

1978). Since such concentrations do not prevail in most body fluids, the functional significance of these inhibitions, measured as they were *in vitro*, is open to question.

Stimulants of CPS II also are known. Of these PRPP is the most important. This compound acts by improving the affinity of the enzyme for ATP, i.e., in a manner that is diametrically opposite to that of UTP. The median stimulatory concentration of PRPP is less than 0.1 mM, a value two to five times greater than its intracellular concentration in tumors (Kensler *et al.*, 1981a). In view of this relationship, it is unlikely that the sugar functions as a regulator of the activity of CPS II *in vivo*. However, since a large number of chemotherapeutic agents, most notably methotrexate, augment the concentration of PRPP many fold (Cadman *et al.*, 1979), their use may serve to promote the generation of carbamyl phosphate.

B. L-Aspartate Transcarbamylase

Like CPS II, ATCase (Table II) catalyzes a reaction whose equilibrium position is strongly in the biosynthetic direction; teleologically speaking, this feature is, of course, conducive to nucleic acid synthesis. Under appropriate conditions, however, the reaction can be demonstrated to be microscopically reversible (Chang and Jones, 1974).

The pH optimum of mammalian ATCase approximates 9. Since the enzyme exhibits only 20–30% of its optimal activity at pH 7.4, it is apparent, other factors being equal, that it does not generate N-carbamyl-L-aspartic acid at a maximal rate *in vivo* (Shoaf and Jones, 1973). One factor abetting this drawback is the pH dependence of the enzyme's Michaelis constant for L-aspartic acid: as the pH falls, the affinity of the enzyme for this substrate improves to a notable degree (Bresnick and Mossé, 1966; Shoaf and Jones, 1973). Despite such an improvement in affinity, it is important to stress that ATCase appears to be markedly undersaturated with its substrates *in vivo*: by factors of 2.5–50 in the case of L-aspartic acid, and by a factor of almost 100 in the case of carbamyl phosphate (assuming the intercellular concentration of this intermediary metabolite to be 0.5 μM). Although such undersaturation would only permit velocities very much lower than the V_{max}, a cautionary note is in order, at least as far as carbamyl phosphate is concerned; this substrate is synthesized on the same polypeptide chain occupied by ATCase; as such, its molarity at the catalytic center of the enzyme might well be dramatically higher than that prevailing elsewhere in the cell sap. In other words, carbamyl phosphate might be channeled from the active site of CPS II to the adjacent active site of ATCase, and in this way the problem of undersaturation treated above might be circumvented. It follows that agents

TABLE II

L-ASPARTATE TRANSCARBAMYLASE (ATCASE)

L-Aspartic acid + carbamyl phosphate $\rightleftharpoons$ *N*-carbamyl-L-aspartic acid + phosphate

			References
a. Source: Ehrlich ascites cells			Bresnick and Mossé (1966)
b. pH optima: 8.5–9.2			Bresnick and Mossé (1966)
c. Michaelis constants for substrates:			
Substrate	K_m (μM)	Concentration of substrate in the cell (μM)	
L-Aspartic acid	2000–5000	100–2000	Shoaf and Jones (1973); Williamson and Brosnam (1974)
Carbamyl phosphate	3.5–50	1	Shoaf and Jones (1973); Huisman *et al.* (1979)
Phosphate	N.D.[a]	2680	Passonneau and Schulz (1974)
d. Specific activity: 1200 nmoles/mg protein/hour			Shoaf and Jones (1973)
e. Molecular weight: (carbamyl transferase fragment, see text) 145,000			Mori and Tatibana (1978)
f. Equilibrium position: strongly in the biosynthetic direction			Chang and Jones (1974)
g. Substrate specificity: β-OH-L-aspartic acid can replace L-aspartic acid; arsenate can replace phosphate; acetyl phosphate is not utilized by the mammalian enzyme			Jones (1974)

[a] Not determined.

TABLE III

L-DIHYDROOROTASE (DHOASE)

N-Carbamyl-L-aspartic acid + $H^+ \rightleftharpoons$ L-5,6-dihydroorotic acid + H_2O

			References
a. Source: Ehrlich ascites tumor cells			Shoaf and Jones (1973)
			Christopherson and Jones (1980)
b. pH optima: biosynthetic 4.4			Shoaf and Jones (1973)
degradative 8–9			Christopherson and Jones (1980)
c. Michaelis constants for substrates:			
Substrate	K_m (μM)	Concentration of substrate in the cell (μM)	
N-Carbamyl-L-aspartate (pH 7.4)	1000	N.D.[a]	Christopherson and Jones (1980)
L-Dihydroorotic acid (pH 7.4)	4.1	N.D.[a]	Christopherson and Jones (1980)
d. Specific activity: 13 nmoles/mg protein/hour			Shoaf and Jones (1973)
e. Molecular weight: 43,000–197,000			Mori and Tatibana (1978)
f. Equilibrium position: strongly in the degradative direction at pH 7.4			Shoaf and Jones (1973)
g. Substrate specificity: *N*-carbamyl-D-aspartic acid and D-5,6-dihydroorotic acid are also substrates			Christopherson and Jones (1980)

[a] Not determined.

which alter tertiary structures of this multifunctional enzyme ought to alter the efficiency of such channeling; 4 *M* urea, although it may be acting by other means, nearly abrogates the catalytic activity of ATCase from rat liver (Bresnick and Mossé, 1966).

Unlike CPS II, and more importantly unlike its counterpart in bacteria [which, as is well known, experiences extensive allosteric controls from the end-products of pyrimidine biosynthesis (Smith, 1977)], mammalian ATCase is refractory to inhibition by pyrimidine or purine nucleotides (Bresnick and Mossé, 1966; Shoaf and Jones, 1973). On the other hand, the reaction product, phosphate, is a good inhibitor of the enzyme, especially when the carbamyl phosphate concentrations are kept at or below the K_m, as they may be in the cytoplasm (Shoaf and Jones, 1973). In this case, 1 m*M* phosphate [a concentration one-third that occurring intracellularly (Passonneau and Schulz, 1974)] engenders approximately 50% inhibition of the enzyme.

Bresnick and Mossé (1966) have also observed that the substrate analogs succinate and oxaloacetate are competitive inhibitors of ATCase, with K_is of 3.3 and 6.8–6.9 m*M*, respectively; fumaric and malic acids were noninhibitory under comparable conditions. Since these constants reflect comparatively feeble inhibition, it is likely that dicarboxylic acids would assume regulatory importance toward ATCase only under conditions of L-aspartate depletion, such as can occur during starvation (Williamson and Brosnam, 1974).

C. L-DIHYDROOROTASE

DHOase (Table III) is the least well-studied of the first three enzymes of the pyrimidine pathway, but Mary Ellen Jones and her colleagues have published substantial contributions toward the characterization of this enzyme's activity in the recent biochemical literature. These workers have upset certain earlier, tentative contentions concerning mammalian DHOase, and confirmed others, such as the influence of pH on the catalytic activity of this enzyme and the role of naturally occurring thiols as inhibitors of it; they have also demonstrated that the ratio of reactants and products present after equilibrium is reached is remarkably pH dependent: thus, after equilibrium is reached at pH 4.4, which is the optimum of the biosynthetic or forward reaction, L-dihydroorotate predominates. However, at pH 7.4, *N*-carbamyl-L-aspartate is present at a concentration between 6 and 16 times that of L-dihydroorotate; and at pH 9.5, which is the optimum of the degradative or reverse reaction, the concentration of L-dihydroorotate at equilibrium is exiguous (Christopherson and Jones, 1980). It is noteworthy that the rates of the forward and reverse reaction, while both suboptimal, are equal at pH 7.1. This observation is consistent with the presence of a catalytic residue on the enzyme–substrate complex having a pK_a of 7.1; L-histidine appears to be the residue in question (Christopherson and Jones, 1980). Noteworthy, too, is the observation that the Michaelis constants of DHOase are also strongly and dramatically pH dependent, especially in the biosynthetic direction, where the affinity of the enzyme for *N*-carbamyl-L-aspartate falls two logs as the pH is raised from 7 to 8.3 (Christopherson and Jones, 1980). In brief, pH is crucially important to the functioning of DHOase for two reasons: it reflects a depression in the concentration of a true cosubstrate (H^+) as it is raised; and, it alters the ionization of the reactants, thereby modulating catalysis. Since small changes in the physiologic range of pH produce large changes in the biosynthesis of L-dihydroorotate, it is obvious that perturbations of acid–base balance might well trigger commensurate changes in pyrimidine biosynthesis at the level of DHOase. However, once again, a cautionary note is in order. As has been mentioned, DHOase and its two precursors exist as a complex with a molecular weight close to one million; since the microenvironment of such a huge molecule is bound to be various, it is difficult to extrapolate from pH effects observed *in vitro* to the case *in vivo*.

It is similarly difficult to assess the degree of saturation of DHOase *in vivo*, and this difficulty is enhanced by the paucity of information available on the concentrations of L-dihydroorotic and *N*-carbamyl-L-aspartic acids in either normal or neoplastic tissues. The one study providing data on the parameter used Ehrlich ascites carcinoma cells treated *in vitro* with 6-azauridine (see Section III,F,3) and so cannot be considered representative of the normal situation (Chen and Jones, 1979). (In the Appendix the problem of measuring these two intermediary metabolites is treated in greater detail.)

Of the normal body constituents known to interact with DHOase, L-cysteine and orotic acid are the most important. L-Cysteine at supraphysiological concentrations (100 m*M*) effects a time-dependent, irreversible inactivation of the enzyme. Christopherson and Jones (1980) suggest that this phenomenon is attributable to chelation of zinc from its active center. Inhibition by orotic acid is equally complicated: at pH 7.27, the apparent K_i for orotate, with *N*-carbamyl-L-aspartic acid as the variable substrate was 170 μM, but with L-dihydroorotate as the substrate, this value fell to approximately 10 μM (Christopherson and Jones, 1980). To reconcile these two disparate constants, it has been suggested that DHOase exists in radically different forms in the presence of substantial concentrations of its two major substrates. Although the intracellular concentration of orotic acid is ordinarily well below 10 μM, and so inconsequential as far as modulation is concerned, under certain pathologic and pharmacologic conditions this concentration is handily exceeded; in these instances at least, orotic acid might well act to retard the biologically counterproductive conversion of L-dihydroorotic acid to *N*-carbamyl-L-aspartic acid.

The specific activity of DHOase is, under certain conditions of analysis at least, numerically the lowest of any enzyme in the pyrimidine pathway (Shoaf and Jones, 1973). Although few students of the field have characterized it as rate-limiting in pyrimidine biosynthesis, during the state of orotic acid buildup, it very well might so function.

D. L-Dihydroorotate Dehydrogenase

The fourth enzyme of the pyrimidine biosynthetic pathway is unique in that it is particulate. Situated on the outer face of the inner mitochondrial membrane, DHO deHase is somewhat cloistered from the soluble complex which precedes it and that which follows it (see below). For efficient function, it is dependent on diffusion of its principal substrate and product through the mitochondrial membrane encasing it. Fortunately this outer membrane is freely permeable to both molecules and energy is not required for the translocations in question (Chen and Jones, 1976). The hydrogen ions abstracted from L-dihydroorotic acid by DHO deHase are conveyed to the mitochondrial respiratory chain in mammals; oxygen alone, in certain cases, is competent acceptor and superoxide anion is the product of this reaction (Forman and Kennedy, 1975). It follows that the function of this enzyme is linked to respiration, and that disruptions of respiration will ultimately perturb pyrimidine biosynthesis. This connection is elaborated on in Section III,D,2. For the moment, it is sufficient to observe that the identity of the proximate acceptor of the protons abstracted from L-dihydroorotate is probably a compound of the ubiquinone family (Kennedy, 1973) in mammals.

Table IV indicates that the specific activity of DHO deHase is rather low. In fact, on account of its topography in the cell, and its comparatively feeble specific activity, the enzyme might well participate in the regulation of the rate of flux through the pyrimidine biosynthetic pathway.[2]

In Ehrlich ascites carcinoma cells, the pH optimum of DHO deHase in the forward reaction centers about pH 8.3, but its pH profile is sufficiently sharp that only 35% of this optimal activity is expressed at pH 7.4. Since the exact pH of the membrane spaces wherein the enzyme resides is

[2] Indeed, in a recent review of the six pyrimidine biosynthetic enzymes, DHO deHase was denoted as exhibiting the lowest specific activity (Jones, 1980).

TABLE IV

L-DIHYDROOROTATE DEHYDROGENASE (DHO DEHASE)
L-5,6-Dihydroorotic acid ⟶ orotic acid + 2 H^+

			References
a. Source: Ehrlich ascites cells			Shoaf and Jones (1973)
b. pH optimum: 8.3			Shoaf and Jones (1973)
c. Michaelis constants for substrates:			
Substrate	K_m (μM)	Concentration of substrates *in vivo* (μM)	
L-5,6-Dihydroorotic acid	5	N.D.[a]	Kennedy (1973)
Orotic acid	N.D.[a]	Undetectable	Moyer and Handschumacher (1979)
d. Specific activity: 48 nmoles/mg protein/hour			Shoaf and Jones (1973)
e. Molecular weight: N.D.[a]			
f. Equilibrium position: irreversibly in the biosynthetic direction with the mitochondrial enzyme			Kennedy (1973)
g. Substrate specificity: D-5,6-dihydroorotic acid is probably not a substrate			Chen and Jones (1976)

[a] Not determined.

unknown, this feature may or may not be of relevance; for example, because enzyme activity falls dramatically and linearly as the pH is lowered (Shoaf and Jones, 1973) if the enzyme's domain is acidic, or acidified, it might cease to function in the biosynthetic direction.

The Michaelis constants of the enzyme for its substrates are low: 5 μM for L-dihydroorotic acid and about 8 μM for orotic acid. To put these values in perspective, it would be desirable to present the concentrations of both molecules in the cell sap, or better still, in the intermembranous space. This cannot as yet be done for L-5,6-dihydroorotate as was mentioned earlier; but there are suggestions in the literature that the concentration of orotic acid is, under ordinary circumstances, kept close to zero in the cell (Moyer and Handschumacher, 1979). Since the latter metabolite is a very potent inhibitor of the forward reaction, with a K_i of about 8 μM, the intracellular paucity of it serves to promote biosynthesis of the pyrimidine ring. In this connection, it is worthwhile stressing that virtually no other pyrimidine or purine nucleosides, nucleotides, or bases repress the function of DHO deHase to an important degree at physiologically attainable concentrations (Kennedy, 1973); D-DHO, however, is a feeble competitive inhibitor with a K_i of about 1 mM (Chen and Jones, 1976).

E. Orotate Phosphoribosyl Transferase

Fifth, in position of the enzymes of pyrimidine biosynthesis, is orotate (pyrimidine) phosphoribosyl transferase. Like the first three enzymes of the pathway (*pyr* 1–3), this protein coexists with its successor, orotidine-5′-monophosphate decarboxylase, as a soluble complex in the cytoplasmic space, and is designated *pyr* 5,6 (Jones, 1980).

In vivo, its equilibrium position is strongly in the biosynthetic direction (Jones *et al.*, 1978), but when the complex is digested into its constituent parts with the proteolytic enzyme, elastase, reversibility is readily demonstrable *in vitro*. The phosphoribosyl transferase activity exhibits a pH optimum in the vicinity of 7.75; at physiologic pH, about 75% of this optimal activity is expressed (Shoaf and Jones, 1973). In the biosynthetic reaction, both organic substrates are bound with affinities in the 2–16 μM range; however, if it is assumed that the intracellular concentration of orotic acid is close to zero (Moyer and Handschumacher, 1979) the enzyme will nevertheless be markedly undersaturated with respect to this substrate *in vivo*, unless orotic acid is somehow concentrated at the catalytic center. Conversely, the cytoplasmic concentration of PRPP is about $3 \times K_m$ in most tissues, thus permitting catalysis at a rate near the V_{max} (Kensler *et al.*, 1981a).

Of the physiologic agents capable of moderating the activity of OPRTase, pyrophosphate is the most potent, engendering 50% inhibition of the enzyme's activity at a concentration of 100 M (Jones *et al.*, 1978). No other physiologic phosphate ester, including the pyrimidine nucleoside mono-, di-, or triphosphates, exerts significant inhibition at physiologically meaningful concentrations; the same can be said of the purine nucleotides and bases (Jones *et al.*, 1978). As can be seen from Table V, the specific activity of OPRTase, at least in Ehrlich ascites carcinoma cells, is low—lower even than that of CPS II, which is customarily considered to be the rate-limiting step in the pathway. For this reason, Shoaf and Jones have suggested that the transferase may, in fact, regulate flux through the pathway, and that variations in the concentrations of its substrate, PRPP, may effect such regulation (Shoaf and Jones, 1973; Jones, 1980).

F. Orotidine-5′-Monophosphate Decarboxylase

OMP deCase can be coinduced and copurified with its predecessor in the pyrimidine pathway, and so is felt to exist as a physical complex with it in mammalian cells (Jones *et al.*, 1978). As can be appreciated from Table VI, this complex is substantially smaller than the multienzyme

TABLE V

OROTATE PHOSPHORIBOSYL TRANSFERASE (OPRTASE)

$$\text{Orotic acid} + \text{PRPP} \cdot Mg^{2+} \rightleftharpoons \text{OMP} + \text{pyrophosphate} \cdot Mg^{2+}$$

			References
a. Source: Ehrlich ascites cells			Shoaf and Jones (1978)
b. pH optimum: 7.75			Shoaf and Jones (1978)
c. Michaelis constants for substrates:			
Substrate	K_m (μM)	Concentration of substrates in the cell (μM)	
Orotic acid	2	Negligible	Jones *et al*. (1978); Moyer and Handschumacher (1979)
PRPP	16	50	Jones *et al*. (1978); Kensler *et al*. (1981a)
Mg^{2+}	2000–5000	25000	Jones *et al*. (1978); Guyton (1971)
OMP	N.D.[a]	0.05–0.10	Jones *et al*. (1978)
Pyrophosphate	N.D.[a]	10–15	Williamson and Brosnan (1974)
d. Specific activity: 10 nmoles/mg protein/hour			Jones *et al*. (1978)
e. Molecular weight of complex *pyr* 5,6: 55,000–110,000 (solvent dependent)			Jones *et al*. (1978)
f. Equilibrium position: Strongly in the biosynthetic direction when coupled to OMP deCase			Jones *et al*. (1978)
g. Substrate specificity: 5-Fluoroorotate is an alternative substrate for the yeast enzyme, whereas neither uracil nor 5-fluorouracil is accepted as substrates			Möllering (1975)
The mammalian enzyme, in contrast, can utilize both 5-FU and uracil			Reyes and Guganig (1979)

[a] Not determined.

TABLE VI

OROTIDINE-5′-MONOPHOSPHATE DECARBOXYLASE (OMP DECASE)
Orotidine-5′-monophosphate + Mg^{2+} ⟶ uridine-5′-monophosphate + CO_2

	References
a. Source: Ehrlich ascites cells	Jones *et al.* (1978)
b. pH optima: 7.0–7.5	Jones *et al.* (1978)
c. Michaelis constants for substrates:	
Substrate — K_m (μM) — Concentration of substrate in the cell	
OMP — 0.3 — <0.1 μM	Jones *et al.* (1978)
d. Specific activity: 150 nmoles/mg protein/hour	Jones *et al.* (1978)
e. Molecular weight of complex *pyr* 5,6: 55,000–110,000 (solvent dependent)	Reyes and Guganig (1975)
f. Equilibrium position: irreversibly in the biosynthetic direction	Jones *et al.* (1978)
g. Substrate specificity: 5-Fluoroorotidine-5′-monophosphate is decarboxylated	Möllering (1975)

complex *pyr* 1–3. The decarboxylase exhibits a pH optimum squarely in the physiologic range.

For all practical purposes, the reaction catalyzed by this enzyme is irreversible, a feature, which, barring blockages, makes flux through the antecedent steps inevitable, although it does not determine the rate of that flux. The enzyme exhibits a very high affinity for orotidine-5′-monophosphate (0.3 μM, although values 1 log higher than this also appear in the literature) and it is therefore believed to be responsible for maintaining the molar concentration of this nucleotide below 0.1 μM in the cell (Jones *et al.*, 1978). Once again, however, the concentration of orotidine-5′-monophosphate at the catalytic centers of the complex is unknown.

Endogenous regulators of the activity of OMP deCase are comparatively abundant: pyrophosphate and UMP are among the most potent, engendering about 70% inhibition at 1×10^{-4} M; CMP and the 5′-monophosphoric acid esters of the naturally occurring purine nucleosides are only somewhat less potent than this (Jones *et al.*, 1978). In general, the higher the degree of phosphorylation of this family of nucleotides, the lesser the inhibition exerted.

G. SUMMARY

In order that the relative velocities of the six enzymes of pyrimidine biosynthesis may be compared most easily in the context of the chemotherapeutic inhibitors about to be discussed, a compilation of their specific activities in four widely used murine tumors and four normal tissues sometimes susceptible to toxic damage from antimetabolites is presented in Table VII. It can be appreciated that all of the velocities are reasonably comparable in the neoplastic samples, but that each normal organ exhibits a rather distinctive profile of activity of the two complexes and the particulate enzyme. This suggests that a step rate-limiting in one type of cell may not so function in another. On the basis of the whole foregoing discourse, too, it might be suggested that there may be one or more rate-limiting steps in the pathway, depending on the physiologic and pharmacologic status of the organism; these might include CPS II, DHO deHase, and OPRTase. However, in view of the problem it could experience with substrate saturation, even ATCase, whose specific activity is most vigorous on the face of it, might act as a bottleneck to pyrimidine synthesis *in vivo*.

III. Inhibitors

A. Carbamyl Phosphate Synthetase II

Inasmuch as the synthesis of carbamyl phosphate is a critical, and very likely rate-limiting step in pyrimidine biosynthesis, the role of inhibitors of CPS II in chemotherapeusis merits attention, particularly in view of the fact that the substrates of CPS II are involved in many other cellular reactions and thus will not accumulate to toxic levels behind a blockade as can occur later in this pathway. Although a relative plethora of L-glutamine antagonists have been developed, none are specific for the L-glutamine-utilizing amidotransferase that synthesizes carbamyl phosphate. Several members of this class of drugs have been in clinical or experimental use for decades; versus human neoplasia they have generally proven to be inefficacious. One new drug, however, acivicin, is an exceptionally potent antagonist of L-glutamine, and may hold some therapeutic potential.

1. *Acivicin*

Acivicin (L-[αS,5S]-α-amino-3-chloro-4,5-dihydro-5-isoxazoleacetic acid) (Fig. 2) is an amino acid antibiotic elaborated by *Streptomyces sviceus*. Cooney *et al.* (1974) and Jayaram *et al.* (1975) have demonstrated that acivicin is a powerful inhibitor of many mammalian and bacterial reactions involving the transfer of nitrogen from the γ-carboxamide of L-glutamine: a concentration of 1 mM totally inhibited purified *E. coli* carbamyl phosphate synthetase and several mammalian amidotransferase

TABLE VII

SPECIFIC ACTIVITIES OF *de Novo* PYRIMIDINE BIOSYNTHETIC ENZYMES IN NORMAL AND NEOPLASTIC TISSUES OF THE MOUSE[a]

Enzyme	Tissue							
	Spleen	Liver	Duodenal mucosa	Bone marrow	L1210	P388	Lewis lung	B16 melanoma
Carbamyl phosphate synthetase II	1.5	5.7	0.2	2.2	4.2	6.2	1.0	1.7
L-Aspartate transcarbamylase	252	151	31	456	479	467	127	340
L-Dihydroorotase	28.4	6.8	7.2	40	67	73	22	47
L-Dihydroorotate dehydrogenase	0.7[b]	1.2[b]	0.1[b]	1.1[b]	113[c]	183[c]	41[c]	11[c]
Orotate phosphoribosyl transferase	7.0	7.3	0.3	8.3	4.9	14.5	4.3	7.5
Orotidine-5′-monophosphate decarboxylase	13.9	9.7	1.2	40.4	15	25	14	10

[a] nmoles/mg protein/hour.
[b] These values were obtained using whole homogenates.
[c] These values were obtained with isolated mitochondria.

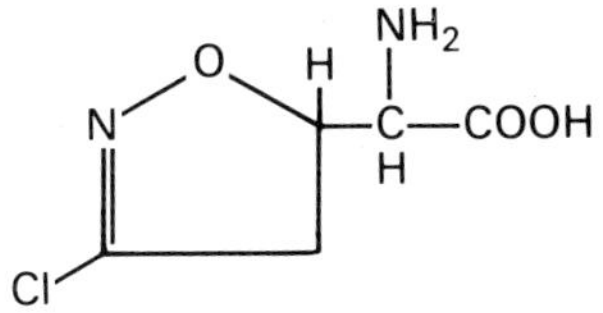

ACIVICIN

FIG. 2.

reactions involved in pyrimidine and purine biosynthesis, most notably: CTP synthetase, XMP aminase, and *N*-formylglycinamidine ribonucleotide synthetase. The cytostatic effects of acivicin on the growth of L1210 leukemia in culture can be reversed by the addition of L-glutamine, but not by other amino acids (Jayaram *et al.*, 1975).

The locus of action of acivicin remains ambiguous. Several studies suggest that inhibition of carbamyl phosphate synthetase may not be of primary importance for the therapeutic activity of this drug. For example, Jayaram *et al.* (1975) infer that the antibacterial activity of acivicin is not due to carbamyl phosphate synthetase inhibition by virtue of the observation that the ring-hydroxylated derivative of the drug, (αS,4S,5R)-α-amino-3-chloro-4-hydroxy-4,5-dihydro-5-isoxazolacetic acid, which lacks bacteriocidal activity, is an equally effective inhibitor of *E. coli* carbamyl phosphate synthetase. Neil *et al.* (1979) also present evidence that carbamyl phosphate synthetase is not a primary site for the antitumor activity of acivicin against L1210 leukemia. Following exposure of L1210 cells to acivicin, these workers observed a dramatic increase in UTP pools, rather than the expected decrease if *de novo* pyrimidine biosynthesis were markedly inhibited. CTP pools, on the other hand, decreased by 30%, leading to the suggestion that inhibition of CTP synthetase is the primary mode of action of the drug. However, addition of cytidine or deoxycytidine to acivicin-treated cultures does not reverse the inhibition of cell growth.

In contrast to the aforementioned studies, Kensler *et al.* (1981b) have investigated the effects of acivicin on mammalian CPS II activity directly. Administration of therapeutic doses of acivicin (10 to 100 mg/kg) to mice bearing Lewis lung carcinomas inhibits tumor CPS II activity up to 90%. Additionally, these doses inhibit the pyrazofurin-provoked accumulation of orotate and orotidine to a comparable degree, indicating that *de novo* pyrimidine biosynthesis is substantially compromised by treatment with acivicin *in vivo* (pyrazofurin is a fradulent nucleoside, that, after phosphorylation, inhibits OMP deCase: see Section III,E,1). Evaluation of a series of L-glutamine antagonists against either carbamyl phosphate synthetase from *E. coli* or partially purified from tumor also showed acivicin to be an exceptionally potent inhibitor *in vitro* (see Table IX). Clearly then, acivicin has a multiplicity of enzymic targets. CPS II is an important one of these, but cannot be considered unique in this regard.

An interesting aspect of acivicin activity is its age and sex-related toxicity in mice: younger mice and females are considerably more sensitive than adult male mice (Neil *et al.*, 1979). Coadministration of testosterone alleviates this toxicity, and serves to improve the therapeutic index. Perhaps not coincidently, 3-azauridine, an inhibitor of CTP synthetase, exhibits similar toxicologic characteristics. In mice, acivicin causes cumulative toxicity which is particularly marked in the gastrointestinal tract; however, repetitive dosing protocols are most carcinostatic. Repetitive dosing protocols may be therapeutically optimal because plasma clearance of acivicin in mice following a single administration is rapid (Jayaram *et al.*, 1981) and inhibition of tumor CPS II is transient (Kensler *et al.*, 1981b). Acivicin is presently undergoing phase I clinical trial.

2. *CONV, DON, and other* L*-Glutamine Antagonists*

CPS purified from *E. coli* consists of two nonidentical polypeptide chains; a heavy subunit which can catalyze the synthesis of carbamyl phosphate from ammonia, but not from L-glutamine, and a light subunit designed for the binding and hydrolysis of L-glutamine (Fig. 3). L-Glutamine binds to the light subunit and the amide nitrogen is then transfered to the heavy subunit where it is used for the synthesis of carbamyl phosphate (see Trotta *et al.*, 1973). In the course of studies on the reaction mechanism for bacterial CPS, Khedouri *et al.* (1966) synthesized a reagent that could react with the L-glutamine binding site of the enzyme without interfering with other catalytic functions. This agent, CONV (L-2-amino-4-oxo-5-chloropentanoic acid) (Fig. 3), severely impedes the ability of CPS to utilize L-glutamine as the nitrogen donor, while the utilization of ammonia remains unimpaired. Inhibition of L-glutamine-dependent CPS activity (CPS II) could be prevented by addi-

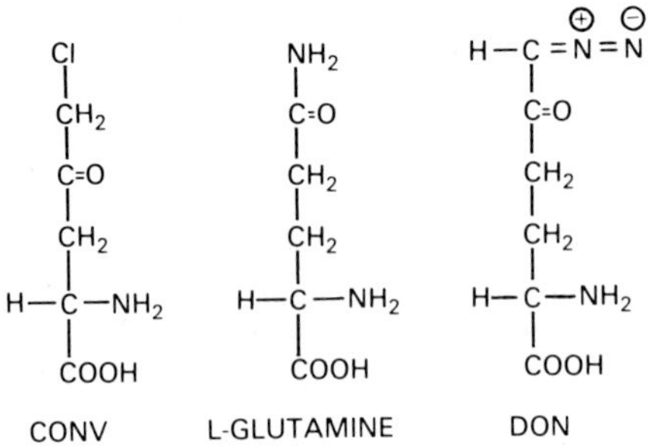

CONV	L-GLUTAMINE	DON
Cl	NH_2	$H-C=\overset{\oplus}{N}=\overset{\ominus}{N}$
CH_2	C=O	C=O
C=O	CH_2	CH_2
CH_2	CH_2	CH_2
$H-C-NH_2$	$H-C-NH_2$	$H-C-NH_2$
COOH	COOH	COOH

FIG. 3.

tion of L-glutamine, L-glutamyl-γ-hydroxamate, L-glutamate, and albizzin, another L-glutamine analog (Pinkus and Meister, 1972). Thus, CONV selectively reacts at the enzymic site on the light subunit that normally accepts L-glutamine, probably by alkylation of a cysteine residue. Sulfhydryl reagents such as the maleimides are also effective inhibitors of CPS II (Pinkus and Meister, 1972; and Section III,G). In a comparison of several L-glutamine antagonists as inhibitors of amidotransferase reactions, Jayaram *et al.* (1975) report that 1 m*M* CONV inhibits *E. coli* CPS activity by 61%. Acivicin (*supra*) totally inhibited activity at this concentration, whereas L-6-diazo-5-oxo-norvaline (DON) (Fig. 3) showed activity comparable to CONV; azaserine was inactive. While not characterized, the activity of CONV against mammalian CPS II has been observed (Jayaram *et al.*, 1976; Kensler *et al.*, 1981b; and Section III,G).

A number of L-glutamine antagonists have been developed as possible chemotherapeutic agents (for review, see Livingston *et al.*, 1970). As can be perceived from Table VIII, most of these agents are not profound inhibitors of CPS II, although, they are very effective inhibitors of other L-glutamine utilizing amidotransferase reactions. The two most studied drugs, biochemically and clinically, are DON and azaserine. Both have been shown to be effective inhibitors of *de novo* purine biosynthesis by blocking the conversion of *N*-formylglycinamide ribotide to *N*-formylglycinamidine ribotide (Moore and LePage, 1957). *N*-Formylglycinamide ribotide accumulates in tumors of drug-treated mice. Azaserine and DON also impinge upon pyrimidine biosynthesis, primarily at the amination step in the biosynthesis of cytidine nucleotides. However, in this instance, the concentration of DON required to inhibit completely the CTP synthetase reaction was at least 10 times the concentration required to inhibit completely *de novo* purine biosynthesis (Moore and Hurlbert, 1961), implying that the therapeutic activity of this drug was likely not a consequence of pyrimidine starvation. Of biochemical interest, though, Hager and Jones (1965) evaluated the effectiveness of DON, azaserine, and *O*-carbamyl-L-serine (a clinically unevaluated drug) as inhibitors of uridine nucleotide synthesis from [^{14}C]bicarbonate in Ehrlich ascites carcinoma cells. *O*-Carbamyl-L-serine was a particularly strong inhibitor when either no external nitrogen source was added or when ammonia was added. Inhibition was largely overcome when L-glutamine was added, suggesting that *O*-carbamyl-L-serine competes with L-glutamine for the same enzymic binding site. The relative potencies of these three drugs as inhibitors of amidotransferase reactions is DON > azaserine > *O*-carbamyl-L-serine; however, against CPS II from Ehrlich ascites cells the order is *O*-carbamyl-L-serine > DON > azaserine. (From the data presented in Table IX, it can be appreciated that *O*-carbamyl-L-serine is not a potent inhibitor of this enzyme from other murine tumors.) The specificity of *O*-carbamyl-L-serine is illustrated by the fact that its growth-inhibitory effects against *Lactobacillus arabinosus* are reversed by L-citrulline and uracil, products of the CPS I and II pathways (Ravel *et al.*, 1958). Preincubation of DON or azaserine for 5 minutes with the L-glutamine utilizing mammalian enzyme produced much more effective inhibition. Additionally, inhibition was irreversible, suggesting alkylation of the enzyme. By contrast, inhibition by *O*-carbamyl-L-serine was invariant with or without preincubation, implying a true competition with L-glutamine. Jayaram *et al.* (1976) evaluated the activity of CONV, DON, and DONV (5-diazo-4-oxo-L-norvaline), the next lower homolog to DON, as inhibitors of several fetal rat liver amidotransferases including CPS II. In these studies, at 1 m*M* concentrations, DON and CONV exerted similar inhibitory activities (~60%); DONV was nearly devoid of activity.

B. L-Aspartate Transcarbamylase

Although ATCase in *E. coli* catalyzes the first committed step in pyrimidine biosynthesis, this is not the case in mammalian cells. Unlike the bacterial enzyme, mammalian ATCase is not particularly sensitive to feedback or product inhibition by pyrimidines (Curci and Donachie, 1964). As a consequence, the most effective inhibitors of mammalian ATCase are analogs of the two substrates, carbamyl phosphate and L-aspartic acid, and, in particular, of the reaction transition-state intermediate.

1. *N-(Phosphonacetyl)-L-Aspartic Acid*

PALA [*N*-(phosphonacetyl)-L-aspartic acid] (Fig. 4) is a recently devised pyrimidine inhibitor and, in certain regards, the most distinctive. PALA was synthesized as a stable analog of the transition-state in the reaction catalyzed by ATCase (Collins and Stark, 1971) and, as such, combines the structural features of the two natural substrates, carbamyl phosphate and L-aspartic acid. Transition-state analogs offer attractive potentials as metabolic inhibitors because they can bind to their target enzymes with high affinity and specificity. In this instance, as best is known, ATCase is the only enzyme directly affected by PALA.

PALA produces competitive inhibition with carbamyl phosphate as the variable substrate, but is noncompetitive with respect to L-aspartic acid. The apparent K_i versus carbamyl phosphate is reported at 10^{-8} to 10^{-10} M for enzyme prepared from a variety of mammalian cell types (Hoogenraad, 1974; Kempe *et al.*, 1976; Kensler *et al.*, 1980b, 1981a; Jayaram *et*

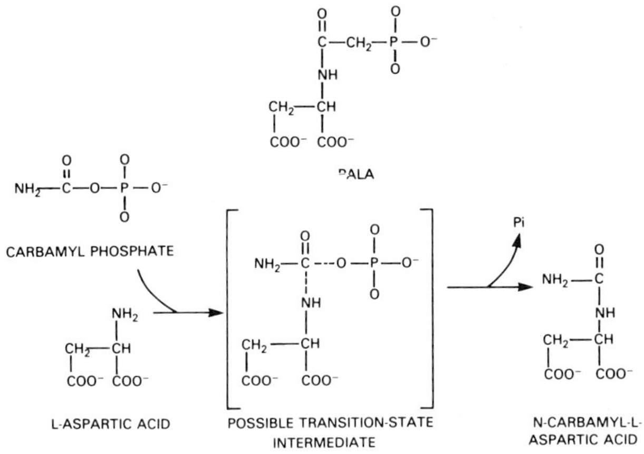

PALA

CARBAMYL PHOSPHATE

L-ASPARTIC ACID

POSSIBLE TRANSITION-STATE INTERMEDIATE

Pi

N-CARBAMYL-L-ASPARTIC ACID

FIG. 4.

al., 1979). Not only is inhibition potent, it is also persistant *in vivo*. Although enzyme inhibition by PALA is reversible, ATCase from mouse spleen (Yoshida *et al.*, 1974; Jayaram and Cooney, 1979), tumors (Jayaram *et al.*, 1979), and human leukocytes (Kensler *et al.*, 1980b) is inhibited for up to 2 weeks following PALA administration. This effect is probably a reflection of the slow terminal elimination phase of PALA. Mice treated with a single therapeutic dose (200 mg/kg) show PALA plasma concentrations well in excess of the K_i toward tissue ATCase for over 3 weeks after administration (Kensler *et al.*, 1980a). A similar protracted rate of clearance of PALA has been observed in humans (Kensler *et al.*, 1980b).

Micromolar concentrations of PALA exert cytostatic/cytotoxic effects on cell growth in culture. For example, continuous exposure to 20 μM PALA completely blocks the growth of Lewis lung carcinoma cells (Moyer and Handschumacher, 1979); ID_{50} concentrations against a variety of murine tumor lines grown *in vitro* are in the 2–50 μM range (Johnson *et al.*, 1978). PALA has an unusual spectrum of antitumor activity against transplantable murine tumors *in vivo*, particularly for an antimetabolite: it is curative against the Lewis lung carcinoma and very effective against other solid tumors, but is ineffective against murine leukemias (Johnson *et al.*, 1976, 1978). The effects of PALA on growth of cells in culture can be reversed by uridine (Swyryd *et al.*, 1974; Tsuboi *et al.*, 1977); moreover, the toxicity and antitumor activity of the drug can be reversed by uridine or *N*-carbamyl-DL-aspartate in mice (Johnson, 1977), showing, in both cases, that the effects of PALA are due specifically to blockade of *de novo* pyrimidine biosynthesis.

A number of biochemical observations reinforce this mode of action for

PALA. PALA has been shown to deplete UTP pools of cultured hepatoma cells (Keppler, 1977), transformed hamster cells (Johnson *et al.*, 1978), and Lewis lung cells (Moyer and Handschumacher, 1979). Substantial depressions in pyrimidine nucleotide pool sizes have also been described following PALA treatment of Lewis lung carcinomas *in vivo* (Moyer and Handschumacher, 1979; Kensler *et al.*, 1981a). Treatment of tumor cells in culture with PALA also reduces the incorporation of $NaH[^{14}C]CO_3$ into pyrimidine nucleotides and intermediates (Tsuboi *et al.*, 1977; Kensler *et al.*, 1981a). In another dynamic approach, Moyer and Handschumacher (1979) have used the accumulation of orotate and orotidine provoked by pyrazofurin as a monitor of *de novo* pyrimidine biosynthesis. Concurrent treatment with PALA of mice bearing Lewis lung carcinomas abrogates this pyrazofurin-provoked accumulation of orotate and orotidine in tumor while substantial accumulation continues in host tissues such as spleen. The basis for this differential tissue susceptibility to PALA remains undefined, though it undoubtedly relates to the biochemical parameters that control PALA sensitivity and resistance in tumors discussed *infra*.

In cultured hamster cells continuously exposed to PALA, the emergence of resistant variants is associated with elevation of the target enzyme (Kempe *et al.*, 1976). Coleman *et al.* (1977) have purified the CPS II–ATCase–DHOase oligomer (*pyr* 1–3) from one of these mutant lines and find it to represent nearly 10% of the total cellular protein: an approximately 100-fold overaccumulation. This increase in ATCase activity is due to an increase in its rate of synthesis which is accompanied by an increase in the amount of a single mRNA which directs the production of this oligomer *in vitro* (Padgett *et al.*, 1979).

A comparison of cultured cell lines from PALA-sensitive solid tumors and PALA-refractory leukemias suggests that naturally occurring resistance to the drug is also associated with high ATCase activity (Johnson *et al.*, 1978). A similar evaluation in transplantable murine tumors growing *in vivo* shows that ATCase activity is significantly higher in PALA-refractory as opposed to PALA-sensitive tumors (Jayaram *et al.*, 1979). However, among tumors sensitive to PALA, there is no clearcut relationship between target enzyme activity and degree of sensitivity to PALA. Additionally, Kensler *et al.* (1981a) have described the emergence of a resistant variant of the Lewis lung carcinoma that has an ATCase activity identical to that of the parent, PALA-sensitive, line. A comprehensive evaluation of parameters in addition to ATCase activity likely to influence PALA sensitivity *in vivo* suggest that uptake and metabolism of PALA, kinetics of inhibition of ATCase, kinetics of uridine uptake and catabolism of pyrimidines or pyrimidine nucleosides are not important determinants. Activities of the salvage pathway, which could influence the response of tumors to PALA by reducing the dependence on the *de novo* pyrimidine pathway for nucleic acid synthesis, and of CPS II, which could serve to diminish ATCase inhibition by producing augmented levels of the competitive substrate carbamyl phosphate, have been suggested as contributing modifiers to PALA response (Jayaram *et al.*, 1979; Kensler *et al.*, 1981a).

PALA is presently undergoing clinical trial; phase I studies demonstrate dose-limiting toxicities in the skin and gastrointestinal tract, while little myelosuppression is observed (Erlichman *et al.*, 1979). However, the antineoplastic utility of PALA, at least as a single agent, appears limited. As an antimetabolite of well-defined specificity, the role of PALA in drug combination protocols is beginning to receive attention. At present, there are no other clinical uses for PALA, but the finding of Ardalan *et al.* (1981) demonstrating the tremendous avidity of bone for the drug, suggests that PALA may have utility toward the management of proliferative diseases of bone.

2. *Analogs of Carbamyl Phosphate*

Porter *et al.* (1969) have evaluated a series of carbamyl phosphate analogs as inhibitors of *E. coli* ATCase. All analogs with a phosphate or phosphate dianion were competitive inhibitors, albeit not potent. For example, *N,N'*-dimethylcarbamyl phosphate, *N*-methylcarbamyl phosphate, acetylphosphate, and phosphonoacetic acid (Fig. 5) have K_is in the 0.1 to 0.5 m*M* range. Inhibition of ATCase by phosphonoacetic acid is of particular interest because this drug is a specific and potent ($ID_{50} = 1\ \mu M$) inhibitor of herpes virus replication (Overby *et al.*, 1974). However, antiviral activity is apparently accomplished by direct binding of phosphonoacetic acid to viral-induced DNA polymerase (Leinback *et al.*, 1976); uninfected host cell polymerases are up to 1000-fold less sensitive to inhibition by the compound (Overby *et al.*, 1977). Because of its dual sites of action, phosphonoacetic acid might be a valuable tool for deranging nucleic acid metabolism in tumors. To date, however, the agent has been used only in a small number of cases where it proved to exhibit limited activity (Table VIII).

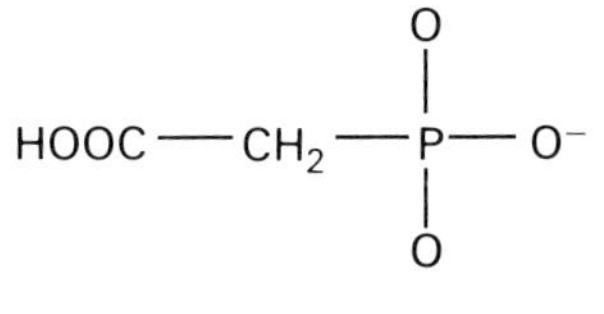

$$HOOC-CH_2-\overset{\overset{\displaystyle O}{|}}{\underset{\underset{\displaystyle O}{|}}{P}}-O^-$$

PHOSPHONOACETIC ACID

FIG. 5.

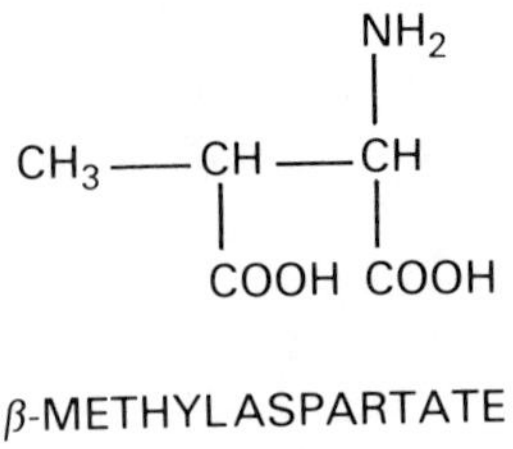

FIG. 6.

3. *Analogs of L-Aspartic Acid*

Several natural analogs of L-aspartic acid have been reported as inhibitors of ATCase in *E. coli*. β-Methylaspartate (Fig. 6) is a natural metabolite formed by the vitamin B_{12}-catalyzed isomerization of glutamic acid (Barker *et al.*, 1958). Isenberg *et al.* (1960) demonstrated that this amino acid could be a substrate for thymine biosynthesis in certain thymine-requiring microorganisms. By contrast, Woolley (1960) found β-methylaspartate to be an inhibitor of the growth of *E. coli* at micromolar concentrations. This inhibition was reversed competitively and completely by L-aspartic acid and those amino acids which readily yield L-aspartic acid: L-glutamine, L-histidine, and L-asparagine. Growth inhibition could also be overcome by addition of the pyrimidine precursors *N*-carbamyl-L-aspartate and L-dihydroorotate, findings which implicate ATCase in the site of inhibitory action. In our hands, β-methylaspartate is a poor inhibitor of murine tumor ATCase, *in vitro* (Table IX).

Using purified ATCase from *E. coli*, Porter *et al.* (1969) reported that several dicarboxylic acids were competitive inhibitors with respect to L-aspartic acid; succinate and maleate were the strongest of these with K_is in the range of 0.5 to 5 m*M*. Similar results have been observed with partially purified rat liver ATCase (Bresnick and Mossé, 1966). The chemotherapeutic activities of several other analogs of L-aspartate have been recently reviewed (Jayaram and Cooney, 1979); however, most analogs discussed therein, such as L-alanosine and PA_2LA [3-(phosphoacetylamido)-L-alanine], are inactive *in vitro* as inhibitors of mammalian ATCase (Table IX), although L-alanosine is carbamylated by the enzyme.

4. *Heavy Metals*

Heavy metals (Fig. 7) inhibit the activity of enzymes containing sulfhydryl groups. Bresnick and Mossé (1966) demonstrated that rat liver ATCase could be inhibited by Ag^+, Hg^{2+}, or Zn^{2+} and that this inhibition could be

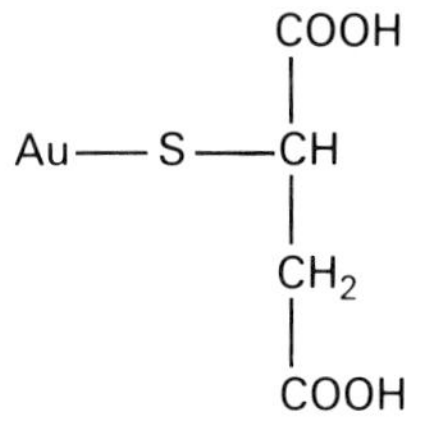

COOH
|
Au—S—CH
|
CH_2
|
COOH

AUROTHIOMALATE

FIG. 7.

prevented by mercaptoethanol. Westwick *et al*. (1974) found that sodium aurothiomatate was an effective inhibitor of ATCase activity in extracts of human peripheral granulocytes. Gold salts are beneficial in the treatment of rheumatoid arthritis; however, neutropenia is a toxic manifestation of therapy. These investigators suggested that this aurothiomatate-induced neutropenia was a consequence of inhibition of pyrimidine biosynthesis.

C. L-DIHYDROOROTASE

The cyclization of *N*-carbamyl-L-aspartate to L-dihydroorotate is accomplished through dehydration by DHOase, the third enzyme of the cytosolic complex that initiates pyrimidine biosynthesis. Study of the regulation of this enzyme and, in particular, the generation of effective and specific inhibitors is notably lacking. As a result, the array of DHOase inhibitors has essentially remained static for two decades. Several classes of compounds are discussed with respect to their activities against DHOase, but in no case are they specific antagonists of this enzyme. Additionally, their utility as chemotherapeutic inhibitors of pyrimidine biosynthesis remains largely untested.

1. *5-Substituted Analogs of Orotic Acid*

Bresnick and Hitchings (1961) reported the inhibition of DHOase activity in high-speed supernatants of Ehrlich ascites tumor cells by a large number of pyrimidines and pyrimidine analogs. Orotic acid, orotidine, and 5-fluoroorotate were relatively effective inhibitors. Pyrimidine nucleosides, and to a limited degree nucleotides, were also reported as feedback inhibitors of this enzyme. The activities of the endogenous regulators of DHOase activity have been discussed in Section II,C.

In view of the pronounced activity of fluorinated pyrimidines as inhibitors of nucleic acid biosynthesis, Smith and Sullivan (1960) evaluated the

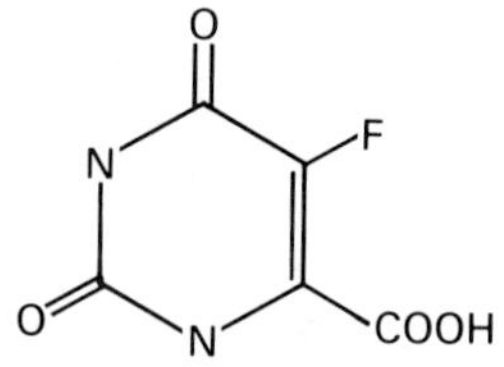

5-FLUOROOROTIC ACID

FIG. 8.

activity of 5-fluoroorotic acid (Fig. 8) as an inhibitor of *E. coli* DHOase and found it to be about 8-fold more potent than orotic acid; inhibition was competitive against *N*-carbamyl-L-aspartic acid, with an apparent K_i of 1.5 m*M*. Christopherson and Jones (1980) have undertaken a very systematic evaluation of the inhibitory effects of 5-substituted analogs of orotate, including 5-fluoroorotate, against mammalian enzyme. They tabulated the apparent K_i values (micromolar) using either *N*-carbamyl-L-aspartate or L-dihydroorotate as variable substrate. The 5-fluoro, 5-amino, and 5-methyl derivatives of orotate are more effective inhibitors of DHOase than unsubstituted orotate. 5-Bromoorotate is a more effective inhibitor than orotate when *N*-carbamyl-L-aspartate is substrate, but less effective than orotate when L-dihydroorotate is substrate; 5-iodoorotate is a less effective inhibitor than orotate using either substrate. As seen with orotate, the apparent K_i values for these inhibitors are considerably lower when L-dihydroorotate is the variable substrate, as opposed to *N*-carbamyl-L-aspartate. Additionally, they note that the apparent K_i values for the orotate derivatives increase with a corresponding increase in the size of the 5-substituent, indicating some steric hindrance to binding with bulky substituents.

At variance with some of the findings of Bresnick and Hitchings (1961), both Kennedy (1974) and Christopherson and Jones (1980) found that orotic acid was the only natural pyrimidine to inhibit DHOase activity. Toward their respective purified rat liver and Ehrlich ascites enzymes, the following pyrimidines and analogs have been reported as ineffective inhibitors: orotidine, OMP, cytosine, cytidine, CMP, CDP, CTP, thymine, thymidine, TMP, TDP, TTP, UMP, UDP, UTP, 5-fluorouracil, barbituric acid, dihydrouracil, dihydrothymine, and 6-azauracil.

2. *Analogs of N-Carbamyl-L-Aspartate*

Smith *et al.* (1960) synthesized five analogs of *N*-carbamyl-L-aspartate for evaluation as inhibitors of DHOase from a number of bacterial and

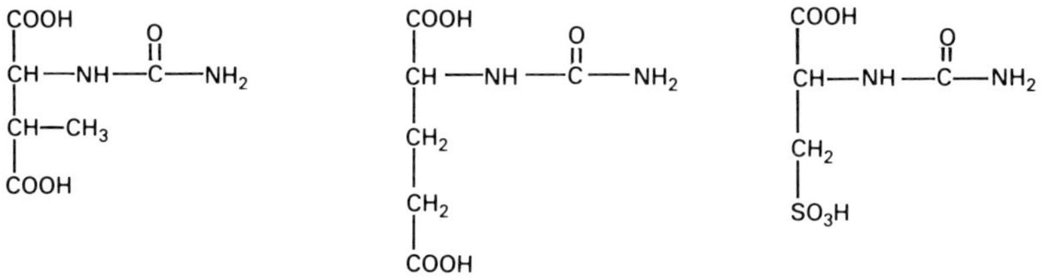

$HOOC{-}CH(CH_3){-}CH(COOH){-}NH{-}C(=O){-}NH_2$ — α-UREIDO-β-METHYLSUCCINATE

$HOOC{-}CH_2{-}CH_2{-}CH(COOH){-}NH{-}C(=O){-}NH_2$ — CARBAMYLGLUTAMATE

$HO_3S{-}CH_2{-}CH(COOH){-}NH{-}C(=O){-}NH_2$ — CARBAMYLCYSTEIC ACID

FIG. 9.

mammalian sources. α-Ureido-β-methylsuccinate, carbamylglutamate, and carbamylcysteic acid (Fig. 9) were of approximately equal inhibitory activity against the rat liver enzyme: however, millimolar concentrations were required for 50% inhibition. When measured in extracts of *E. coli*, inhibition of DHOase activity by these three analogs was competitive with *N*-carbamyl-L-aspartate as variable substrate, and the apparent K_i for α-ureido-β-methylsuccinate was 1.7×10^{-5} *M*. The other two synthetic analogs, carbamylcysteine-sulfinic acid and carbamylasparagine, were considerably less active. Christopherson and Jones (1980) have reported that the following *N*-carbamyl-L-aspartate analogs were inactive as DHOase inhibitors when tested at 5 m*M* against purified DHOase from Ehrlich ascites carcinoma: *N*-carbamyl-β-alanine, *N*-carbamyl-L-α-alanine, *N*-carbamyl-L-glutamate, *N*-acetyl-L-aspartate, fumarate, maleate, malonate, and succinate. The effectiveness of any of the analogs of *N*-carbamyl-L-aspartate as inhibitors of nucleic acid biosynthesis *in vivo,* or as carcinostatic agents, remains undefined.

3. *Sulfonamides*

The sulfonamides were the first effective chemotherapeutic drugs to be systematically utilized for the cure of bacterial infections in man; even with the advent of the fungal antibiotics, they continue to hold a prominent role in the modern pharmacopeia. The bacteriostatic activity of the sulfonamides is thought to result from competitive antagonism with *p*-aminobenzoic acid; thus, they are inhibitors of folic acid biosynthesis (Woods, 1962). However, the sulfonamides can also interfere with other enzymatic reactions. In cell-free extracts of *E. coli*, sulfonamides inhibit formation of dihydropteric acid from *p*-aminobenzoic acid and 2-amino-4-hydroxy-6-hydroxy-methyldihydropteridine in the presence of ATP-Mg^{2+} (Brown, 1962). Substituted sulfonamides with the general structure, $R_1{-}SO_2{-}NH_2$ also inhibit carbonic anhydrase, presumably by binding within

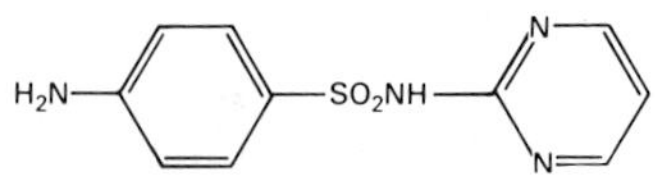

FIG. 10.

the coordination sphere of the Zn^{2+} cation at the active site of the enzyme (Maren, 1963). Inhibition constants are in the micromolar range (Taylor *et al.*, 1970).

Pradham and Sander (1973) have reported that substituted sulfonamides inhibit semipurified DHOase from *Zymobacterium oroticum*. Inhibition was noncompetitive with respect to *N*-carbamyl-L-aspartate; K_is ranged from 0.2 to 5 m*M*. Sulfadiazine (Fig. 10), one of the clinically more prominent sulfonamides, was the most potent inhibitor. Interestingly, this was the only derivative tested to contain a pyrimidine substituent on the sulfonamide nitrogen. The mechanism of inhibition is unclear, although the authors suggest that, as in the case of carbonic anhydrase, the sulfonamides may add a coordinating ligand to the Zn^{2+} atom of DHOase, thus competing with water and/or hydroxide ion at the active site. As was discussed earlier, recent work by Christopherson and Jones (1980) suggests that the mammalian enzyme also contains Zn^{2+} at its active site, inasmuch as dialysis against L-cysteine, a particularly effective zinc chelator, eliminates enzyme activity. However, with the exception of *p*-nitrobenzenesulfonamide, which these workers found to be inactive, the influence of sulfonamides on mammalian DHOase is as yet, largely untested. It is noteworthy in this context, that sulfadiazine was virtually inert as an inhibitor of DHOase from four murine tumors (Table IX).

D. L-DIHYDROOROTATE DEHYDROGENASE

Inhibition of the mitochondrial enzyme involved in *de novo* pyrimidine biosynthesis, DHO deHase, is accomplished by two general classes of compounds. In common with other enzymes of this pathway, DHO deHase is subject to product inhibition; orotic acid and some of its analogs are effective inhibitors (cf. Section II). Additionally, naphthoquinones have been recently identified as potent inhibitors of DHO deHase. These drugs may act as analogs of the cofactor, ubiquinone, and serve as electron acceptors that alter electron flow. Other inhibitors of electron transfer such as cyanide, thenoyltrifluoroacetone, antimycin, and 2,4-dinitrophenol can also interfere with DHO deHase activity, but in nonspecific manners (Miller and Curry, 1969; Forman and Kennedy, 1975;

Chen and Jones, 1976). As such, the therapeutic utility of these latter metabolic inhibitors is limited.

1. *Orotic Acid and Analogs*

DHO deHase from rat liver mitochondria is strongly inhibited by the enzymic product, orotate; inhibition is competitive, with a K_i of 8.4 μM, and is specific for this pyrimidine intermediate (Chen and Jones, 1976). Among all the possible intermediates of pyrimidine biosynthesis and pyrimidine nucleotides, only orotate inhibits DHO deHase. Interestingly, 5-fluoroorotate, which is an effective inhibitor of DHOase and OPRTase, was without inhibitory activity against DHO deHase prepared from *Zymobacterium oroticum*. In fact, use of 5-fluoroorotate as substrate increased the V_{max} by 50% for the reverse or reductive activity of the enzyme, although little differences were observed in the K_is for either 5-fluoroorotate or orotate (Friedmann and Vennesland, 1958). These authors also demonstrated enzyme inhibition by the analogs 2,4-dihydroxy-6-methyl pyrimidine and barbituric acid (Fig. 11). Several investigators (Wuu and Krooth, 1968; Chen and Jones, 1976; and Potvin *et al*., 1978) have subsequently shown inhibition of mammalian DHO deHase by barbituric acid to be competitive and potent: $K_i = 56\ \mu M$ for rat liver enzyme. Barbiturates, such as barbital, are inactive.

Santilli *et al.* (1968) synthesized dihydro-5-azaorotate from 5-azaorotate as a possible analog of L-dihydroorotate. An evaluation of this analog was made by incubating L-[^{14}C]dihydroorotic acid with mouse liver homogenate and measuring the generation of radiolabeled *N*-carbamyl-L-aspartate and orotate. The addition of dihydro-5-azaorotate at concentrations of 10^{-4} to 10^{-3} *M* inhibited the conversion to [^{14}C]orotic acid, but was without affect on *N*-carbamyl-L-[^{14}C]aspartate formation, indicating that the drug was an inhibitor of DHO deHase, but not DHOase. Additionally, in contrast to the parent compound, 5-azaorotate, the dihydro derivative was without effect on the OPRTase and OMP deCase steps. Dihydro-5-azaorotate inhibited the growth of *Agrobacterium*

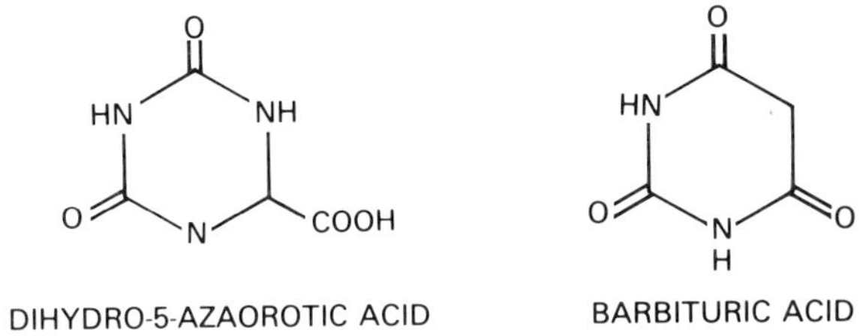

FIG. 11.

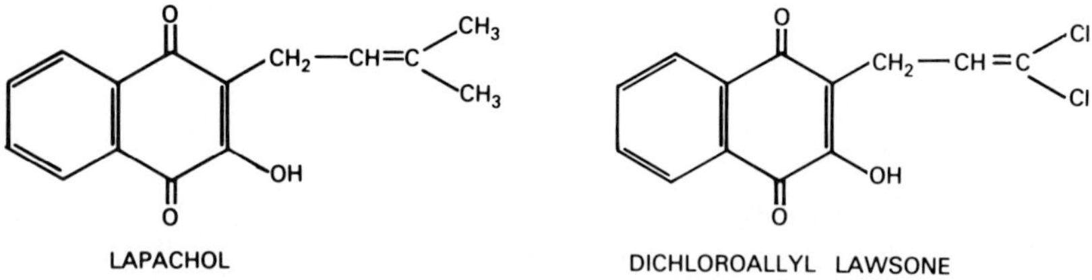

LAPACHOL

DICHLOROALLYL LAWSONE

FIG. 12.

tumefaciens and *E. coli* ($ID_{50} \simeq 2$ mM), and this inhibition could be reversed by the addition of preformed pyrimidines.

2. *Naphthoquinones*

A number of naphthoquinones are known to possess antimalarial (Fieser *et al*., 1948), antitrypanosomal (Lopes *et al*., 1978), and antitumor activity (Rao *et al*., 1968; Driscoll *et al*., 1974; Sieber *et al*., 1976). Lapachol [2-hydroxy-3-(3-methyl-2-butenyl)-1,4-naphthoquinone] (Fig. 12), an extract of the Indian plant *Stereospermum suavolens,* inhibited growth of the Walker 256 tumor. However, lapachol is without antitumor activity in humans, apparently because gastrointestinal toxicity becomes dose-limiting at subtherapeutic plasma concentrations (Loo *et al*., 1978). An extensive search has been conducted for other quinones that possess antitumor activity (Driscoll *et al*., 1974). Acetylglucosylation of lapachol results in a compound which, unlike the parent, is effective against P-388 murine leukemia (da Consolacão *et al.,* 1975). Dichloroallyl lawsone (Fig. 12), a synthetic analog of lapachol containing chlorine atoms in place of methyl groups, has received expanded attention as a congener of lapachol. It was hoped that the increased lipophilicity of dichloroallyl lawsone would offer some pharmacokinetic advantages over the parent compound. In fact, in experimental systems, dichloroallyl lawsone has greater activity and a better therapeutic index than lapachol (Chadwick and Chang, 1973; Chadwick *et al*., 1976). Dichloroallyl lawsone is not myelosuppressive and shows little gastrointestinal toxicity. However, high doses of dichloroallyl lawsone induce acute cardiotoxicity in primates which may limit the therapeutic usefulness of this drug (McKelvey *et al*., 1979).

Many naphthoquinones including both lapachol and dichloroallyl lawsone interfere with electron transport and act as respiratory poisons (Ball *et al.,* 1947; Gosálvez *et al.,* 1976). These drugs cause intense respiratory inhibition in Ehrlich ascites tumor *in vivo* (Gosálvez *et al.,* 1976). Other studies by these investigators using mitochondria isolated from rat liver demonstrate that lapachol and dichloroallyl lawsone behave as oligomycin-type inhibitors of respiration. Lapachol has also been shown to uncouple oxidative phosphorylation (Howland, 1963a) and to inhibit succinate oxidation (Howland, 1963b) and 3α-hydroxysteroid-mediated transhydrogenase (Koide, 1962).

Bennett *et al.* (1979) have presented compelling evidence to suggest that, although many enzymes may be inhibited, the primary mode of antitumor activity for dichloroallyl lawsone is inhibition of pyrimidine biosynthesis, at the level of DHO deHase. Conducting experiments in cultured L1210 cells, they demonstrated that dichloroallyl lawsone stimulates the utilization of [^{14}C]uridine, reduced UTP pools, inhibits pyrazofurin-induced accumulation of orotate and orotidine, and exerts cytotoxicity that can be reversed (80–85%) by addition of uridine to the cultures. The inhibition of pyrimidine nucleotide biosynthesis in intact cells was confirmed in homogenates, where dichloroallyl lawsone inhibited the conversion of [^{14}C]carbamyl phosphate to orotate, but not its conversion to L-dihydroorotate. These findings collectively pointed to DHO deHase as the site of pyrimidine blockade. Studies with isolated mitochondria from mouse liver demonstrated that inhibition of DHO deHase was uncompetitive with respect to L-dihydroorotate; the apparent K_i was 2.7×10^{-8} *M*. A similar, though less potent action was also established for lapachol; in this instance the K_i was 2.1×10^{-6} *M*. Dehydrogenase from *Zymobacterium oroticum* was not inhibited by dichloroallyl lawsone, presumably because the mammalian enzyme uses ubiquinone as an electron acceptor, whereas the *Z. oroticum* enzyme utilizes NAD. Postulating the role of dichloroallyl lawsone as a ubiquinone analog, these authors suggest that other ubiquinone analogs known to possess antitumor activity and to inhibit nucleic acid synthesis *in vitro* (Folkers *et al.*, 1978) may act in a manner similar to dicholoroallyl lawsone. This possibility awaits experimental verification.

Westwick *et al.* (1972) have demonstrated that the antiinflammatory agent phenylbutazone, which like lapachol uncouples oxidative phosphorylation (Whitehouse, 1965), is also a potent inhibitor of DHO deHase. Enzyme activity assayed in disrupted human granulocytes was inhibitable by micromolar concentrations of phenylbutazone: however, the kinetics of this inhibition were not investigated.

E. Orotate Phosphoribosyl Transferase

OPRTase exists as a soluble multienzyme complex with OMP deCase in mammalian cells. As a result, it becomes a difficult task to segregate the actions of inhibitors on one enzyme from the other. Nonetheless, a num-

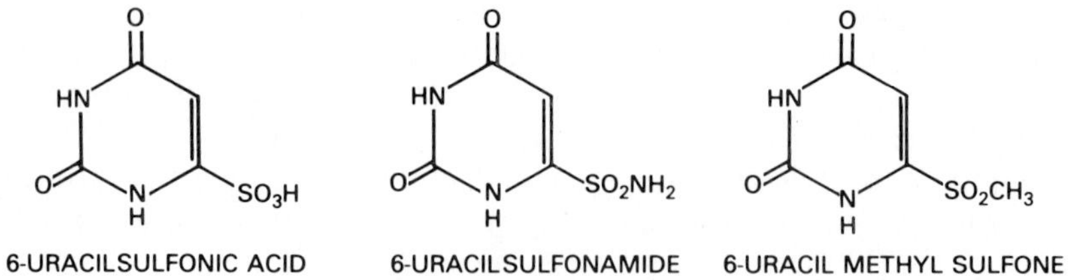

6-URACILSULFONIC ACID 6-URACILSULFONAMIDE 6-URACIL METHYL SULFONE

FIG. 13.

ber of orotic acid analogs have been described as OPRTase inhibitors; many are also substrates for this enzyme. The fraudulent ribotides so formed can be potent inhibitors of the second enzyme in the complex.

1. *6-Uracilsulfonic Acids*

The earliest antagonists of OPRTase were the 6-uracilsulfonic acids. 6-Uracilsulfonic acid ($K_i = 7 \times 10^{-6}\ M$), 6-uracilsulfonamide ($K_i = 3.9 \times 10^{-4}\ M$), and 6-uracil methyl sulfone ($K_i = 7.1 \times 10^{-4}\ M$) (Fig. 13) are competitive inhibitors of yeast OPRTase (Holmes, 1956). No anabolism to phosphate derivatives has been demonstrable. The rationale for the synthesis of these compounds was based on the established antimetabolic activity of sulfonic acids, sulfonamides, and substituted sulfones analogous to certain naturally occurring carboxylic acids; in this instance, the correlate was orotic acid. These orotic acid analogs inhibited microbial growth (Holmes and Welch, 1956), but showed limited carcinostatic activity due to host toxicity (Jaffee and Cooper, 1958).

2. *5-Substituted and Other Orotic Acid Analogs* (*Fig. 14*)

In a comprehensive approach to the study of OPRTase inhibitors, Traut and Jones (1977a,b) examined a series of natural purines and pyrimidines

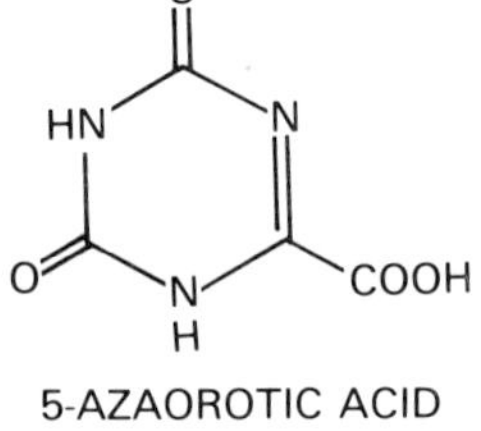

5-AZAOROTIC ACID

FIG. 14.

as well as synthetic analogs against enzyme prepared from mouse Ehrlich ascites cells. Of particular merit in this report was the attempt to approximate physiological substrate concentrations and the use of an OMP deCase-independent assay that would be kinetically uncompromised for the inhibition measurements. 5-Fluoroorotate was the most potent inhibitor tested: 50 μM 5-fluoroorotate inhibited activity by 75%. Dahl *et al.* (1959) had previously described 5-fluoroorotate as an excellent competitive substrate for yeast OPRTase. Other 5-substituted derivatives, bromo-, chloro-, amino-, nitro-, and methylorotate, were not active against the yeast enzyme. Stone and Potter (1957) observed that 5-fluoroorotate inhibited the conversion of orotic acid to orotidine-5′-monophosphate in rat liver supernatants; 5-bromo and 5-chloroorotate were also active. Halogenated derivatives of uracil were weak inhibitors in the Traut and Jones study. Concordantly, Reyes and Guganig (1975) report 5-fluorouracil to be a competitive inhibitor of OPRTase, but with a K_i of only 1.9 mM. Those synthetic pyrimidine and purine base analogs, which following ribotide formation are extremely potent OMP deCase inhibitors (Section III,F), are, in general, inhibitors of OPRTase: i.e., allopurinol, oxipurinol, 6-azauridine, 6-azauracil, barbituric acid, and 5-azaorotate (Traut and Jones, 1977a,b; Potvin *et al.*, 1978; Rubin *et al.*, 1964). The activity of these base analogs is not particularly profound, although, in the instance of 5-azaorotate, notable potency is observed ($K_i = 5 \times 10^{-7}\ M$) (Rubin *et al.*, 1964). In large measure, the impact of these OPRTase inhibitors on pyrimidine biosynthesis is likely to be a consequence of subsequent anabolism to highly potent ribotide inhibitors of the adjacent enzyme, OMP deCase. As a result the segregated use of these drugs as specific biochemical tools must be approached cautiously.

F. Orotidine-5′-Monophosphate Decarboxylase

The inhibitors of the last of the *de novo* biosynthetic enzymes, OMP deCase, are comparatively well studied, reflective, in part, of the well-defined clinical utility of several of these drugs. Evaluations of the mechanisms of action, metabolism and drug resistance for the OMP deCase inhibitors seem to reiterate a common theme of action, namely, the anabolism of a pyrimidine analog to the 5′-monophosphate derivative which, in turn, is a competitive inhibitor of OMP deCase.

1. *Pyrazofurin*

Pyrazofurin (3-β-D-ribofuranosyl-4-hydroxypyrazole-5-carboxamide) (Fig. 15), an isolate from the fermentation broth of a strain of *Streptomyces*

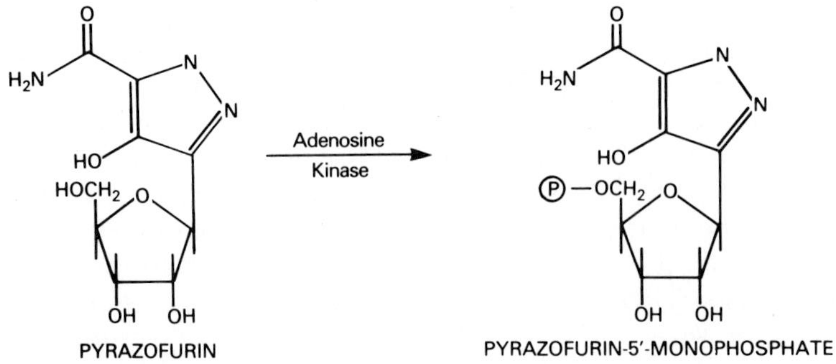

FIG. 15.

candidus, shows a limited antifungal activity *in vitro* but exhibits considerable activity against vaccinia virus and Friend leukemia virus *in vitro* and in mice (DeLong *et al.*, 1971; and Streightoff *et al.*, 1969). The presence of the pyrazole nucleus in this C-nucleoside apparently confers additional activities, for although C-nucleosides, in general, have some antifungal and antibacterial activities, few have antitumor activity (Gerzon *et al.*, 1971). Pyrazofurin is very active against several transplantable murine tumors, most notably, Walker 256 carcinosarcoma, mammary carcinoma 755, Gardner lymphosarcoma, and X5563 plasma cell myeloma. However, in contrast to the situation with another OMP deCase inhibitor, 6-azauridine, the murine leukemias are quite refractory to this agent (Sweeney *et al.*, 1973). Clinical trials in man have also indicated a limited antitumor effect (Gutowski *et al.*, 1975; Ohnuma *et al.*, 1977; and Cadman *et al.*, 1978). Dose-limiting toxicities primarily affect the oral mucosa, but not the bone marrow or intestinal mucosa.

Pyrazofurin, at concentrations as low as 0.1 μM, inhibits the replication of mammalian cells in culture (Plagemann and Behrens, 1976). Inhibition of Novikoff rat hepatoma cell replication was reversible by the addition of uridine or the combination of deoxyuridine and deoxycytidine, implying that *de novo* pyrimidine biosynthesis was blocked by pyrazofurin, and that inhibition of DNA, as opposed to RNA, synthesis was responsible for inhibition of growth. Sweeney *et al.* (1973) demonstrated that addition of pyrazofurin to Ehrlich ascites or Walker 256 cells *in vitro* markedly inhibited the conversion of [carboxy-^{14}C]orotic acid to [^{14}C]CO_2 and UMP. Streightoff *et al.* (1969) had previously suggested that pyrazofurin may inhibit growth through inhibition of OMP deCase. Cadman *et al.* (1978) have described the occurrence of extensive conversion to the 5′-monophosphate as well as higher phosphorylated derivatives in murine tumors. The 5′-monophosphate derivative of pyrazofurin is a competitive inhibitor of purified OMP deCase with an apparent K_i of 5×10^{-9} M;

pyrazofurin, and the di- and triphosphate derivatives are inactive (Dix *et al.*, 1979). The initial phosphorylation of pyrazofurin appears to occur via adenosine kinase since (1) adenosine, but not other nucleosides, inhibits the formation of pyrazofurin-5′-monophosphate, (2) adenosine kinase activity copurifies with pyrazofurin kinase activity, and (3) pyrazofurin inhibits adenosine phosphorylation (Dix *et al.*, 1979). Pyrazofurin-5′-monophosphate (Fig. 15) has also recently been demonstrated to be an inhibitor of *de novo* purine biosynthesis. Rat liver AICAR formyltransferase is inhibited *in vitro*; the apparent K_i is 3×10^{-5} *M*. Additionally, 5-aminoimidazole-4-carboxamide excretion in urine increases following pyrazofurin administration to rats *in vivo* (Worzalla and Sweeney, 1980). Thus, pyrazofurin inhibits the *de novo* biosynthesis of both purines and pyrimidines, although inhibition of the latter is much more potent.

Treatment of cells or mice with pyrazofurin leads to dramatic alterations in pyrimidine intermediate and nucleotide pool sizes. Cadman *et al.* (1978) observed a pronounced and persistant depression of UTP and CTP pools in L5178Y leukemia cells in culture treated with pyrazofurin; ATP and GTP pools rose transiently. Similarly, administration of 8 mg/kg pyrazofurin to mice bearing colon 38 tumors produced a 50% depression of uridine nucleotide pools for several days. Concurrently, orotate and orotidine levels rose dramatically; however, orotidine-5′-monophosphate did not accumulate behind the blockade (Brockman *et al.*, 1977). Moyer and Handschumacher (1979) and Handschumacher *et al.* (1979) have utilized the pyrazofurin-provoked accumulation of orotate and orotidine, in urine and tissues, as a means for assessing drug-induced (e.g., PALA) alterations in pyrimidine metabolism. Kensler *et al.* (1981b) have extended this approach by utilizing the kinetics of drug inhibition of pyrazofurin-provoked tumor orotate and orotidine accumulation as a means for optimizing drug-treatment schedules.

Evaluation of the mechanisms of resistance to pyrazofurin has suggested several possibilities. Metabolic deficiencies have been implicated in a line of L5178Y developed for resistance to pyrazofurin because this line did not concentrate radiolabeled pyrazofurin and its phosphate derivatives even though the cells were freely permeable to the drug. Since the intracellular concentration of pyrazofurin depends on the degree of its phosphorylation, pyrazofurin resistance, in this case, involved a loss of adenosine kinase activity, which was undetectable in extracts of these resistant cells (Dix *et al.*, 1979). In naturally sensitive (Walker 256) and resistant (L5178Y) murine tumors, anabolism of pyrazofurin is comparable; however, the L5178Y leukemia has a greater capacity to utilize uridine to effect its rescue from pyrimidine starvation (Cadman *et al.*, 1978). Another mode for resistance is suggested by the results of Suttle and Stark (1979) who developed a series of hamster cell lines resistant to

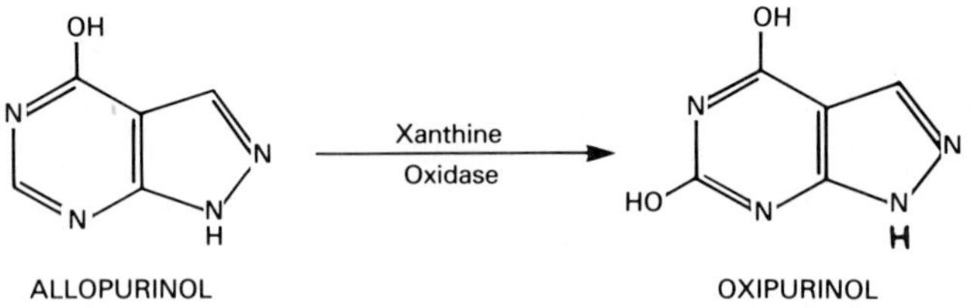

OH N N N N H ALLOPURINOL — Xanthine Oxidase → OH N HO N N N H OXIPURINOL

FIG. 16.

pyrazofurin and/or 6-azauridine. In each instance, the activity of the target enzyme was elevated 10- to 60-fold, but whether these resistant lines show differential susceptibility to decarboxylase inhibition by pyrazofurin-5′-monophosphate, when compared to their sensitive progenitors, has not been evaluated.

2. *Allopurinal and Oxipurinol*

Allopurinol [4-hydroxypyrazolo(3,4-*d*)pyrimidine] (Fig. 16) is a synthetic isomer of the xanthine oxidase substrate, hypoxanthine. As such, allopurinol is a competitive inhibitor of this enzyme and an extremely useful therapeutic agent for the treatment of the primary hyperuricemia of gout as well as the secondary hyperuricemias associated with malignancies (Rundles *et al.*, 1963). However, allopurinol has no antitumor activity (White, 1959; and Shaw *et al.*, 1960). The actions and metabolism of allopurinol have been the subjects of several recent reviews (O'Sullivan, 1974; Elion, 1978). In addition to inhibition of xanthine oxidase, allopurinol and/or its metabolites are also reported as inhibitors of xanthine dehydrogenase (Fhaolain and Coughlan, 1978), PRPP amidotransferase (McCollister *et al.*, 1964), tryptophan oxygenase (Badawy and Evans, 1973), and OMP deCase (Beardmore and Kelley, 1971).

Allopurinol is rapidly metabolized by xanthine oxidase to oxipurinol (Fig. 16), which is also an inhibitor of this enzyme. 1-Ribosylallopurinol-5′-monophosphate, 1-ribosyloxipurinol-5′-monophosphate, and 7-ribosyloxipurinol-5′-monophosphate have been identified in nanomolar concentrations in rat liver and kidney following [^{14}C]allopurinol administration. Higher phosphates, the di- or triphosphate ribonucleotides of allopurinol and oxipurinol, were not detected (Nelson *et al.*, 1973), findings consonant with the lack of incorporation of allopurinol into nucleic acids *in vivo* (Elion, 1966).

The presumption that treatment with allopurinol was also interfering with pyrimidine metabolism arose from the report of mild orotate and orotidinuria in patients (Fox *et al.*, 1970). The urinary appearance of orotidine which arises from the irreversible dephosphorylation of orotidine-5′-monophosphate, is suggestive of an inhibition of OMP deCase activity. Additionally, allopurinol and oxipurinol inhibit the *in vivo* conversion of [carboxyl-^{14}C]orotic acid to UMP (Beardmore and Kelley, 1971). These investigators also suggested that the ribonucleotide metabolites of oxipurinol were the inhibitory species *in vivo*. Fyfe *et al*. (1973) subsequently established that the 1- and 7-ribosyl-5′-monophosphates of oxipurinol were potent competitive inhibitors of rat liver and yeast OMP deCase. Substrate and inhibition kinetics show bimodal characteristics, presumably due to enzyme aggregation; the low K_i values for rat liver enzyme were 0.5 and 40 nM for the two derivatives, respectively. Allopurinol, oxipurinol, and 1-ribosylallopurinol-5′-monophosphate were relatively ineffective inhibitors. Similar kinetics of inhibition have also been reported for human erythrocyte OMP deCase (Brown and O'Sullivan, 1977). Thus, apparently, oxipurinol is metabolically activated by condensation with PRPP through the activity of OPRTase, and this species, in turn, inhibits the adjacent enzyme, OMP deCase. Interestingly, administration of allopurinol to rats and man leads to an elevation of the activities of OPRTase and OMP deCase (Brown *et al*., 1972; Tax *et al*., 1976) manifested by the formation of a more stable aggregated state of the enzymes. In spite of the marked elevations in urinary and tissue orotate and orotidine concentrations that can be provoked by allopurinol, alterations in uridine nucleotide pool sizes are small and transient (Nelson *et al*., 1973) suggesting that effective impediment to *de novo* pyrimidine biosynthesis *in vivo* is minor.

3. *6-Azauridine and Other Pyrimidine Analogs*

6-Azauridine (Fig. 17), a clinically useful drug in the treatment of psoriasis, mycosis fungoides, and neoplasms such as chronic myelogenous and acute leukemias (Handschumacher *et al*., 1962; and Hernandez *et al*., 1969), is an anabolite of 6-azauracil—a synthetic 1,2,4-triazine analog of uracil. In contrast to 6-azauridine, 6-azauracil is toxic to the central nervous system and, consequently, is not used clinically (Welch *et al*., 1960). Furthermore, 6-azauridine is a much more potent antitumor agent than 6-azauracil, both *in vivo* (Šorm and Keilová, 1958) and *in vitro* (Schindler and Welch, 1957).

6-Azauridine, synthesized by Schindler and Welch (1957), was one of the first pyrimidine analogs to be described as an inhibitor of OMP deCase (Handschumacher and Pasternak, 1958). Phosphorylation to the monophosphate derivative has been observed in many bacterial and mammalian systems; it is this derivative of 6-azauridine that is the

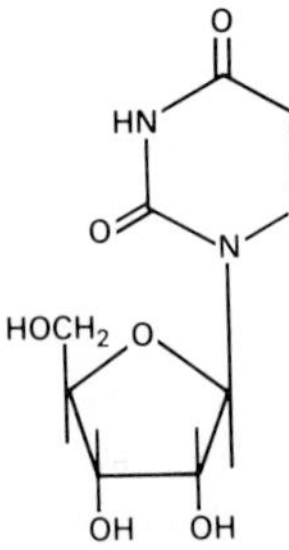

6-AZAURIDINE

FIG. 17.

most effective enzymic inhibitor. Competitive inhibition with 6-azauridine-5′-monophosphate has been reported against partially purified yeast OMP deCase ($K_i = 7 \times 10^{-7}$ M) (Handschumacher, 1960) and murine tumor enzyme ($K_i = 10^{-7} M$) (Traut and Jones, 1977a,b). Enzyme inhibition is reversible and is specific for the mononucleotide. Although structurally different, 6-azauridine-5′-monophosphate closely mimics the conformational properties of the enzyme substrate orotidine-5′-monophosphate (Saenger *et al.*, 1979). An interesting application of this high affinity competitive inhibition is the use of 6-azauridine-5′-monophosphate coupled to agarose as a means for purifying the *pyr* 5,6 complex from Ehrlich ascites carcinoma (McClard *et al.*, 1980).

The growth inhibitory effects of 6-azauridine appear to be due to the suppression of *de novo* pyrimidine biosynthesis, even though a number of other enzymic reactions are affected by this drug and/or its derivatives [e.g., uridine kinase (Škoda, 1963; Schumm and Webb, 1975), aminoacylation of transfer RNA (Kalousek *et al.*, 1962), RNA polymerase (Goldberg and Rabinowitz, 1963), and polynucleotide phosphorylase (Brockman and Anderson, 1963)]. Bruemmer *et al.* (1962) and Conn *et al.* (1967) demonstrated that the spectrum of antitumor effects of 6-azauridine in a series of murine ascites and plasma cell tumors corresponded with inhibition of orotic acid metabolism in tumor slices. Additionally, orotate and orotidinuria occur in animals and man following 6-azauridine treatment (Habermann, 1960; Skoda, 1963). L5178Y cells in culture exposed to 5 μM 6-azauridine exhibit pronounced alterations in nucleotide content. Uridine and cytidine nucleotides diminish within hours to less than 10% of control levels, whereas adenine nucleotide levels more than double during the same time-frame; GTP levels remain relatively unchanged. Intracellular orotate and orotidine levels also rise markedly; orotidine-5′-monophosphate does not, presumably because of catabolism to orotidine by phosphatases (Janeway and Cha, 1977). Chen and Jones (1979) have examined the effect of 6-azauridine (20 m*M*) on the incorporation of $NaH[^{14}C]CO_3$ into pyrimidine intermediates in logarithmically growing Ehrlich ascites cells. Orotidine, orotic acid, L-dihydroorotic acid, and *N*-carbamyl-L-aspartate accumulate, the latter to the greatest abundance. As was expected, little radiolabeled UMP was generated.

Several mechanisms of resistance to 6-azauridine have been described. In a situation typical of OMP deCase inhibitors, 6-azauridine resistant variants of L5178Y leukemia have been developed that exhibit very limited anabolism of 6-azauridine to the 5′-monophosphate (Pasternak *et al.*, 1961). Direct addition of the nucleotide to extracts of sensitive or resistant cells provoked equal inhibition of OMP deCase activities, demonstrating a lack of alteration in the target enzyme. Alteration in the activity of uridine kinase is not the only mechanism of resistance to 6-azauridine. May *et al.* (1977) have reported on the selection of a mouse fibroblast clone that grows in the presence of 6-azauridine. Despite the resistance of this variant cell line to 6-azauridine, these cells are killed by 5-fluorouridine, implying that uridine kinase is not deficient. Direct measurement of this enzyme in cell lysates substantiates this point. The resistant cells synthesize both purines and pyrimidines *de novo* at twice the rate of the sensitive cells; however sensitive and resistant cells have comparable activities of OPRTase and OMP deCase. In other circumstances, growth of mammalian cells in the presence of 6-azauridine can lead to the increased synthesis and activity of OMP deCase (Pinsky and Krooth, 1967). The aforementioned resistant mouse fibroblasts did have elevated (45% higher) levels of PRPP, a metabolite important to the promotion of flux through both synthetic pathways, and this fact may account for the enhanced synthetic rates. The expanded pool of PRPP might also increase the concentration of orotidine-5′-monophosphate at the active site of OMP deCase, which could then diminish the competitive inhibition of the enzyme by 6-azauridine-5′-monophosphate. Interestingly, augmented PRPP pools have also been described in several PALA-resistant variants of the Lewis lung carcinoma (Kensler *et al.*, 1981a). In both instances, the biochemical basis for elevation of PRPP is undefined.

A number of other pyrimidine analogs have been reported as inhibitors of OMP deCase. Administration of 5-azaorotate to mice substantially inhibits OMP deCase activity measured in liver homogenates; 5-azauracil is also inhibitory, but to a lesser degree (Čihák and Šorm, 1972). The difference in the activities of these 5-azapyrimidines is attributed to differences in the phosphoribosyl transferases involved in their metabolic transformation, in the former case, synthesis of 5-azaorotidine-5′-monophosphate is accomplished by OPRTase, and in the latter case, 5-azauridine-5′-monophosphate by uridine phosphoribosyl transferase.

5-Azacytidine, following formation of the ribotides, is incorporated into

RNA where it, in particular, appears to perturb message translation. However, the monophosphate derivative is also an effective inhibitor of *de novo* pyrimidine biosynthesis through OMP deCase inhibition (Veselý *et al.*, 1968). Similarly, 5-hydroxyuridine (Smith and Visser, 1965) and 5-aminouridine (Smith *et al.*, 1966), following phosphorylation, are specific inhibitors of OMP deCase. Both of these analogs are also incorporated into nucleic acids. Barbituric acid inhibits the last three enzymes of the pathway (Potvin *et al.*, 1978). The ribotide of barbituric acid is a competitive inhibitor of OMP deCase: the apparent K_i in rat brain is 4 nM. Levine *et al.* (1980) report that 1-ribosylbarbituric-5′-monophosphate has an apparent K_i of 9×10^{-12} M against purified yeast OMP deCase and a half-time of dissociation at 4°C of about 10 hours. This inhibition is one of the strongest protein–synthetic ligand interactions that has been measured. The anionic form of this inhibitor may represent a transition state analog of OMP deCase. By contrast, barbiturates, the hydrocarbon substituted derivatives of barbituric acid, do not impede *de novo* pyrimidine biosynthesis, leading Potvin *et al.* (1978) to suggest that those substituents, critical to barbiturate activity, serve to divest barbituric acid of its potency as an inhibitor of UMP synthesis.

G. Chemotherapeutic Summary

The chemotherapeutic activity of many of the aforementioned pyrimidine inhibitors against several murine tumors have been summarized in Table VIII. This summary is a compilation of information contained in the drug-screening data bank of the Developmental Therapeutics Program, Division of Cancer Treatment, National Cancer Institute. The transplantable murine tumor lines chosen represent a spectrum of tumor types: three leukemias—L1210, P388, and L5178Y are included as are three solid tumors—Lewis lung carcinoma, B16 melanoma, and colon 26 carcinoma. Cumulatively, these tumor lines tend to reflect the diverse range of therapeutic responses to developmental oncolytics. In general, the leukemias are the more responsive tumor class; very few drugs are effective against all lines. Indeed, of the listed drugs, only 5-fluorouracil is active against all six tumor lines.

Summarized in Table IX are the effects of inhibitors on pyrimidine biosynthetic enzyme activity *in vitro*. Most of the inhibitors listed in Table VIII as well as other agents suggested in the literature to have activity were systematically evaluated *in vitro* against crude extracts of target enzymes prepared from four murine tumor lines. Inhibitors were added at a final concentration of 1 mM and the data are presented as percentage inhibition of control (no inhibitor) enzyme activity. (Specific activities for these tumor enzymes are included in Table VII.) Methods for enzymatic assays are discussed in the Appendix and were conducted as described elsewhere (Kensler *et al.*, 1981a). Our findings are in overall good accord with the literature reviewed in the antecedent subsections. A few specific comments are in order, however. For the extensive series of L-glutamine antagonists evaluated, only CONV and acivicin show appreciable activity, indicating that CPS II is not particularly susceptible to inhibition by this type of antimetabolite. Sulfhydryl reactants, such as *N*-methyl maleimide, are good inhibitors, but since maleimides exhibit a strong delayed toxicity (Cooney *et al.*, 1978), they are not clinically useful. PALA was by far the most effective inhibitor of ATCase; analogs of either L-aspartate or carbamyl phosphate were relatively inactive, although this might be partially reflective of the high substrate concentrations used in the assay. Sulfadiazine was found to be inactive against mammalian DHOase. Taken together with the findings of Christopherson and Jones (1980) it would appear that the sulfonamides may only be effective against prokaryotic DHOase. Of merit is the novel observation that several triazine derivatives (see Table X for structures) that were previously reported as respiratory inhibitors (Gosálvez *et al.*, 1976) are quite active as inhibitors of DHO deHase. Whether these compounds are as specific in their action as the naphthoquinones remains to be determined. The inactivity of several pyrimidine analogs, notably 5-fluoroorotate, against OPRTase, may also reflect the use of high substrate levels in the assay, although the pronounced activity of barbituric acid does not support this notion. Finally, the inactivity of the OMP deCase inhibitors reflects the inability of the assay homogenates to phosphorylate these drugs to the ultimate inhibitory species, the 5′-monophosphate derivatives. Addition of exogenous 6-azauridine-5′-monophosphate, for example, is completely inhibitory.

IV. Combination Chemotherapy with Pyrimidine Inhibitors

Current principles governing the selection of drug combinations used against human neoplasms include use of drugs with (1) activity against the target tumor, (2) different sites of dose-limiting toxicities, and (3) different mechanisms of action (Carter, 1977). The last of these criteria, which have been developed empirically, would preclude the use of drugs that act as sequential blockers of a pathway, such as the *de novo* pyrimidine pathway. There exists pertinent experimental data that argue this point, *pro* and *contra*. The therapeutic activity of several "antipyrimidine" sequential drug combinations against common murine tumors is presented in

TABLE VIII

CHEMOTHERAPEUTIC ACTIVITY OF PYRIMIDINE INHIBITORS AGAINST SELECTED MURINE TUMORS[a]

Compound	NSC number	Tumor line					
		L1210	P388	L5178Y	Lewis lung	B16	Colon 26
Azaserine	742	++	++	+	–	–	–
DON	7365	++	++		–	–	+
S-Carbamyl-L-cysteine	102498	–					
DONV	117613	+	+				
CONV	124412	+	+			–	
O-Carbamyl-L-serine	128373	–					
Albizzin	132089			No test records			
δ-OH-L-lysine	132938	–					
Acivicin	163501	++	++		+	–	+
β-Methylaspartate	118508			No test records			
Phosponoacetic acid	138745	–	–		+	++	–
PALA	224131	–	–	–	++	++	++
5-Fluoroorotate	31712	++	++	+	–	–	

5-Bromoorotate	34493	−					
Sulfadiazine	35600	−					
5-Aminoorotate	43249	−	++				
Carbamylglycine	49417	−					
5-Methylorotate	52390	−					
Barbituric acid	7889	−					
Lapachol	11905	+	+		−	−	
Dichloroallyl lawsone	126771	−	−		+	+	−
Dihydro-5-azaorotate	320932	−	−		−	−	
Triazine	123461	+	++			−	
Triazine	127755	+	++			+	
Triazine	128570	−	++			−	
Triazine	128571	−	++			−	
Triazine	135764	+	++			+	
5-Fluorouracil	19893	++	++	++	++	+	++
6-Uracilsulfonamide	41963	−	−				
Allopurinol	1390	−	−				
Oxypurinol	76239			No test records			
6-Azauridine	32074	++	+	+	+	−	
Pyrazofurin	143095	+	+	−	−	+	−

[a] Drug sensitivity *in vivo* is expressed as: ++, >90% tumor inhibition and/or >75% increase in lifespan; +, 70–90% tumor inhibition and/or 40–75% increase in lifespan; and −, <70% tumor inhibition and/or <40% increase in lifespan.

TABLE IX

EFFECTS OF INHIBITORS ON PYRIMIDINE BIOSYNTHETIC ENZYME ACTIVITY IN MURINE TUMORS *in Vitro*

Inhibitor (1 m*M*)	NSC number	Tumor			
		L1210 leukemia	P388 leukemia	Lewis lung carcinoma	B16 melanoma
Carbamyl phosphate synthetase II					
Azaserine	742	0	3	12	8
DON	7365	0	6	24	7
γ-Glutamate hydrazide	7786	0	7	23	9
S-Carbamyl-L-cysteine	102498	0	16	25	30
DONV	117613	0	3	6	9
CONV	124412	34	57	59	79
O-Carbamyl-L-serine	128373	7	3	15	8
Albizzin	132089	2	17	8	5
δ-OH-L-lysine	132938	0	9	3	14
Acivicin	163501	46	33	67	73
Maleic hydrazide		6	12	24	3
L-Methionine-DL-sulfoximine		10	11	24	0
N-Methyl maleimide		100	100	100	100
Monomethyl phosphate		4	20	47	46
γ-Thiocyano-α-aminoisobutyrate		14	24	47	54
L-Aspartate transcarbamylase					
β-Methyl-DL-aspartate	118508	0	0	10	10
PALA	224131	97	98	96	97
Phosphonoacetic acid	138745	0	0	14	5
PA_2LA		0[a]	0[a]	0[a]	0[a]
L-Alanosine	153353	0	0	0	0

L-Dihydroorotase					
5-Fluoroorotate	31712	58	55	58	58
5-Iodoorotate		9	47	13	14
5-Methylorotate	52390	98	69	65	69
5-Aminoorotate	43249	19	5	0	0
Sulfadiazine	35600	10	0	0	0
L-Dihydroorotate dehydrogenase					
Lapachol	11905	91	86	77	100
Dichloroallyl lawsone	126771	93	81	86	95
Dihydro-5-azaorotate	320932	100	100	100	100
Barbituric acid	7880	0	32	33	22
Phenylbutazone		28	32	25	28
Triazine[b]	123461	67	74	82	87
Triazine[b]	127755	85	87	79	76
Triazine[b]	128570	90	89	82	84
Triazine[b]	128571	89	91	86	76
Triazine[b]	135764	85	91	90	73
Orotate phosphoribosyl transferase					
Allopurinol	1390	0	0	0	7
5-Fluorouracil	19893	4	0	0	0
5-Fluoroorotate	31712	0	0	1	2
6-Uracilsulfonamide	41963	0	0	0	2
Barbituric acid	7889	91	85	86	92
Orotidine-5′-monophosphate decarboxylase					
Allopurinol	1390	2	4	0	6
Pyrazofurin	143095	7	3	2	0
6-Azauridine	32074	8	10	0	0
6-Azauridine-5′-monophosphate		98	100	96	98
Barbituric acid	7889	0	0	0	0

[a] Stimulates 20–25%.

[b] See Table X for structures.

TABLE X

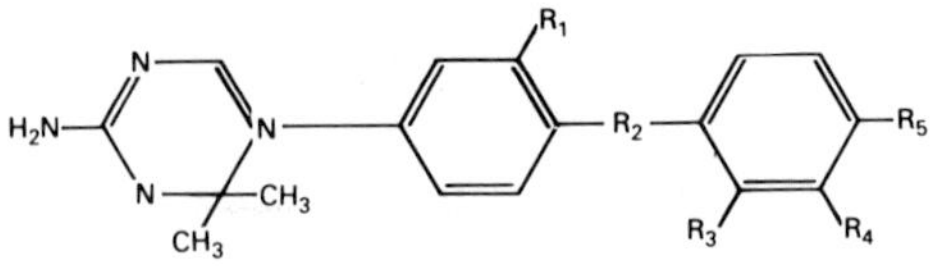

Triazine Derivatives	R_1	R_2	R_3	R_4	R_5
NSC–123461	Cl	$-(CH_2)_2-CO-NH-$	H	H	$-SO_2F$
NSC–127755	Cl	$-(CH_2)_4-$	Cl	H	$-SO_2F$
NSC–128570	Cl	$-(CH_2)_4-$	H	$-SO_2F$	H
NSC–128571	Cl	$-(CH_2)_4-$	H	$-SO_2F$	Cl
NSC–135764	Cl	$-O-CH_2-C_6H_4-CO-NH-$ 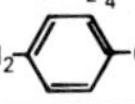	H	$-SO_2F$	H

Table XI. Although many antipyrimidine combinations appear to offer no therapeutic advantages, this is not always the case (e.g., PALA and acivicin: Kensler *et al.*, 1981b).

Webb (1963) has argued, on theoretical grounds, that "multiple inhibition of simple monolinear chains would seem generally to be incapable of producing an effect much greater than a single inhibitor, and a marked potentiation would be out of the question." Essentially, the rate of formation of a product of a sequence of reactions can never be any slower than the rate of the one slowest reaction in that pathway. This argument suggests that inhibition of an ordinarily non-rate-limiting enzyme in the pathway would affect the rate of production of the end product only when the reaction catalyzed by the target enzyme becomes the new rate-limiting step; addition of a second inhibitor would not affect the rate of formation of the end product until added in sufficient concentration to make the inhibited step rate-limiting, and in this case the overall inhibition would be the same whether the first inhibitor was present or not. Kinetic data presented by Rubin *et al.* (1964), using 5-azaorotate and 6-azauridine as sequential inhibitors of crude rat liver OPRTase and OMP deCase, respectively, substantiate this viewpoint. The therapeutic failure of other "antipyrimidine" combinations, such as PALA and pyrazofurin (Johnson *et al.*, 1978), might be construed as confirmation of this thesis.

However, as stressed in Section II, the control of flux through the pyrimidine pathway is a very interdependent process. Pathologic or pharmacologic perturbations can alter product and intermediate pool sizes and consequently provoke large alterations in reaction rates at various enzymic sites, thus serving to redefine rate-limiting steps. In consider-

TABLE XI

CHEMOTHERAPEUTIC SUMMARY OF EFFICACIOUS ANTIPYRIMIDINE DRUG COMBINATIONS EVALUATED AGAINST TRANSPLANTABLE MURINE TUMORS[a]

Drug	Dose (mg/kg)	Protocol/route	T/C
5-Fluorouracil + PALA (colon 26 carcinoma)			
5-FU	36	qd × 3, ip	173
PALA	108	qd × 3, ip	183
5-FU +	60	qd × 3, ip	236
PALA	500		
5-FU +	36	qd × 3, ip	346
PALA	500		
5-Fluorouracil + PALA (M5076 ovarian carcinoma)			
5-FU	100	qd 1–4, ip	154
PALA	833	qd 1–4, ip	216
5-FU +	60	qd 1–4, ip	242
PALA	500		
Dichloroallyl lawsone + PALA (colon 26 carcinoma)			
DCL	16	qd 5–13, ip	101
PALA	128	qd 5–13, ip	116
DCL +	16	qd 5–13, ip	154
PALA	256		
Acivicin + PALA (P388/ara C leukemia)			
Acivicin	3	qd 1–9, ip	202
PALA	240	qd 1–9, ip	205
Acivicin +	1.3	qd 1–9, ip	235
PALA	140		
Acivicin +	1.3	qd 1–9, ip	242
PALA	160		

[a] The data in this table summarize the chemotherapeutic activities of combinations of pyrimidine inhibitors that have been shown to have significantly better activity than the single drugs alone. These data were obtained from the drug-screening data bank of the Developmental Therapeutics Program, Division of Cancer Treatment, National Cancer Institute. For the sake of brevity, only optimal drug responses for agents administered singly and in combination are given.

ing the design of multiple therapeutic interventions, this pathway should more profitably be viewed in a dynamic perspective than a static or steady-state one.

Additionally, as argued by Potter (1951) and Black (1963) among others, sequential inhibition can lead to a synergistic response. Several studies (Skipper *et al.*, 1954; Hitchings, 1955) have demonstrated that blockade along a sequential pathway produces synergistic antineoplastic responses in terms of growth inhibition and animal survival. Furthermore, Kensler *et al.* (1981b) have demonstrated a pronounced synergism between acivicin and PALA in a biochemically designed trial against a PALA-resistant variant of the Lewis lung carcinoma. In this case, the exploited rationale was that acivicin inhibition of CPS II would reduce the concentration of carbamyl phosphate at the PALA binding site on ATCase, thus ameliorating the competitive displacement of PALA by carbamyl phosphate and serving to enhance inhibition. Utilizing treatment protocols that were determined on the basis of the effects of single drugs and combinations on pyrazofurin-provoked accumulation of orotate and orotidine in tumors, the use of PALA and acivicin (which are inactive as single agents against this tumor) leads to significant increases in life-span.

As a general strategy it is probably imprudent to expect much advantage from sequential blockade of the *de novo* pathway. But, as the biodynamics of this pathway become better defined and therapeutic agents with specific sites of action are developed, the rational (biochemical) approach to combination chemotherapy will undoubtedly provide useful treatment modalities.

V. Prospects

The present generation of drugs described—by serendipity or design—as inhibitors of the enzymes of *de novo* pyrimidine biosynthesis is for the most part without significant therapeutic value in man. The notable exception is allopurinol and, in this case, the valuable mode of action is against a different pathway. Paradoxically, allopurinol is without antineoplastic activity, for it is the search for such an activity that has been the driving force underlying the development of most of the drugs discussed in this treatise. It is false to imply though that inhibition of pyrimidine biosynthesis is a tactically improper approach to oncolytic therapy. What will be required is a more rational approach to the synthesis of new inhibitory drugs—drugs that possess great specificity of action. PALA, in this regard, represents a useful new approach to the problem, although, hindsight might suggest that ATCase is not the best point to attack pyrimidine biosynthesis. Transition-state analogs are fulfilling an expanding role as therapeutically useful agents (Wolfenden, 1979). Perhaps such an approach directed to the synthesis of carboxy phosphate analogs or other derivatives of the transition-state of CPS II will yield therapeutically useful drugs. Additionally, the judicious use of these drugs in combination offers still further possibilities, either when they are applied sequentially against the *de novo* pathway or perhaps used in combination with agents that inhibit the salvage pathway, thus effecting a total pyrimidine deprivation. It is hoped that this compendium will serve to stimulate work along these lines.

VI. Appendix: Strategies for Measuring the Enzymes and Substrates of the Pyrimidine Biosynthetic Pathway

Although extensive information is available in the literature on techniques for measuring the activities of the enzymes of the pyrimidine biosynthetic pathway, it is the purpose of the present Appendix to evaluate these techniques critically, to suggest improvements and alternative analytical strategies, and to outline means for assessing the concentrations of the substrates or products of the six reactions under consideration in normal as well as neoplastic tissues. Succinctly put, it is hoped that this Appendix will serve as a compendium of analytical data on the pyrimidine biosynthetic pathway.

A. Carbamyl Phosphate Synthetase II

1. *Enzyme*

Because of the susceptibility of carbamyl phosphate to chemical and biochemical decomposition (Diederick *et al.*, 1971), most of the suggested strategies for measuring the enzymes which synthesize this molecule either rely on prompt trapping of it, or else assess the consumption of one of the other more stable cosubstrates of the reaction. The traps used to date are of two general types: chemical and biochemical. In the first approach, radioactive carbamyl phosphate, synthesized from [^{14}C]CO_2 through the action of CPS II, is decomposed to cyanate in an alkaline environment; the cyanate is simultaneously condensed with ammonia (Williams and Davis, 1978) or hydroxylamine (Ingraham and Abdelal, 1978) to yield urea or hydroxyurea. After the dissipation of unused [^{14}C]CO_2, the radiolabeled residue is either isolated or subjected to enzymatic decomposition with urease to yield a new crop of [^{14}C]CO_2, which can be distilled and trapped with alkali in the usual manner (Cooney *et al.*, 1971b). The urea can also be measured colorimetrically, if quantities permit (Williams and Davis, 1978).

In the second general approach to the measurement of CPS II, an excess of L-aspartate (Kensler *et al.*, 1981a), or L-ornithine transcarbamylase (Mori and Tatibana, 1978) is used to condense any newly synthesized carbamyl phosphate with L-aspartate or L-ornithine. The resultant *N*-carbamylamino acids are completely stable to acid, and so serve as indices of the quantity of carbamyl phosphate synthesized, after dissipation of unreacted bicarbonate with HCl. In variants of this approach, the amino acids used to trap the newly synthesized carbamyl phosphate can be radiolabeled.

Both of the foregoing general strategies suffer from a severe drawback: dilution of the $[^{14}C]CO_2$ used in the assay (often ~0.01 *M*) by $[^{12}C]CO_2$ in the atmosphere or that generated metabolically (often ~0.01 *M*, Guyton 1971). For this reason, all measurements made by these techniques underestimate CPS II activity, often to an unpredictable degree.[3]

Three expedients might be suggested for overcoming this problem: (1) use of a vast excess of radiolabeled bicarbonate, so that dilution is minimized; this expedient would be expensive and dangerous; (2) use of a high concentration of $[^{13}C]CO_2$ as substrate; this expedient is practicable, but requires derivitization of the product and mass spectrophotometric analyses; thus it might be unsuitable for routine use; (3) measurement of the consumption or generation of one or more of the other cosubstrates of the reaction. In fact, Meister has quantitated the generation of ADP by CPS II from *E. coli* using a standard enzyme-based assay (Boettcher and Meister, 1980). Such a strategy is desirable because 2 moles of this nucleotide are generated during each of the enzyme's catalytic cycles. Nevertheless, in crude extracts, the presence of autochthonous ADP, coupled to the nonspecific hydrolysis of ATP by phosphatases and related enzymes, would render it somewhat less satisfactory.

Other workers have measured the appearance of L-[^{14}C]glutamic acid arising from the amido donor, L-[^{14}C]glutamine, by means of a purified L-glutamic decarboxylase and a standard $[^{14}C]CO_2$ trapping system (Jayaram *et al.*, 1975). Since the mammalian enzyme has a low K_m for L-glutamine (~5 μM), this approach is kinetically sound; i.e., the isotopic L-glutamine can be present at a concentration sufficient to saturate the enzyme. However, for its successful deployment, it is mandatory that the radioactive L-glutamine used be free of any L-glutamic acid since only a very small percentage of the substrate will be hydrolyzed in the case of

[3] The actual specific activity of bicarbonate can, in fact be measured by diffusing all the $[^{14}C]O_2$ and $[^{12}C]O_2$ present in a reaction vessel into a saturated solution of barium hydroxide, and by washing, drying, and weighing the resultant precipitate of barium carbonate. This expedient is, however, tedious, cumbersome, and impractical when 10–20 μl reaction volumes are being used.

analyses of mammalian CPS II in crude extracts. It is also mandatory that the L-glutamic acid decarboxylase be essentially free of L-glutaminase (less than 0.001%) or else prohibitively high blanks will ensue, and mask the ordinarily minor activities of the synthetase. These constraints notwithstanding, the assay using L-[^{14}C]glutamine has found limited use in monitoring the first step of pyrimidine biosynthesis in select tissues, such as fetal mouse liver (Jayaram *et al.*, 1975).

2. *Substrates*

The techniques for measuring the concentrations of the substrates and products of the CPS II reaction in tissues are mainly enzymatic, and have been well described elsewhere. For the purposes of this article, it will be sufficient to sketch briefly the theoretical features of these approaches.

ATP is most frequently measured spectrophotometrically with hexokinase and glucose-6-phosphate dehydrogenase using NADP as the pyridine nucleotide indicator (Gruber *et al.*, 1974). ADP is also measured spectrophotometrically using pyruvate kinase, phosphoenol pyruvate, lactate dehydrogenase, and NADH (Gruber *et al.*, 1974). Neither method is absolutely specific for adenine nucleotides, so that the concentrations of the reagent enzymes should be controlled in such a way as to minimize the use of aberrant or alternate substrates (Gruber *et al.*, 1974).

Ammonia and L-glutamine can both be measured spectrophotometrically via the L-glutamate dehydrogenase reaction, the latter after amidohydrolysis by crystalline L-asparaginase from *E. coli.* (Cooney *et al.*, 1971a). Once again, NADH is the pyridine nucleotide indicator. It should be pointed out that the Tris buffers suggested originally for these assays promote the irreversible denaturation of L-glutamate dehydrogenase, and so should be supplanted by 0.1 *M* KPO_4 in 20% (v/v) glycerin.

Magnesium ions can be conveniently assessed by atomic absorption spectrometry or any of a number of wet chemical reactions (Brooks *et al.*, 1979).

Of the substrates and products of CPS II, only carbamyl phosphate cannot be measured by standard means. Nevertheless, several experimental techniques are available for quantifying this labile metabolite. These will be presented here in greater detail, and their applicability to samples of biologic origin reviewed critically. In the first experimental approach, developed in the authors' laboratory, crystalline alkaline phosphatase is used to hydrolyze carbamyl phosphate to inorganic phosphate, carbon dioxide, and ammonia, which is then quantitated via the L-glutamate dehydrogenase reaction. Insofar as is known, this is the only reaction catalyzed by alkaline phosphatase to yield ammonia, and it is this feature

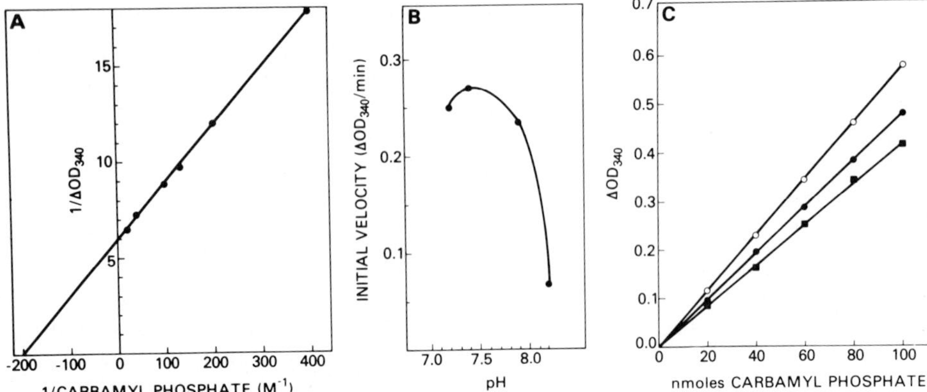

FIG. 18. Characteristics of the spectrophotometric assay for carbamyl phosphate. Ten milligrams of NADP and of α-ketoglutaric acid were dissolved in 5 ml of 20% glycerin (v/v) in 0.1 *M* potassium phosphate pH 7.5. In glass cuvettes were admixed 100 μl of this solution, 50 μl of L-glutamate dehyrogenase in glycerin (Boehringer), 940 μl of H_2O, and the appropriate concentrations of a fresh aqueous solution of carbamyl phosphate in a volume of 10 μl. The *A* was read at 340 nm, whereafter 10 μl, IU of dialyzed ammonium-free alkaline phosphatase from *E. coli* (Type IIIR) was added to initiate the reaction. After the -ΔA had stabilized, a second reading of absorbance was taken. Computations were made on the basis of the equation: -ΔA_{340} of 0.00575 = 1 nmole carbamyl phosphate decomposed. (A) Affinity of alkaline phosphatase from *E. coli* for carbamyl phosphate. (B) pH optimum for the hydrolysis of carbamyl phosphate by alkaline phosphatase from *E. coli*. The concentration of carbamyl phosphate was 10 × K_m; 0.1 *M* potassium phosphate was the buffer. (C) Dose–response of the spectrophotometric assay for carbamyl phosphate using alkaline phosphatases from *E. coli*. Theoretical curve, ○; freshly dissolved carbamyl phosphate, ●; carbamyl phosphate aged 15 minutes, ■.

which invests the method with unique specificity. The K_m of alkaline phosphatase for carbamyl phosphate approximates 1×10^{-4} *M* (Fig. 18A) and the pH optimum has been found to lie between pH 7 and 8 (Fig. 18B). This first method responds in a linear way to amounts of carbamyl phosphate between 5 and 100 nmoles (Fig. 18C). Due to its relative insensitivity and the ubiquitous presense of ammonia in biologic specimens, it finds its greatest utility in situations requiring the *in vitro* analysis of stock solutions of carbamyl phosphate intended for kinetic analyses, or in experiments aimed at assessing the rate of decomposition of this labile metabolite at various pHs or in various solvents.

The second strategy utilizes purified ATCase from *E. coli* to catalyze the condensation of carbamyl phosphate with L-[U-^{14}C]- or L-[2,3-^{3}H]aspartic acid of high specific activity. In the case of the ^{14}C-labeled substrate, the carbon skeleton of any unused radioactive L-aspartic acid is dismantled and volatilized enzymatically (Kensler *et al.*, 1980a) and the residual radioactivity is taken as a measure of the amount of *N*-carbamyl-L-

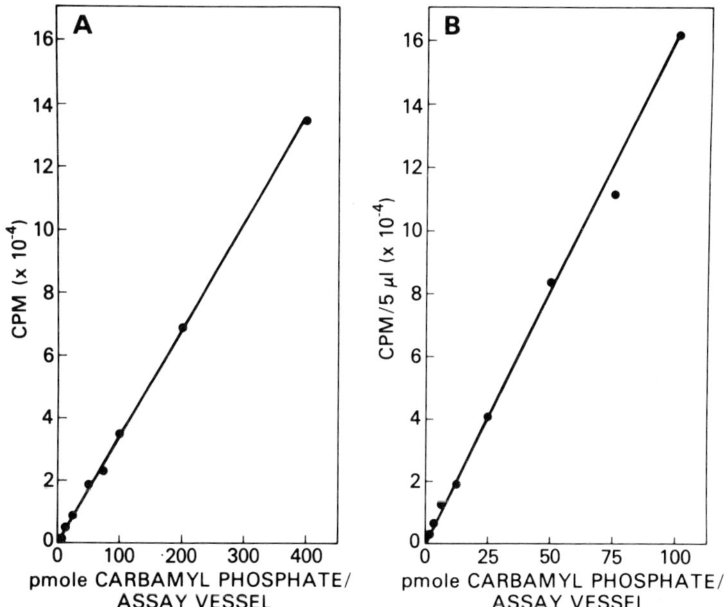

FIG. 19. Response of the radiometric assays with [^{14}C]- or [^{3}H]aspartic acids to graded concentrations of carbamyl phosphate. To quintuplicate vessels were added the amounts of carbamyl phosphate indicated on the abscissas, in a volume of 5 μl, followed by 5 μl, 0.25 μCi of L-[4-^{14}C]aspartic acid (A), or 5 μl, 0.25 μCi of L-[2,3-^{3}H]aspartic acid (B); 5 μl of ATCase from *E. coli* (3 mg/ml) was added last to initiate the reaction. After 1 hour at 37°C, the unreacted L-aspartic acid was either dissipated by enzymatic volatilization (A), or separated from *N*-carbamyl-L-[2,3-^{3}H]aspartic acid by ascending chromatography with butanol : acetic acid : water, 4/1/1, as solvent (B).

[U-^{14}C]aspartic acid formed. This method responds in a linear way to amounts of carbamyl phosphate ranging from 3 to 1000 pmoles (Fig. 19A). It can be used to check carbamyl phosphate concentrations *in vitro* in large numbers of samples, such as those intended for kinetic analyses, but is not applicable to measurements of the compound in tissues because of high blank values. With the tritiated substrate, greater sensitivity is attained (Fig. 19B) but the product must be separated by paper chromatography (Table XII), a step which can become cumbersome.

In a third approach radioactive L-aspartic acid and ATCase are replaced by prepurified L-[U-^{14}C]ornithine, and L-ornithine transcarbamylase (OCTase) from *Streptococcus faecalis*. Any labeled L-citrulline formed will reflect the concentration of carbamyl phosphate present in the reaction vessel. Precusor is separated from product on a 8 × 700-mm column of JEOL AR-50 resin equilibrated and developed with 0.3 *M* lithium citrate

TABLE XII

MIGRATION VALUES OF SOME PYRIMIDINE BIOSYNTHETIC PRECURSORS[a]

Molecule	*n* BuOH : HAc : H_2O 1:1:1 (R_f)	*n* BuOH : HAc : H_2O 4:1:1 (R_f)	EtOH : 1 *M* NH_4Ac 70:30 (R_f)	tBuOH : HAc : H_2O 1:1:1 (R_f)	HVE $NaPO_4$ pH 2.0	HVE $NaPO_4$ pH 7.0
L-Aspartic acid	0.55	0.34	0.28	0.67	−35	+75
N-Carbamyl-L-aspartic acid	0.65	0.55	0.28	0.77	+5.0	+130
L-Dihydroorotic acid	0.55	0.43	0.44	0.66	+5.0	+70
Orotic acid	0.60	0.28	0.48	0.70	+42	+75
OMP	0.47	0.09	0.09	0.57	+72	+105
UMP	0.50	0.23	0.21	0.60	+45	+58

[a] Ascending paper chromatography [or high-voltage electrophoresis (HVE)] in the solvents (or buffers) shown was carried out on Whatman 3M paper for 16 hours at room temperature, or for 1 hour at 4°C, respectively.

TABLE XIII

REPORTED CONCENTRATIONS OF CARBAMYL PHOSPHATE (CP) IN TISSUE AND TUMORS

Tissue	Trapping agent	Denaturant	[CP] (nmoles/gm)	Recovery of exogenous CP (%)	Reference
Rabbit blood	ATCase	PCA	0	62–75	Jones *et al.* (1978)
Lewis lung carcinoma	OCTase	PCA[a]	0	5	Present workers
Rat liver	OCTase	PCA	100–120[b]	75	Raijman (1974)
Neurospora crassa	OCTase	PCA	6[c]	45	Williams *et al.* (1971)
Human lymphoblasts	OCTase	PCA	1	80	Huisman and Becker (1980)
Human fibroblasts	OCTase	PCA	1.5–2	80	Huisman and Becker (1980)

[a] Added after conversion of CP to L-citrulline.

[b] In our laboratory, using an identical technique for tissue preparation, but ATCase as the trapping agent, less than 1 μM carbamyl phosphate was demonstrable in rat liver.

[c] Per gram, dry weight.

at pH 8.0. Separation is excellent, L-citrulline eluting at 35 minutes, L-ornithine at 220 minutes.

In practice, the organ or tumor to be analyzed has been extirpated with dispatch and homogenized with a Polytron sonic disrupter in a medium containing all the requisite substrates and trapping enzymes in large excess. After 1 minute of further incubation, the preparation is deproteinized with 5% PCA, neutralized with KOH, clarified by centrifugation, and loaded on the long column of an amino acid analyzer, equilibrated and developed as described. For verification of the nature of the product, an aliquot of the neutralized extract is exposed again to OCTase in the presence of sufficient arsenate to facilitate the arsenolysis of any L-citrulline present in it; the difference in radioactivity in the appropriate fractions of the native versus the arsenolyzed samples provides a reliable index of the amount of L-citrulline present.

Variations of the second and third method have been used by several workers to measure carbamyl phosphate in rabbit blood, *Neurospora crassa*, rat liver, tumor cells, and fibroblasts. In most cases, 5% perchloric acid was used to extract and denature freeze-clamped, percussion-pulverized material, and the resultant suspensions were in contact with acid for 5 or 10 minutes, then in solution, near neutrality, for an additional half-hour prior to condensation. Recoveries of exogenous carbamyl phosphate were reported to be 75%; the molar concentrations found are listed in Table XIII.

Several caveats should be tendered in regard to those studies in which perchloric acid was used as a denaturant prior to the condensation of carbamyl phosphate with either L-aspartate of L-ornithine. The pH of 5% PCA is 0.6. According to Allen and Jones (1964), at this pH, the rate constant (K_{ob}s) for the decomposition of carbamyl phosphate would approximate 0.04; at neutrality it was nearly 0.1. This means that in the net time which elapsed prior to neutralization, approximately 25% of a 1 m*M* solution of carbamyl phosphate would have decayed; after neutralization an additional fraction of 25% might be expected to decompose. Inexplicably, such major decomposition was not ordinarily observed. One explanation for this finding is that the ice-cold temperatures used successfully retarded the decomposition of carbamyl phosphate.

Also evident from Table XIII is the conclusion that homogenization of tissue (Lewis lung carcinoma) in a medium containing the trapping enzymes leads to notably lower recoveries of exogenous carbamyl phosphate than are observed when acid denaturation is deployed first; this may be attributable to the competing action of phosphatases in the intact homogenate; these enzymes are known to decompose carbamyl phosphate vigorously. Alternatively it is possible in these, and most of the other studies recapitulated above, that the presence of cold L-aspartate and L-ornithine (both of which occur in liver at concentrations between 200 and 1000 μM) (Williamson and Brosnam, 1974; Matsuzawa *et al.*, 1980) diluted the specific activity of the isotopes used to an important degree. This problem is not easy of solution, because extensive manipulations are precluded when one is dealing with a labile molecule such as carbamyl phosphate, whose $t_{1/2}$ at 37°C, even at pH 7.0, is rather rapid: ~45 minutes.

In summary, although techniques for measuring carbamyl phosphate have been published and used, they should be viewed as provisional until the problem of breakdown is overcome, and unless stringent assessment of recoveries *per primum* is included. The problem of the dilution of the specific radioactivity of the trapping species is also a major hurdle to be negotiated in most cases.

B. L-Aspartate Transcarbamylase

1. *Enzyme*

As the enzyme of the pyrimidine pathway whose specific activity is ordinarily the highest, L-aspartate transcarbamylase poses no undue analytical problems. Two general approaches have been taken to measure it: colorimetric or radiometric assessment of the carbamyl-L-aspartate produced. The colormetric procedures capitalize on the reactivity of the ureido functionality with one of several chromogenic reagents; the antipyrine–diacetyl monoxime reagent pair is the most widely used of these (Adair and Jones, 1978). The sensitivity of this method ordinarily extends to the detection of 10 nmoles of product per vessel. Using it, careful attention must be paid to the diverse conditions of color development prescribed in the literature. Moreover, if other ureido groups—for example urea—are present in the extracts used, they often must be removed, or unduly high blanks will result. In fact, blank values, in our hands, tend to be a problem with this whole family of assays when the specific activity of ATCase is measured in crude homogenates of tissues with modest activity. In this circumstance, radiometric methodology finds its greatest utility. The optimal radiometric assays use L-[^{14}C]aspartic acid of low specific activity in order to saturate the enzyme (cf. above) and cold carbamyl phosphate. At the term of an appropriate incubation period, unused L-[^{14}C]aspartate is either dissipated enzymatically or separated chromatographically from the newly synthesized *N*-carbamyl-L-aspartate (Table XII). The enzymatic dissipation techniques, which can selectively detach the β-carboxyl as [^{14}C]O_2 in the case of

L-[4-^{14}C]aspartate (Milman and Cooney, 1974), or dismantle the whole carbon skeleton of the substrate (2[^{14}C]O_2↑ + 1[^{14}C]H_3–[^{14}C]HO↑) in the case of L-[U-^{14}C]aspartate (Kensler *et al.*, 1980a), are exceptionally well suited to the handling of large batteries of samples—such as those generated in organ surveys, etc.; however, relying as they do on the residual radioactivity in vessels receiving and lacking the cosubstrate, carbamyl phosphate, they can exhibit troublesome blanks. This is partly because L-aspartate can experience a large number of metabolic fates in addition to transcarbamylation even in otherwise unfortified crude extracts (Jones, 1975). This problem is exacerbated by radiochemical impurities (about 1% usually) in the substrates used; these impurities generally are resistant to enzymatic volatilization.

Chromatographic separations of the product solve both of these problems, but are also time-consuming. They fall into three classes: (a) chromatographic and electrophoretic separations; (b) ion-exchange thin layer chromatography, and (c) miniature column ion-exchange chromatography. High voltage electrophoresis on paper at pH 7.0 in 0.1 *M* sodium phosphate clearly separates L-aspartate from *N*-carbamyl-L-aspartate; capacity: approximately 10 samples/sheet. Ascending paper chromatography is similarly efficient (Table XII). Ion-exchange thin layer chromatography is most frequently conducted on polyethyleneimine sheets developed with 0.19–0.34 *M* LiCl; substrate is well separated from product; capacity: 10–20 samples/sheet (Christopherson *et al.*, 1978). Miniature ion-exchange columns can be used in series; these capitalize on the fact that L-aspartic acid in neutral solutions is nearly quantitatively (98%) retained on Dowex-50, H^+ form, while *N*-carbamyl-L-aspartic acid is not; the 2% contaminating L-aspartic acid can be removed from product on a second battery of columns of Dowex-1-formate at pH 3.2. Under these conditions, L-aspartic acid, bearing no net charge, elutes in or near the void volume, while *N*-carbamyl-L-aspartate, bearing a strong net negative charge, requires substantial volumes of 0.1 *M* formic acid for its elution; capacity: 1 sample/column (Jones, 1975).

Perhaps the most widely adopted radiometric assay for ATCase uses [^{14}C]carbamyl phosphate as substrate. Since the K_m of mammalian ATCase for carbamyl phosphate is low, it is possible to saturate it with the radioactive species alone if 5–10 μl reaction volumes are used. At the term of the requisite incubation, unused ^{14}C-labeled substrate is decomposed to [^{14}C]CO_2 with acid, and the radioactivity of the residue assessed by scintillation spectrometry (Kempe *et al.*, 1976). This method offers the practical advantage of ease and applicability to numerous samples, but the substrate is expensive and less than optimally pure from a radiochemical standpoint (ca. 90%) which makes mandatory its purification via recrystallization from ethanol to remove contaminating cyanate, a potent chemical carbamylating agent. Used with care, however, the [^{14}C]carbamyl phosphate assay would appear to be the method of choice for measuring ATCase in most laboratories.

2. *Substrates*

L-Aspartate poses no analytical problems: it can be quantified with excellent reliability by automatic amino acid analyses as well as by spectrophotmetric or radiometric enzymatic techniques; the latter approach offers sensitivity down to 200 pmoles (Cooney and Milman, 1972).

The measurement of *N*-carbamyl-L-aspartic acid in tissues and cells however, is by no means as easy; this is so because of the insensitivity of the colormetric assays treated above, and the presence in crude extracts of materials capable of interfering with color development. In fact, few if any reliable estimates of the concentration of *N*-carbamyl-L-aspartate in physiologic specimens have appeared in the biochemical literature, as was discussed earlier.

In attempting to counteract this deficiency, we have initiated studies which have as their aim the facile conversion of *N*-carbamyl-L-aspartate to the more readily measurable parent compound, L-aspartic acid. Two approaches have been used. In the first, advantage has been taken of the observation of Duschinsky *et al.* (1975) and Pausch *et al.* (1975) that nitrous acid at pH < 1 will decarbamylate *N*-carbamyl-L-aspartate without any significant destruction of the α-amino functionality. This phenomenon has been called the "anti-Van Slyke" reaction. Practically speaking, the "anti Van Slyke" reaction can be carried out by exposing pure *N*-carbamyl-L-aspartic acid to 0.6% sodium nitrite in 0.5 *N* H_2SO_4 for 10 minutes. After quenching unreacted nitrous acid with glycine, the yield of L-aspartic acid, measured by an enzymatic spectrophotometric assay, averages 75%. However, efforts to apply this interesting approach to extracts of biological origin have not, so far, met with success, most likely because of the presence therein of numerous alternative substrates competing with *N*-carbamyl-L-aspartate for attack by nitrous acid.

The second approach to measuring *N*-carbamyl-L-aspartate is also experimental. It capitalizes on the observation of Jones and others that the reaction catalyzed by ATCase can be reversed if an enzymatic trapping agent is included to collect and remove the carbamyl phosphate so generated; these workers used L-ornithine and OCTase for this purpose (Chang and Jones, 1974). We have extended these studies with the observation that ATCase will also function retrograde if arsenate is used to replace phosphate. Like many arsenate esters, it may be presumed that carbamyl arsenate undergoes prompt irreversible decomposition. Large quantities of ATCase (final concentration: 5–8 mg/ml) are needed to catalyze this effect, however, within a practicable time-scale. Nevertheless, if volumes are kept to a minimum, and with a radioactive substrate, it has been observed that 80% of a 0.001 *M* solution of *N*-carbamyl-L-[4-^{14}C]aspartic acid was converted to L-[4-^{14}C]aspartic acid within 10 hours at pH 6 (0.01 *M* sodium acetate) in the presence of 0.01 *M* arsenate and ATCase (8 mg/ml).

With this in mind, a strategy is being developed along the following lines: flash frozen, percussion-pulverized tissue is homogenized in 0.1 *M* acetic acid containing 10 IU of L-aspartic acid β-decarboxylase/ml. This enzyme can function tolerably well in such acidic environments (Tate and Meister, 1968). After 5 minutes at 25°C, the homogenate is chilled to 4°C, centrifuged at 12,000 *g* for 10 minutes, and the supernatant acidified to approximately pH 1 with 1/20th volume of HCl; this step destroys the reagent enzyme instantly. The supernatant is frozen at once, lyophilized with a KOH pellet trap, and reconstituted in 0.1 *M* sodium acetate rendered 0.01 *M* in sodium arsenate. An equal volume of ATCase (16 mg/ml) is added. After 10 hours at 37°C, the mixtures are deproteinized by heating at 95°C for 2 minutes and the new crop of L-aspartic acid is measured on the amino acid analyzer using orthophthalaldehyde detection. Attempts to apply this technique to the tumors of mice given pyrazofurin are, at present, underway in our laboratory.

C. L-Dihydroorotase

1. *Enzyme*

L-Dihydrootase is perhaps the most difficult enzyme of the pyrimidine biosynthetic pathway to measure accurately. This difficulty has kinetic and technical origins. As was discussed earlier, the affinity of L-DHOase for its substrates is sharply and strongly pH dependent; the same is true of the enzyme's V_{max}, and the ultimate ratio of reactants to products achieved. These three features conspire to make control of pH and substrate concentration critical in the assay, because what was a saturating concentration of *N*-carbamyl-L-aspartate at pH 6 will be substantially insufficient to promote a V_{max} at pH 7.5. These kinetic features also cause a quandary in the matter of the exact pH to be used in the assay of this bidirectional enzyme. It will be recalled that only at pH 7.1 will the forward and reverse reactions proceed at equal rates; since this pH is close to physiological, it might appear to be well-suited to the assay. However, although the specific activities measured at this pH might appear to be physiologically representative, they are far from maximal. In fact, it is also doubtful if they are representative: *in vivo*, any L-5,6-dihydroorotic acid formed will be further metabolized by the action of DHO deHase, a feature which will displace the "equilibrium" of the DHOase reaction in the biosynthetic direction regardless of pH. *In vitro*, no such "drain" has been used by the majority of investigators studying this enzyme. This feature will be returned to below.

Because L-dihydroorotic acid is difficult to quantify, there are technical, as well as kinetic problems with the assay. This compound has a feeble ultraviolet absorption, and its chemically reactive ureido function has been masked by the cyclization which attends its synthesis. Thus, most workers have either elected to study the reverse reaction, knowing that *N*-carbamyl-L-aspartate could be measured—albeit without great sensitivity—by one or the other of the analytical techniques outlined earlier, or, when use of the biosynthetic reaction was inevitable, have, at the term of an incubation, separated the newly synthesized L-dihydroorotate, hydrolyzed it back to *N*-carbamyl-L-aspartic acid with alkali, and measured it colorimetrically.

For general purposes, at present, the best overall analytical techniques for L-DHOase use *N*-carbamyl-L-[^{14}C]aspartic or L-[^{14}C]dihydroorotic acids synthesized in the investigators' laboratory by one of several techniques, and purified either by recrystallization or by ion-exchange chromatography. Since these two substrates are unavailable commercially, a brief description of these syntheses is in order here.

N-Carbamyl-L-[^{14}C]aspartic acid can be conveniently synthesized from L-[4-^{14}C]aspartic acid and carbamyl phosphate by the action of crystalline ATCase. To 1 ml of 0.01 *M* carbamyl phosphate, pH 7.4, are added: 100 μCi of L-[4-^{14}C]aspartic acid (specific activity 50 μCi/mole) and 2 IU of pure bacterial ATCase. After 10 minutes at 37°C, the reaction mixture is loaded directly onto an 8 × 200-mm column of Aminex A-14 resin (or its equivalent) in the bicarbonate form. (Note: extensive washing with 1 *M* NH_4HCO_3 is required to convert this resin to the ionic form specified; after conversion, and just prior to use, the column is washed with water until the effluent is Nessler's negative.) The column is developed with a gradient of 0–1 *M* ammonium bicarbonate at its native pH; fractions of 3.67 ml are collected. Salts are removed by four lyophilizations of the active peak. The product is free of L-aspartic acid and homogeneous on paper electrophoresis at pH 2.0 and 7.2.

Chemical techniques, using cyanate, are also available for an analogous synthesis; the LiCl used in the chromatographic purification of the resultant product has sometimes been removed by washing with organic solvents; e.g., a binary mixture of acetone and ethanol. This step, in our hands, is occasionally precarious, and large losses of the radiolabeled *N*-carbamyl-L-aspartate can ensue during it.

The preparation of L-[^{14}C]dihydroorotate capitalizes on the ability of DHO deHase from *Zymobacterium oroticum* to reduce orotic acid in the presence of an excess of NADH.[4] In practice, 25 μCi of carboxyl-[^{14}C]orotate is incubated with 10 μmoles of NADH, 500 μmoles of ethanol, 1 μmole of dithiothrietol, 1.67 IU of DHO deHase, and 10 IU of alcohol dehydrogenase in a final volume of 1 ml. After 2 hours at 37°C the entire reaction mixture is chromatographed on an 8 × 200 column of Aminex A-14 resin in the bicarbonate form, using isocratic elution with 0.2 *M* ammonium bicarbonate. Excess ammonium bicarbonate in the fractions containing L-dihydroorotate is then dissipated by lyophilization.

When large amounts of enzyme are used, a second peak of radioactivity appears (Kensler *et al.,* 1981c). Based on chromatographic and electrophoretic evidence, the peak is concluded to be *N*-carbamyl-L-aspartic acid. In fact, direct enzymatic analysis of the dehydrogenase preparation reveals substantial concentrations of DHOase (Table XIV). Because of this fortuitous contamination, both commercially unavailable pyrimidine precursors can be obtained from a single incubation mixture (Kensler *et al.*, 1981c).

With these syntheses as background, the conduct of the assays for DHOase can now be discussed. In older approaches, using the reverse reaction, any *N*-carbamyl-L-aspartic acid produced was assessed colorimetrically, most frequently with the antipyrine diacetylmonoxime reagents; in fact, as a recent compendium shows, this approach is still widely used (Hoffee and Jones, 1978). However, for augmented sensitivity and specificity, radiolabeled substrates have gained in use; they are, as indicated, somewhat troublesome to synthesize, but where precision is a concern, of far greater utility than their "cold" counterparts. After incubation, *N*-carbamyl-L-[^{14}C]aspartate can be separated from L-[^{14}C]dihydroorotic acid either by high voltage electrophoresis (Table XII), by ion-exchange thin layer chromatography (Smithers *et al.*, 1978), or by paper chromatography (Table XII).

2. *Substrate*

Virtually nothing is known about the concentration of L-dihydroorotic acid in tumors or tissues under physiologic conditions. The present sec-

[4] Unlike the mammalian enzyme (cf. Table IV) the bacterial DHO dehydrogenase catalyzes a freely reversible reaction.

TABLE XIV

CROSS-CONTAMINATION OF BACTERIAL PYRIMIDINE REAGENT ENZYMES[a]

Reagent enzyme		Contaminant activities(%)					
Specific activity (nmole/mg/minute)	Enzyme/source	CPS II	ATCase	DHOase	DHO deHase	OPRTase	OMP deCase
1100	CPS II *E. coli*		+ (0.2)	+ (0.2)	−	−	−
365000	ATCase *E. coli*	−		+ (trace)[b]	+ (trace)	−	−
6400	DHO deHase *Z. oroticum*	−	−	+ (trace)		+ (trace)	+ (trace)
320	ORPTase/OMP deCase yeast	−	−	+ (0.4)	+ (trace)		
1100	OMP deCase yeast	−	+ (0.3)	−	+ (trace)	+ (trace)	

[a] Pyrimidine reagent enzymes were assayed as described in Kensler *et al.* (1981a) and contaminant activities are expressed as percentage of specific activity.

[b] Trace is <0.1% contamination.

tion will suggest approaches to such measurements, but it must be stressed that a great deal of work remains to be done before these approaches can be deployed with assurance.

In the first approach, tissues are flash frozen and extracted with 0.1 *M* acetic acid; acid is removed by lyophilization, with an alkali trap. After reconstitution and clarification, the extract from the equivalent of 1 gm of liver is subjected to automatic chromatography on a Hamilton HA × 4 resin using lithium citrate-chloride buffers at pH 2.65–2.72 (Tyagi *et al.*, 1979). Most pyrimidine intermediates are well resolved in this system, but L-dihydroorotic acid and orotic acids coelute (Table XV). Fractions are collected and those containing these two acids are pooled, concentrated, brought to pH 13 with sodium hydroxide, and then subjected to colorimetric assay for *N*-carbamyl-L-aspartate. Orotic acid is nonreactive under these conditions. Using this technique, no alkali-generated ureido functionalities were detected in the appropriate fractions derived from 1 gm of mouse liver. Since the level of detection of the assay is around 10 nmoles, this negative result would suggest that L-5,6-dihydroorotic acid is normally present in liver at a concentration of less than 10 μM.

In the second approach, a concentrated acetic acid extract or neutralized 5% PCA extract of tissue is subjected to a spectrophotometric assay for L-5,6-dihydroorotic acid using NAD as pyridine nucleotide indicator

TABLE XV

RETENTION TIMES OF THE PYRIMIDINES[a]

	Time (minutes)
Carbamyl phosphate	20
N-Carbamyl-L-aspartate	15
L-Dihydroorotate	175
Orotic acid	170
Orotidine	115
OMP	233–240
UMP	87
UDP	233
UTP	325
CMP	9
CDP	106
CTP	232
TMP	102
TDP	240
TTP	348

[a] The chromatographic system used is that described by Tyagi *et al.* (1979).

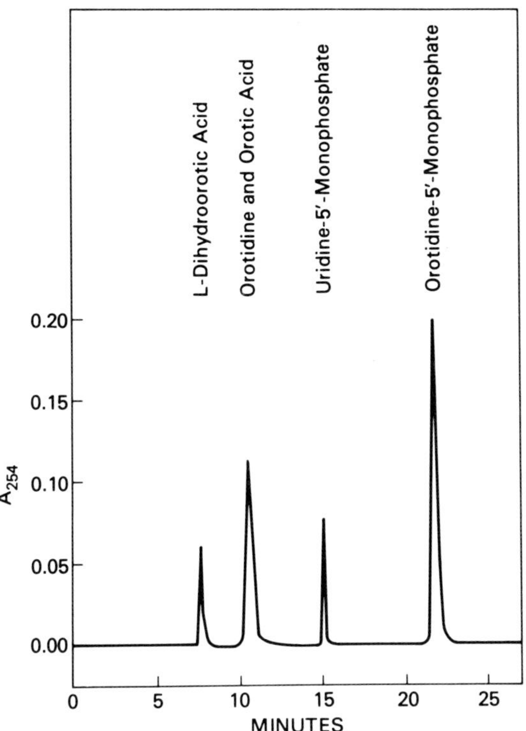

FIG. 20. High pressure liquid chromatographic separation of select pyrimidine precursors. Conditions of the run are described in detail by Kensler *et al.* (1981a). The load consisted of 500 nmoles of L-dihydroorotic acid, 5 nmoles of orotic acid, and 2 nmoles each of orotidine, uridine-5′-monophosphate, and orotidine-5′-monophosphate.

and DHO deHase as reagent enzyme. The increase in absorbance at 340 nm on addition of enzyme is taken as an index of the presence of substrate. In practice, the following reactants are admixed in a quartz cuvette with a 1 cm light path: 1 ml of neutralized, clarified extract, equivalent to 0.1–1.0 gm of tissue and 100 μl of 0.5 *M* Tris–HCl pH 8.4, containing 1 μmole of NAD. When optical stability is assured, 0.1 IU of DHO deHase is added to initiate the reaction and the $+\Delta A$ at 340 nm is measured continuously. Under these conditions, a final change in absorbance of 0.115 is equivalent to 20 nmoles of L-dihydroorotate. Performed as prescribed, this assay suffers from several drawbacks: the concentrated extracts used often interfere with the rate, and perhaps extent of the dehydrogenation. Moreover, the reagent enzyme, at least as presently marketed, is impure and so cannot be considered specific for L-dihydroorotate (Table XIV).

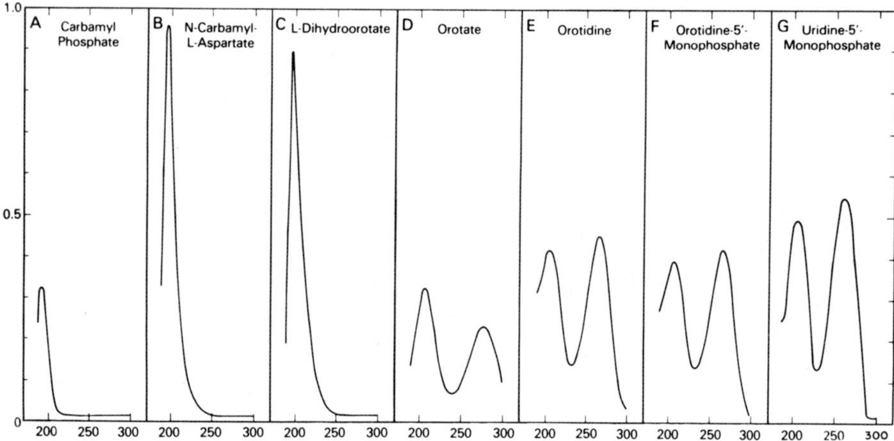

FIG. 21. Ultraviolet spectra of selected pyrimidines and pyrimidine percursors. Spectra were recorded on a Beckman DBG recording spectrophotometer.

This method, too, failed to detect L-dihydroorotate in the extract equivalent to 1 gm of liver.

High pressure liquid chromatography is an obvious choice for the measurement of L-dihydroorotate (Fig. 20), but the feeble extinction coefficient of this metabolite (Fig. 21) tends to mitigate against the routine use of this technique. However, because of the comparatively intense extinction of orotic acid (Fig. 21), it should be theoretically possible to measure the content of L-dihydroorotate in an extract before and after exposure to the action of DHO deHase from *Zymobacterium oroticum,* the increase being taken as an index of its L-dihydroorotate content. Work along these lines is, at present, underway in several laboratories.

D. L-DIHYDROOROTATE DEHYDROGENASE

1. *Enzyme*

Unlike the bacterial dehydrogenase discussed in Section II, DHO deHase from mammals cannot use NAD as its cofactor; rather, as was discussed, ubiquinone is felt to fill this function. Two general approaches have been taken for the analysis of DHO deHase. In the first, orotic acid production is measured spectrophotometrically either directly or after deproteinization; this latter expedient must be adopted in laboratories lacking instruments capable of accepting turbid samples because of the optical disturbances resulting from the addition of mitochondria. In the second analytical strategy, L-[carboxy-^{14}C]dihydroorotate is used as a substrate, and the product is either separated by electrophoresis (Table XII) or else, after incubation, is further metabolized to [^{14}C]CO_2, by the addition of bacterial OPRTase and OMP deCase in non-rate-limiting amounts. This last approach offers the advantage of ease and precision. For this reason it will be described in detail.

Mitochondria, prepared by the technique of Schnaitmann and Greenawalt (1968), are resuspended in 0.01 *M* HEPES buffer, pH 7.4, containing 0.25 *M* sucrose, to a concentration of approximately 1 mg of protein/ml; 5 μl of L-[carboxyl-^{14}C]dihydroorotate is then incubated for 10 minutes at 37°C with 20 μl of mitochondrial suspension. The reaction is arrested by 2 minutes of heating at 95°C and any [carboxyl-^{14}C]orotate generated is converted to UMP by the addition of 50 μl of 0.01 *M* Mg^{2+} · PRPP prepared in a solution of the mixed OPRTase–OMP deCase from yeast (1 mg/ml); a droplet of 40% KOH on the underside of the lid serves to trap the released [^{14}C]CO_2. After 12 hours at 25°C the radioactivity so trapped is counted by scintillation spectrometry.

Since this assay is carried out in two discrete stages, the second of which is allowed to run to completion independent of the first, it is not necessary that the processing enzymes (which are far from homogeneous) be used at 10–100 times their K_ms as is theoretically desirable in simultaneously coupled enzyme assays entailing the use of two reagent enzymes, in series. As a consequence of this advantage, the quantities of OPRTase and OMP deCase can be kept to a minimum, thus also minimizing contamination from any (variable) bacterial DHO deHase possibly present therein (Table XIV).

Inasmuch as it is the 2 and 3 hydrogens of the L-aspartic acid skeleton which are ultimately labilized by DHO deHase (Fig. 1), an alternative method of assay can be suggested: *N*-carbamyl-L-[2,3-^{3}H]aspartic acid is synthesized enzymatically and converted in acceptable yield to L-[5,6-^{3}H]-dihydroorotate, by means of crude DHOase from mutant BHK cells (Coleman *et al.*, 1977); this substrate is purified by paper chromatography and desalted as described earlier. On incubation with DHO deHase, tritiums are labilized. The resultant [^{3}H]OH can be sublimed or distilled with ease. This assay, while still developmental, will be described in greater detail, because of the facility which it brings to the measurement of DHO deHase.

In a final volume of 10 μl are admixed: 5 μl (~0.5 μCi) of L-[5,6-^{3}H]dihydroorotic acid and 5 μl of mitochondrial suspension prepared as described *supra*. After 4 minutes at 37°C, during which tritium release is verified to be linear (Fig. 22), the vessels are heated at 95°C for 2 minutes, centrifuged at 12,000 *g* to aggregate any condensation, set in a

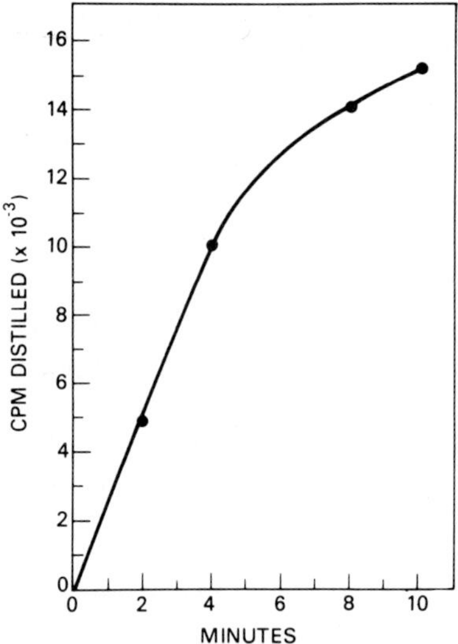

FIG. 22. Time-course of the tritium-release assay for dihydroorotate dehydrogenase. Incubations and distillations were carried out as described in the text.

bed of dry ice and opened; 5 μl of 100% KOH is pipetted onto the underside of the lid which is then closed securely; [^{3}H]OH is allowed to distill overnight whereafter the lids are removed and their radioactivity measured by scintillation spectrometry.

2. *Substrates and Products*

Historically and statistically speaking, orotic acid is perhaps the oldest and most frequently measured of the pyrimidine precursors. Long known to abound in cow's (but not human) milk, this acid later came to be recognized in the serum and tissues of patients treated with any one of the several inhibitors of OMP deCase discussed earlier in this article. Earlier methods of analysis were mainly colorimetric, relying on the interaction of Ehrlich's reagent with orotate (Rogers and Porter, 1968). More recently, however, high pressure liquid chromatographic measurements have supplanted these older techniques. Figure 20 illustrates the kind of resolution possible with high pressure liquid chromatography. Using instrumentation such as this, it has been possible to document that orotic acid and orotidine are ordinarily present in extracts of liver at $<1\ \mu M$, but that they accumulate during pharmacologic blockage of OMP deCase, occasionally to concentrations as high as 0.5 mM (Moyer and Handschmacher, 1979). Two enzymatic strategies have also been published for measuring orotic acid. Both are spectrophotometric. The first takes advantage of the change in absorbance attending the conversion of orotate to orotidine-5′-monophosphate and then to UMP, reactions catalyzed by OPRTase and OMP deCase from yeast (Möllering, 1974). The second makes use of the flavoprotein dehydrogenase from *Z. oroticum* in the presence of excess NADH to catalyze the reduction of orotate to the nonabsorbing product, L-dihydroorotate. Both assays have a common drawback: the impurity of the reagent enzymes required for their utilization. Neither yields stoichiometric or quantitative results (Friedmann and Krakow, 1974) especially when authentic extracts of tumors or normal murine tissues are being examined.

E. Orotate Phosphoribosyl Transferase

1. *Enzyme*

In the presence of PRPP · Mg^{2+}, and the cytoplasmic transferase discussed earlier, orotic acid is converted to the nucleotide, orotidine-5′-monophosphate. Since the enzyme catalyzing this reaction coexists with OMP deCase, its separate activity cannot be analyzed unless and until the decarboxylase is either separated, or more practically, inhibited. Fortunately the trio of exceedingly potent inhibitors of the decarboxylase discussed earlier can be put to use as analytical tools toward this end (Jones *et al.*, 1978). When this is done, any orotidine-5′-monophosphate generated can be analyzed by one of several techniques: (1) spectrophotometric-capitalizing on the ΔA at 280 or 295 which ensues upon the acquisition by orotic acid of the ribose and phosphate functionalities (cf. Fig. 21); (2) chromatographic-capitalizing on the diminished solubility of orotidine-5′-monophosphate vis-à-vis orotic acid in solvents such as ethanol : 1 *M* ammonium acetate (70 : 30, v/v) (Table XII); and (3) electrophoretic-capitalizing on the stronger net negative charge of orotidine-5′-monophosphate at pH 2 (Table XII).

In practice, 5 μl (0.25 μCi) of carboxyl [^{14}C]orotic acid is incubated with 5 μl (50 nmoles) of PRPP · Mg^{2+}, pH 7.5; 5 μl (5 pmoles) of 6-azauridine-5′-monophosphate, and 5 μl of a 12,000 *g* (3 minute) supernatant from the tissue of interest. After 10 minutes at 37°C, and 2 minutes at 95°C, any [^{14}C]orotidine-5′-monophosphate formed is separated from orotate by means of high-voltage electrophoresis in 0.1 *M* sodium phosphate at pH 2 (Table XII). Consequent to the use of such an inhibitor-based analysis of OPRTase, it has been possible to document, as discussed *supra,* that the reaction catalyzed by this enzyme is, in fact, reversible and that it ordinarily channels at least a portion of its product, orotidine-5′-monophosphate, to the catalytic center of its partner enzyme, OMP deCase *in vivo.*

2. *Substrate*

Pure orotidylic acid is easily measurable on account of its intrinsic absorbance in the ultraviolet (Fig. 22); however, since a huge collection of other nucleotides with equivalent or greater absorbance is present in samples of biologic origin, this property is of little direct analytical value. Rather, it is necessary to separate or otherwise resolve orotidine-5′-monophosphate from its congeners, when quantitative measurements are of importance. This can most easily be done nowadays using high-pressure liquid chromatography (Fig. 20).

It is also possible to quantify orotidylic acid in a direct spectrophotometric approach which capitalizes on the substantial change in absorbance which accompanies its conversion to UMP via the action of OMP deCase (Fig. 21). In practice, the absorbance of a neutralized extract of tissue is read at 280 nm before and after the addition of OMP deCase to a final concentration of 0.01 IU/ml; the difference is taken as an index of the amount of orotidine-5′-monophosphate present.

This method, while exceedingly facile, suffers from the drawback of insensitivity; since orotidine-5′-monophosphate is ordinarily present at concentrations of only 50 n*M*, this drawback effectively precludes the use of the direct spectrophotometric assay for samples of biologic origin. Moreover, under pharmacologic circumstances (e.g., following the administration of 6-azauridine, allopurinol, or pyrazofurin, when orotidine-5′-monophosphate can accumulate to concentrations many-fold above its basal level), the nucleotides of the drugs are ordinarily present at concentrations quite sufficient to inhibit the action of the reagent enzyme, OMP deCase.

Numerous viable techniques have been published for estimating the concentration of PRPP; most frequently a radioactive purine or pyrimidine base is incubated with an excess of the appropriate phosphoribosyl transferase in the presence of the unknown or standard amount of PPRP · Mg^{2+}. The resulting nucleotides are then either separated by electrophoretic means (Hisata, 1975), or in the case of [carboxyl-^{14}C]-orotidine-5′-monophosphate, decarboxylated with yeast OMP deCase (May and Krooth, 1976). This last approach has the advantage of being suitable for analytical "mass production."

F. Orotidine-5′-Monophosphate Decarboxylase

1. *Enzyme*

Three principal methods are available for measuring this, the last enzyme in the pyrimidine biosynthetic pathway.

The first such method is spectrophotometric, and utilizes the change in absorbance which ensues upon the decarboxylation of orotidine-5′-monophosphate (see also the previous section). When clear extracts with high activity are being studied, this approach offers the salient virtue of high facility; it also yields continuous measurements of V, a feature which, in theory at least, allows for the computation of kinetic constants from a single reaction progress curve. However, it is not always applicable to crude or opalescent samples, and suffers from comparative insensitivity. The method is also not well suited to the processing of numerous samples.

Paper chromatography, the second method, does satisfy this last requirement. In the system used most frequently, orotidine-5′-monophosphate is well resolved from UMP on Whatman 3M paper developed in the ascending mode with *n*-butanol : acetic acid : H_2O, 4 : 1 : 1 (Table XII). Use of this method with nonradioactive substrate is practicable, but we have observed that as yet unidentified materials present in the crude tissue extracts coelute with UMP, thus compromising the absolute reliability of the method. When radioactive orotidine-5′-monophosphate is used, however, this objection is circumvented.

In point of fact, the third system for analyzing OMP deCase also uses [carboxyl-^{14}C]orotidine-5′-monophosphate but traps the resultant [^{14}C]CO_2 in droplets of alkali. In practice, in order to minimize use of [^{14}C]orotidine-5′-monophosphate, the reaction volumes are kept to a minimum: 10–15 μl. In the authors' laboratory, Eppendorf polypropylene vessels are used in this assay. To the bottom of a battery of such vessels are dispensed 5-μl aliquots of [^{14}C]orotidine-5′-monophosphate; 5 μl of 40% KOH is next pipetted onto the center of the underside of the vessels' lids. At timed intervals, the substrate is overlaid with 10 μl of extract, the assemblies closed at once, and incubated at 37°C for a span over which the reaction has been antecedently verified to be linear. At the term of this time, the bases of the vessels are heated at 95°C for 2 minutes to arrest the reaction, returned to 25°C, and left there for an additional 3 hours to permit the quantitative evolution and collection of the crop of [^{14}C]CO_2.

While manifestly easy and accurate, this method uses a radiolabeled substrate which at present is exceedingly expensive.

2. *Substrate*

High pressure liquid chromatography is the present method of choice for measuring UMP pool sizes; a typical separation on a Partisil SAX column with a mixed pH and ionic strength gradient of potassium phosphate is presented in Fig. 20. Using this technique, we have observed that UMP pools average 30 nmoles/gm wet weight, in the native Lewis lung carcinoma but are significantly elevated in PALA-resistant variant lines (Kensler *et al.*, 1981a).

A second viable approach to the assessment of UMP pools is enzymatic: in this approach UMP is first converted to UDP then to UTP via the action of pyrimidine nucleoside mono- and diphosphate kinases; the UTP is converted to UDP glucose in the presence of UTP and UDP glucose pyrophosphorylase, and the UDP glucose is converted to UDP glucuronic acid in the presence of UDP glucose dehydrogenase; NAD is simultaneously reduced in this process, thus providing a convenient and sensitive optical index of the reaction. The method is cumbersome on paper but manageable in practice; however, using it, cognizance must be taken of UDP glucose, UTP, and UDP which might coexist in any given sample with UMP, because these nucleotides will also reduce NAD in the assay system. In practice, all of the reagent enzymes except UMP kinase are added to the cuvette; after the absorbance at 340 has completely stabilized, an appropriate quantity of the kinase is added in a negligible volume and the absorbance monitored until a new "plateau" has supervened. In those cases where the baseline fails to become horizontal, corrections for the creep upward or downward are made by extrapolation to the time of addition of the UMP kinase. This method can detect about 5 nmoles of UMP in the spectrophotometric mode; if fluorimetric measurement of the NADH generated in it are made, as little as 5 pmoles of the nucleotide can be measured in optimal cases (Keppler *et al.*, 1974).

G. Prospects

It should be clear from the whole thrust of this Appendix that techniques for measuring the enzymes of the pyrimidine biosynthetic pathway are at present well developed and reliable. The same cannot be said of certain of the substrates and products of the path. Three of these especially demand attention: carbamyl phosphate, *N*-carbamyl-L-aspartic, and L-dihydroorotic acids. It should also be clear that assiduous attention must be paid to enzymes used as reagents in any of the analyses recapitulated here; contaminating activities are the rule—not the exception, at present. It is hoped that this compendium and its caveats will serve to stimulate work along these lines.

References

Adair, L. B., and Jones, M. E. (1978). *Methods Enzymol.* **51,** 51.
Allen, C. M., Jr., and Jones, M. E. (1964). *Biochemistry* **3,** 1238.
Ardalan, B., Kensler, T. W., Jayaram, H. N., Morrison, W., Choie, D. D., Chadwick, M., Liss, R., and Cooney, D. A. (1981). *Cancer Res.* **41,** 150.
Badawy, A. A.-B., and Evans, M. (1973). *Biochem. J.* **133,** 585.
Ball, E. G., Anfinsen, C. B., and Cooper, O. (1947). *J. Biol. Chem.* **168,** 257.
Barker, H. A., Weissbach, H., and Smyth, R. D. (1958). *Proc. Natl. Acad. Sci. U.S.A.* **44,** 1093.
Beardmore, T. D., and Kelley, W. N. (1971). *J. Lab. Clin. Med.* **78,** 696.
Bennett, L. L., Jr., Smithers, D., Rose, L. M., Adamson, D. J., and Thomas, H. J. (1979). *Cancer Res.* **39,** 4868.
Black, M. L. (1963). *J. Med. Chem.* **6,** 145.
Boettcher, B. R., and Meister, A. (1980). *J. Biol. Chem.* **255,** 7129.
Bresnick, E., and Mossé, H. A. (1966). *Biochem. J.* **101,** 63.
Bresnick, E., and Hitchings, G. H. (1961). *Cancer Res.* **21,** 105.
Brockman, R. W., and Anderson, E. P. (1963). *Annu. Rev. Biochem.* **32,** 463.
Brockman, R. W., Shaddix, S. C., and Rose, L. M. (1977). *Cancer* **40,** 2681.
Brooks, K. P., Kim, B. D., and Sander, E. G. (1979). *Biochim. Biophys. Acta* **570,** 213.
Brown, G. K., and O'Sullivan, W. J. (1977). *Biochem. Pharmacol.* **26,** 1947.
Brown, G. K., Fox, R. M., and O'Sullivan, W. J. (1972). *Biochem. Pharmacol.* **21,** 2469.
Brown, G. M. (1962). *J. Biol. Chem.* **237,** 536.
Bruemmer, N. C., Holland, J. F., and Sheehe, P. R. (1962). *Cancer Res.* **22,** 113.
Buchanan, J. M. (1973). *Adv. Enzymol.* **39,** 91.
Cadman, E. C., Dix, D. E., and Handschumacher, R. E. (1978). *Cancer Res.* **38,** 682.
Cadman, E., Heimer, R., and Davis, L. (1979). *Science* **205,** 1135.
Carter, S. K. (1977). *Natl. Cancer Inst. Monogr.* **45,** 93.
Chadwick, M., and Chang, C. (1973). *Proc. Am. Assoc. Cancer Res.* **14,** 89.
Chadwick, M., Jaques, D., and Beard, G. (1976). *Proc. Am. Assoc. Cancer Res.* **17,** 178.
Chang, T.-Y., and Jones, M. E. (1974). *Biochemistry* **13,** 646.
Chen, J.-J., and Jones, M. E. (1976). *Arch. Biochem. Biophys.* **176,** 82.
Chen, J.-J., and Jones, M. E. (1979). *J. Biol. Chem.* **254,** 4908.
Christopherson, R. I., and Jones, M. E. (1980). *J. Biol. Chem.* **255,** 3358.
Christopherson, R. I., Matsuura, T., and Jones, M. E. (1978). *Anal. Biochem.* **89,** 225.
Čihák, A., and Brouček, J. (1972). *Biochem. Pharmacol.* **21,** 2497.
Čihák, A., and Šorm, F. (1972). *Biochem. Pharmacol.* **21,** 607.
Coleman, P. F., Suttle, D. P., and Stark, G. R. (1977). *J. Biol. Chem.* **252,** 6379.
Collins, K. D., and Stark, G. R. (1971). *J. Biol. Chem.* **246,** 6599.
Cooney, D. A., and Milman, H. A. (1972). *Biochem. J.* **129,** 953.
Cooney, D. A., Davis, R. D., and Van Atta, G. (1971a). *Anal. Biochem.* **40,** 312.
Cooney, D. A., Milman, H. A., and Truitt, R. (1971b). *Anal. Biochem.* **41,** 583.
Cooney, D. A., Homan, E. R., Cameron, T., and Schaeppi, U. (1973). *J. Lab. Clin. Med.* **81,** 455.
Cooney, D. A., Jayaram, H. N., Ryan, J. A., and Bono, V. H. (1974). *Cancer Treat. Rep.* **58,** 793.
Cooney, D. A., Milman, H. A., Cable, R. G., Dion, R. L., and Bono, V. H., Jr. (1978). *Biochem. Pharmacol.* **27,** 151.
Conn, H. O., Creasey, W. A., and Calabresi, P. (1967). *Cancer Res.* **27,** 618.
Curci, M. R., and Donachie, W. D. (1964). *Biochim. Biophys. Acta* **85,** 338.

da Consolacão, M., Linardi, F., de Oliveria, M. M., and Sampaio, M. R. P. (1975). *J. Med. Chem.* **18,** 1159.
Dahl, J. L., Way, J. L., and Parks, R. E., Jr. (1959). *J. Biol. Chem.* **234,** 2998.
Davis, R. H. (1972). *Science* **178,** 835.
DeLong, D. C., Baker, L. A., Gerzon, K., Gutowski, G. E., Williams, R. H., and Hamill R. L. (1971). *Proc. Int. Congr. Chemother., 7th, Prague.*
Diederich, D., Ramponi, G., and Grisolia, S. (1971). *FEBS Lett.* **15,** 30.
Dix, D. E., Lehman, C. P., Jakubowski, A., Moyer, J. D., and Handschumacher, R. E. (1979). *Cancer Res.* **39,** 4485.
Driscoll, J. S., Hazard, G. F., Jr., Wood, H. B., Jr., and Goldin, A. (1974). *Cancer Chemother. Rep.* **4,** 1.
Dunlap, R. B. (1978). *Methods Enzymol.* **51,** 90.
Duschinsky, R., Walker, H., and Wojnarowski, W. (1975). "Design and Mechanism of Action of Antimetabolites," p. 29. Bulgarian Acad. Sci.
Elion, G. B. (1966). *Ann. Rheum. Dis.* **25,** 608.
Elion, G. B. (1978). *Handb. Exp. Pharmacol.* **51,** 485.
Erlichman, C., Strong, J. M., Wiernik, P. H., McAvoy, L. M., Cohen, M. H., Levine, A. S., Hubbard, S. M., and Chabner, B. A. (1979). *Cancer Res.* **39,** 3992.
Fhaolain, I. N., and Coughlan, M. P. (1978). *FEBS Lett.* **90,** 305.
Fieser, L. F., Berliner, E., Bondhus, F. J., Chang, F. C., Dauben, W. G., Ettlinger, M. G., Fawaz, G., Fields, M., Fieser, M. Heidelberger, G., Heyman, H., Seligman, A. M., Vaughan, W. R., Wilson, A. G., Wilson, E., Wu, M.-I., Leffler, M. T., Hamlin, K. E., Hathaway, R. J., Matson, E. J., Moore, E. E., Moore, M. B., Rapala, R. T., and Zaugg, M. E. (1948). *J. Am. Chem. Soc.* **70,** 3151.
Folkers, K., Porter, T. H., Acton, E., Taylor, D. L., and Henry, D. (1978). *Biochem. Biophys. Res. Commun.* **83,** 353.
Forman, H. J., and Kennedy, J. (1975). *J. Biol. Chem.* **250,** 4322.
Friedmann, H. C., and Krakow, A. (1974). *Methods Enz. Anal.* **4,** 1963.
Friedmann, H. C., and Vennesland, B. (1958). *J. Biol. Chem.* **233,** 1398.
Fox, R. M., Royse-Smith, D., and O'Sullivan, W. J. (1970). *Science* **168,** 861.
Fyfe, J. A., Miller, R. L., and Krenitsky, T. A. (1973). *J. Biol. Chem.* **248,** 3801.
Gerzon, K., DeLong, D. C., and Cline, J. C. (1971). *Int. Pure Appl. Chem.* **28,** 489.
Goldberg, I. H., and Rabinowitz, M. (1963). *Biochim. Biophys. Acta* **72,** 116.
Gosálvez, M., Garcia-Cañero, R., Blanco, M., and Gurucharri-Lloyd, G. (1976). *Can. Chemother. Rep.* **61,** 1.
Gruber, W., Möllering, H., and Bergmeyer, H. U. (1974). *Methods Enzym. Anal.* **4,** 2078.
Gutowski, G. E., Sweeney, M. J., DeLong, D. C., Hamill, R. L., Gerzon, K., and Dyke, R. W. (1975). *Ann. N.Y. Acad. Sci.* **255,** 544.
Gutteridge, W. E., Dave, D., and Richards, W. H. G. (1979). *Biochim. Biophys. Acta* **582,** 390.
Guyton, A. C. (1971). "Textbook of Medical Physiology." Saunders, Philadelphia, Pennsylvania.
Habermann, V. (1960). *Biochim. Biophys. Acta* **43,** 137.
Hager, S. E., and Jones, M. E. (1965). *J. Biol. Chem.* **240,** 4556.
Handschumacher, R. E. (1960). *J. Biol. Chem.* **235,** 764.
Handschumacher, R. E., and Pasternak, C. A. (1958). *Biochim. Biophys. Acta* **30,** 451.
Handschumacher, R. E., Calabresi, P., Welch, A. D., Bono, V., Fallon, H., and Frei, E., III (1962). *Cancer Chemother. Rep.* **21,** 1.
Handschumacher, R. E., Schwartz, P. M., and Moyer, J. D. (1979). *In* "Antimetabolites in Biochemistry, Biology and Medicine" (J. Škoda and P. Langen eds.), pp. 297–303. Pergamon, Oxford.

Hernandez, K., Pinkel, D., Lee, S., and Leone, L. (1969). *Cancer Chemother. Rep.* **53,** 203.
Hisata, T. (1975). *Anal. Biochem.* **68,** 448.
Hitchings, G. H. (1955). *Am. J. Clin. Nutr.* **3,** 321.
Hoffee, P. A., and Jones, M. E., eds. (1978). *Methods Enzymol.* **51.**
Holmes, W. L. (1956). *J. Biol. Chem.* **233,** 667.
Holmes, W. L., and Welch, A. D. (1956). *Cancer Res.* **16,** 251.
Hoogenraad, N. J. (1974). *Arch. Biochem. Biophys.* **161,** 76.
Howland, J. L. (1963a). *Biochim. Biophys. Acta* **77,** 659.
Howland, J. L. (1963b). *Biochim. Biophys. Acta* **77,** 665.
Huisman, W. H., and Becker, M. A. (1980). *Anal. Biochem.* **101,** 160.
Huisman, W. H., Raivio, K. O., and Becker, M. A. (1979). *J. Biol. Chem.* **254,** 12595.
Ingraham, J. L., and Abdelal, A. T. H. (1978). *Methods Enzymol.* **51,** 29.
Isenberg, H. D., Seifter, E., and Berkman, J. I. (1960). *Biochim. Biophys. Acta* **39,** 187.
Jaffee, J. J., and Cooper, J. R. (1958). *Cancer Res.* **18,** 1089.
Janeway, C. M., and Cha, S. (1977). *Cancer Res.* **37,** 4382.
Jayaram, H. N., and Cooney, D. A. (1979). *Cancer Treat. Rep.* **63,** 1095.
Jayaram, H. N., Cooney, D. A., Ryan, J. A., Neil, G., Dion, R. L., and Bono, V. H. (1975). *Cancer Treat. Rep.* **59,** 481.
Jayaram, H. N., Cooney, D. A., Milman, H. A., Homan, E.R., and Rosenbluth, R. J. (1976). *Biochem. Pharmacol.* **25,** 1571.
Jayaram, H. N., Cooney, D. A., Vistica, D. T., Kariya, S., and Johnson, R. K. (1979). *Cancer Treat. Rep.* **63,** 1291.
Jayaram, H. N., Kensler, T. W., and Ardalan, B. (1981). *Cancer Treat. Rep.*, in press.
Jernigan, H. M., Jr., and Kraus, L. M. (1975). *J. Lab. Clin. Med.* **85,** 694.
Johnson, R. K. (1977). *Biochem. Pharmacol.* **26,** 81.
Johnson, R. K., Inouye, T., Goldin, A., and Stark, G. R. (1976). *Cancer Res.* **36,** 2720.
Johnson, R. K., Swyryd, E. A., and Stark, G. R. (1978). *Cancer Res.* **38,** 371.
Jones, M. E. (1974). *Methods Enzym. Anal.* **4,** 1749.
Jones, M. E. (1980). *Annu. Rev. Biochem.* **49,** 253.
Jones, M. E., Kavipurapu, P. R., and Traut, T. W. (1978). *Methods Enzymol.* **51,** 155.
Kalousek, F., Rychlík, I., and Šorm, F. (1962). *Biochim. Biophys. Acta* **61,** 368.
Kempe, T. D., Swyryd, E. A., Bruist, M., and Stark, G. R. (1976). *Cell* **9,** 541.
Kennedy, J. (1973). *Arch. Biochem. Biophys.* **157,** 369.
Kennedy, J. (1974). *Arch. Biochem. Biophys.* **160,** 358.
Kensler, T. W., Jayaram, H. N., and Cooney, D. A. (1980a). *J. Biochem. Biophys. Methods* **2,** 29.
Kensler, T. W., Erlichman, C., Jayaram, H. N., Tyagi, A. K., Ardalan, B., and Cooney, D. A. (1980b). *Cancer Treat. Rep.* **64,** 967.
Kensler, T. W., Mutter, G., Hankerson, J. G., Reck, L. J., Harley, C., Han, N., Ardalan, B., Cysyk, R. L., Johnson, R. K., Jayaram, H. N., and Cooney, D. A. (1981a). *Cancer Res.* **41,** 894.
Kensler, T. W., Reck, L. J., and Cooney, D. A. (1981b). *Cancer Res.* **41,** 905.
Kensler, T. W., Han, N., and Cooney, D. A. (1981c). *Anal. Biochem.* **111,** 49.
Keppler, D. O. R. (1977). *FEBS Lett.* **73,** 263.
Keppler, D., Gawehn, K. and Decker, K. (1974). *Methods Enzym. Anal.* **4,** 2172.
Khedouri, E., Anderson, P. M., and Meister, A. (1966). *Biochemistry* **5,** 3552.
Koide, S. S. (1962). *Biochim. Biophys. Acta* **59,** 708.
Legrain, C., Stalon, V., Glansdorff, N., Gigot, D., Pierard, A., and Crabeel, M. (1976). *J. Bacteriol.* **128,** 39.
Leinbach, S. S., Reno, J. M., Lee, L. F., Isbell, A. F., and Boezi, J. A. (1976). *Biochemistry* **15,** 426.

Levine, R. L., and Kretchmer, N. (1971). *Anal. Biochem.* **42,** 324.
Levine, H. L., Brody, R. S., and Westheimer, F. H. (1980). *Biochemistry* **19,** 4993.
Liebermann, I., and Kornberg, A. (1953). *Biochim. Biophys. Acta* **12,** 223.
Livingston, R. B., Venditti, J. M., Cooney, D. A., and Carter, S. K. (1970). *Adv. Pharm. Chemother.* **8,** 57.
Lopes, J. N., Cruz, F. S., Docampo, R., Vasconcellos, M. E., Sampaio, M. C., Pinto, A. V., and Gilbert, B. (1978). *Ann. Trop. Med. Parasitol.* **72,** 523.
Loo, T. L., Benjamin, R. S., Lu, K., Benvenuto, J. A., Hall, S. W., and McKelvey, E. M. (1978). *Drug Metab. Rev.* **8,** 137.
McClard, R. W., Black, M. J., Livingstone, L. R., and Jones, M. E. (1980). *Biochemistry* **19,** 4699.
McCollister, R. J., Gilbert, W. R., Ashton, D. M., and Wyngaarden, J. B. (1964). *J. Biol. Chem.* **239,** 1560.
McKelvey, E. M., Lomedico, M., Lu, K., Chadwick, M., and Loo, T. L. (1979). *Clin. Pharm. Ther.* **25,** 586.
Maren, T. H. (1963). *J. Pharm. Exp. Ther.* **139,** 129.
Matsuzawa, T., Ito, M., and Ishiguro, I. (1980). *Anal. Biochem.* **106,** 1.
May, S. R., and Krooth, R. S. (1976). *Anal. Biochem.* **75,** 389.
May, S. R., Hashmi, S., Miller, O. J., and Krooth, R. S. (1977). *Somatic Cell Genet.* **3,** 263.
Miller; R. W., and Curry, J. R. (1969). *Can. J. Biochem.* **47,** 725.
Milman, H. A., and Cooney, D. A. (1974). *Biochem. J.* **142,** 27.
Möllering, H. (1974). *Methods Enzym. Anal.* **4,** 1959.
Moore, E. C., and Hurlbert, R. B. (1961). *Cancer Res.* **21,** 257.
Moore, E. C., and LePage, G. A. (1957). *Cancer Res.* **17,** 804.
Mori, M., and Tatibana, M. (1978). *Methods Enzymol.* **51,** 111.
Moyer, J. D., and Handschumacher, R. E. (1979). *Cancer Res.* **39,** 3089.
Neil, G. L., Berger, A. E., McPartland, R. P., Grindey, G. B., and Bloch, A. (1979). *Cancer Res.* **39,** 852.
Nelson, D. J., Buggé, C. J. L., Krasny, H. C., and Elion, G. B. (1973). *Biochem. Pharmacol.* **22,** 2003.
Ohnuma, T., Roboz, J., Shapiro, M. L., and Holland, J. F. (1977). *Cancer Res.* **37,** 2043.
O'Sullivan, W. J. (1974). *Prog. Biochem. Pharmacol.* **9,** 174.
Overby, L. R., Robishaw, E. E., Schleicher, J. B., Reuter, A., Shipkowitz, N. L., and Mao, J. C.-H. (1974). *Antimicrob. Ag. Chemother.* **6,** 360.
Overby, L. R., Duff, R. G., and Mao, J. C.-H. (1977). *Ann. N.Y. Acad. Sci.* **284,** 310.
Padgett, R. A., Wahl, G. M., Coleman, P. F., and Stark, G. R. (1979). *J. Biol. Chem.* **254,** 974.
Passonneau, J. V., and Schulz, D. W. (1974). *Methods Enzyma. Anal.* **4,** 2229.
Pasternak, C. A., Fischer, G. A., and Handschumacher, R. E. (1961). *Cancer Res.* **21,** 110.
Pausch, J., Wilkening, J., Nowack, J., and Decker, K. (1975). *Eur. J. Biochem.* **53,** 349.
Pinkus, L. M., and Meister, A. (1972). *J. Biol. Chem.* **247,** 6119.
Pinsky, L., and Krooth, R. S. (1967). *Proc. Natl. Acad. Sci U.S.A.* **57,** 925.
Plagemann, P. G. W., and Behrens, M. (1976). *Cancer Res.* **36,** 3807.
Porter, R. W., Modebe, M. O., and Stark, G. R. (1969). *J. Biol. Chem.* **244,** 1846.
Potter, V. R. (1951). *Proc. Soc. Exp. Biol. Med.* **76,** 41.
Potvin, B. W., Stern, H. J., May, S. R., Lam, G. F., and Krooth, R. S. (1978). *Biochem. Pharmacol.* **27,** 655.
Pradham, T. K., and Sander, E. G. (1973). *Life Sci.* **13,** 1747.
Prescott, L. M., and Jones, M. E. (1969). *Anal. Biochem.* **32,** 408.
Raijman, L. (1974). *Biochem. J.* **138,** 225.

Rao, K. V., McBride, T. J., and Oleson, J. J. (1968). *Cancer Res.* **28,** 1952.
Ravel, J. M., McCord, T. J., Skinner, C. G., and Shire, W. (1958). *J. Biol. Chem.* **232,** 159.
Reyes, P., and Guganig, M. E. (1975). *J. Biol. Chem.* **250,** 5097.
Rogers, L. E., and Porter, F. S. (1968). *Pediatrics* **42,** 423.
Rubin, R. J., Reynard, A., and Handschumacher, R. E. (1964). *Cancer Res.* **24,** 1002.
Rundles, R. W., Wyngaarden, J. B., Hitchings, G. H., and Elion, G. B. (1963). *Trans. Assoc. Am. Phys.* **76,** 126.
Saenger, W., Suck, D., Knappenberg, M., and Dirkx, J. (1979). *Biopolymers* **18,** 2015.
Santilli, V., Škoda, J., Gut, J., and Šorm, F. (1968). *Biochim. Biophys. Acta* **155,** 623.
Schindler, R., and Welch, A. D. (1957). *Science* **125,** 548.
Schnaitmann, C. S., and Greenawalt, J. W. (1968). *J. Cell. Biol.* **38,** 158.
Schumm, D. E., and Webb, T. E. (1975). *Cell. Immunol.* **15,** 479.
Shambaugh, G. E., III (1979). *Am. J. Clin. Nutr.* **32,** 1290.
Shaw, R. K., Shulman, R. N., Davidson, J. D., Rall, D. P., and Frei, E., III (1960). *Cancer* **13,** 482.
Shoaf, W. T., and Jones, M. E. (1973). *Biochemistry* **12,** 4039.
Sieber, S. M., Mead, J. A. R., and Adamson, R. J. (1976). *Cancer Chemother. Rep.* **60,** 1127.
Skipper, H. E., Thomson, J. R., and Bell, M. (1954). *Cancer Res.* **14,** 503.
Škoda, J. (1963). *Prog. Nucleic Acid Res.* **2,** 197.
Smith, D. A., and Visser, D. W. (1965). *J. Biol. Chem.* **240,** 446.
Smith, D. A., Roy-Burman, P., and Visser, D. W. (1966). *Biochim. Biophys. Acta* **119,** 221.
Smith, G. D. (1977). *Theor. Biol.* **69,** 275.
Smith, L. H., Jr., and Sullivan, M. (1960). *Biochim. Biophys. Acta* **39,** 554.
Smith, L. H., Jr., Sullivan, M., Baker, F. A., and Frederick, E. (1960). *Cancer Res.* **20,** 1059.
Smithers, G. W., Gero, A. M., and O'Sullivan, W. J. (1978). *Anal. Biochem.* **88,** 93.
Šorm, F. A., and Keilová, H. (1958). *Experientia* **14,** 215.
Sperling, O., Baer, P., Brosh, S., Elazar, E., Pinkhas, J., Szeinberg, A., and deVries, A. (1975). *Acta Haematol.* **54,** 75.
Stone, J. E., and Potter, V. R. (1957). *Cancer Res.* **17,** 800.
Streightoff, F. J., Nelson, J. D., Cline, J. C., Gerzon, K., Hoehn, M., Williams, R. H., Gorman, M., and DeLong, D. C. (1969). *Conf. Antimicrob. Ag. Chemother., 9th, Washington, D.C.* p. 8.
Suttle, D. P., and Stark, G. R. (1979). *J. Biol. Chem.* **254,** 4602.
Sweeney, M. J., Davis, F. A., Gutowski, G. E., Hamill, R. L., Hoffman, D. H., and Poore, G. A. (1973). *Cancer Res.* **33,** 2619.
Swyryd, E. A., Seaver, S. S., and Stark, G. R. (1974). *J. Biol. Chem.* **21,** 6945.
Tate, S. S., and Meister, A. (1968). *Biochemistry* **7,** 3240.
Tatibana, M., and Shigesada, K. (1972). *J. Biochem.* **72,** 549.
Tax, W. J. M., Veerkamp, J. H., Trijbels, F. J. M., and Schretlen, E. D. A. M. (1976). *Biochem. Pharmacol.* **25,** 2025.
Taylor, P. W., King, R. W., and Burgen, A. S. V. (1970). *Biochemistry* **9,** 2638.
Traut, T. W., and Jones, M. E. (1977a). *Biochem. Pharmacol.* **26,** 2291.
Traut, T. W., and Jones, M. E. (1977b). *J. Biol. Chem.* **252,** 8374.
Trotta, P. P., Pinkus, L. M., Wellner, V. P., Estis, L., Haschemeyer, R. H., and Meister, A. (1973). *In* "The Enzymes of Glutamine Metabolism" (S. Prusiner and E. R. Stadtman, eds.), pp. 431–482. Academic Press, New York.
Tsuboi, K. K., Edmunds, H. N., and Kwong, L. K. (1977). *Cancer Res.* **37,** 3080.
Tyagi, A. K., Jayaram, H. N., Anandaraj, S., Taylor, B., and Cooney, D. A. (1979). *J. Biochem. Biophys. Methods* **1,** 221.

Veselý, J., Čihák, A., and Šorm, F. (1968). *Biochem. Pharmacol.* **17,** 519.
Webb, J. L. (1963). *In* "Enzyme and Metabolic Inhibitors" (J. L. Webb, ed.), Vol. I, pp. 487–512. Academic Press, New York.
Weinfeld, H., Savage, C. R., Jr., and McPartland, R. P. (1978). *Methods Enzymol.* **51,** 84.
Welch, A. D., Handschumacher, R. E., and Jaffe, J. J. (1960). *J. Pharm. Exp. Ther.* **129,** 262.
Westwick, W. J., Allsop, J., and Watts, R. W. E. (1972). *Biochem. Pharmacol.* **21,** 1955.
Westwick, W. J., Allsop, J., and Watts, R. W. E. (1974). *Biochem. Pharmacol.* **23,** 153.
White, F. R. (1959). *Cancer Chemother. Rep.* **3,** 26.
Whitehouse, M. W. (1965). *Prog. Drug Res.* **8,** 301.
Williams, L. G., and Davis, R. H. (1978). *Methods Enzymol.* **51,** 105.
Williams, L. G., Bernhardt, S. A., and Davis, R. H. (1971). *J. Biol. Chem.* **246,** 973.
Williamson, D. H., and Brosnam, J. T. (1974). *Methods Enzym. Anal.* **4,** 2266.
Wolfenden, R. (1979). *In* "Antimetabolites in Biochemistry, Biology and Medicine" (J. Škoda and P. Langen, eds.), pp. 151–160. Pergamon, Oxford.
Woods, D. D. (1962). *J. Gen. Microbiol.* **29,** 687.
Woolley, D. W. (1960). *J. Biol. Chem.* **235,** 3238.
Worzalla, J. F., and Sweeney, M. J. (1980). *Cancer Res.* **40,** 1482.
Wuu, K.-D., and Krooth, R. S. (1968). *Science* **160,** 539.
Yashphe, J. (1973). *Anal. Biochem.* **52,** 154.
Yip, M. C. M., and Knox, E. (1970). *J. Biol. Chem.* **245,** 2199.
Yoshida, T., Stark, G. R., and Hoogenraad, N. J. (1974). *J. Biol. Chem.* **249,** 6951.

Index

B

C

D

E

F

G

H

I

K

M

N

O

P

Q

R

T